Clinical Handbook of Antipsychotic Drug Therapy

Clinical Handbook of Antipsychotic Drug Therapy

AARON S. MASON, M.D.

*Chief Psychiatrist, Mental Health Branch,
Department of Human Resources, Commonwealth of Kentucky;
Professor of Clinical Psychiatry,
University of Kentucky Medical Center,
Lexington, Kentucky*

and
ROBERT P. GRANACHER, M.D.

*Associate Clinical Professor of Psychiatry,
University of Kentucky Medical Center,
Lexington, Kentucky*

BRUNNER/MAZEL, Publishers • New York

Library of Congress Cataloging in Publication Data

Mason, Aaron S   1912-
  Clinical handbook of antipsychotic drug therapy.

  Bibliography: p.
  Includes index.
  1. Psychopharmacology. 2. Psychoses—Chemotherapy.
I. Granacher, Robert P., 1941-   joint author.
II. Title. [DNLM: 1. Tranquilizing agents,
Major—Handbooks. 2. Lithium—Handbooks. QV77.9
M398c]
RC483.M29   616.89′18   80-11235
ISBN 0-87630-215-0

Copyright © 1980 by Aaron S. Mason and Robert P. Granacher

Published by
BRUNNER/MAZEL, INC.
19 Union Square
New York, New York 10003

MANUFACTURED IN THE UNITED STATES OF AMERICA

Foreword

There are now a growing number of general purpose textbooks in psychopharmacology which contain one or two chapters on the antipsychotic drugs. These generally provide a reasonable abbreviated review of the subject—mechanisms of action, clinical efficacy and side effects, dosage ranges—but none even approaches the thoroughness and detail provided in the present text.

Drs. Mason and Granacher are to be congratulated on the excellence of this most useful and comprehensive book. In contrast to all other texts, it actually gives the junior (or senior) psychiatrist a detailed set of treatment regimens to follow and tells how dosage can and should be adjusted and how side effects should be handled at various stages in therapy. In my experience, this kind of help and guidance is not available anywhere else.

The book also gives an excellent review of the current states of rapid, high dose antipsychotic drug use to control acute psychosis, an area in which I do not have personal experience, but one which is attracting much attention in recent years. Again, the text not only reviews the literature in the area, but provides information on exactly how different experts approach this complicated treatment problem.

Lithium therapy, its uses and side effects, is also well covered. Special newer problems in the use of antipsychotic drugs—tardive dyskinesia with the dopamine blocking agents and renal toxicity with lithium—are intelligently and sensibly handled.

Although I can find an occasional minor point with which I might mildly disagree, the book as a whole should be a very useful and valuable addition to any psychiatrist's library and a necessary possession for anyone practicing inpatient psychiatry or conducting a practice emphasizing the pharmacotherapy of schizophrenic patients. I was delighted to have early access to the volume prior to publication. I found it not only helpful but easy to read.

JONATHAN O. COLE, M.D.
Chief, Psychopharmacology Program
McLean Hospital, Belmont, MA

Preface

There are several dozen books on psychopharmacology and the reader may well ask "why another book—and on only one facet of the subject—antipsychotic drug therapy?" A number of reasons have to be mentioned in reply.

Antipsychotic drugs are primarily responsible for the revolution in mental health care and the change in the concept of mental illness throughout the world. Their advent and use have sparked widespread reforms and changes in mental hospitals, made possible the era of community psychiatry and provided a touchstone for the reentry of psychiatry into medicine. On any one day at least one million patients are taking antipsychotic medication. Yet, to our knowledge, there is no comprehensive or integrated book devoted solely and specifically to the clinical application of these drugs. In fact, one book on psychopharmacology completely omits the subject of antipsychotic drug therapy.

Recently, Dr. Jack Weinberg, President of the American Psychiatric Association, stated "for the first time in the history of medicine, the average psychotic patient receiving the services of a *well-trained* psychiatric physician has a prognosis equal to that of the average patient requiring most other medical treatments." Many physicians in other fields of medical specialization lack sufficient training and skill in some of their therapies. Similarly, it is still quite common to find psychiatrists who are not "well-trained" in the use of antipsychotic drug therapy.

From the analysis and review of thousands of medication regimen for psychiatric patients in a variety of settings during the past decade, it is evident that numerous physicians have not acquired the skill and sophistication to prescribe antipsychotic drugs in the most effective and economical manner. Many psychiatrists (and medical students) are trained at centers where psychopharmacology is considered of minor importance and the curriculum devotes only a few hours to this subject. Often it is looked upon as a therapy that the resident in psychiatry can pick up quickly without formal instruction or any supervision. Many physicians learn about the antipsychotic drugs from the detail men and the glamorous advertisements of the drug companies. The lack of concern about this important therapy is exemplified by the fact that, at the 1977 and 1978 annual meetings of the American Psychiatric Association, of 62 and 84 APA/AMA Category I continuing medical education courses offered, there was not one course dealing specifically with antipsychotic drug therapy or the pharmacotherapy of the psychoses. Little wonder, then, that there are glaring deficiencies in the clinical knowledge of antipsychotic drugs by many physicians and that, all too often, these agents are used unwisely and with little rationale.

The bulk of ideas in this book reflect the works of Frank J. Ayd, Jr., Barry Blackwell, Jonathan O. Cole, Eugene M. Caffey, Jr., John M. Davis, Alberto DiMascio, Donald F. Klein, Gerald L. Klerman, Heinz E. Lehmann, Leo E. Hollister, Robert F. Prien, Richard I. Shader and many other outstanding psychopharmacologists and clinicians who have made valuable contributions to the clinical literature about antipsychotic drugs. To them, grateful acknowledgement is made; indeed, the psychiatric profession owes them a great debt of gratitude. Special mention must be made of Frank J. Ayd, Jr., who, through his numerous articles, books, drug newsletter, lectures and seminars has been the leading educator in the field of rational psychopharmacology during the past two decades.

Our goal is to fill the gap in clinical psychopharmacological literature and to furnish a practical handbook for the student who desires to acquire a fundamental knowledge of antipsychotic drug therapy and for the physicians and psychiatrists who prescribe antipsychotic medication. Efforts have been made to focus on relevant clinical information with a minimum of jargon and theoretical details. Sentences dealing with basic principles or guidelines of antipsychotic drug therapy and related essential clinical data are in bold type. However, it is stressed that antipsychotic drug therapy is as much an art as other forms of psychiatric treatment, necessitating, to a considerable extent, adaption of the therapy to the individual patient—very few firm universal rules can be made that would apply categorically to all patients.

The format of the book results in some repetition and overlapping. These qualities are valuable and purposeful since they serve to highlight and reinforce useful and essential clinical information. In contrast to many ponderous tomes, we have tried to keep the parenthesized references to authors and dates of publications in the text to a minimum, although often numerous bibliographic citations could have been added to the one cited. Where an aspect of a topic or fundamental guideline has an element of controversy or lacks consensus, the minority viewpoint of opinion is included. At times this has been necessary to demolish myths or highlight obsolete clinical practices which may have changed over the years and are at variance with known scientific evidence.

We believe with many others that the classification of psychotropic drugs should be based on the principal therapeutic effect rather than any physiological property or propensity to cause specific side effects. Thus, we prefer the term "antipsychotic" rather than "neuroleptic." The subject of rapid tranquilization is discussed fully since it is highly probable that this procedure will be the treatment of choice for the majority of acute psychoses if the current trend portends the future.

It is our hope that this handbook will provide a practical guide for therapists with a need to develop greater skill and effectiveness in the use of the antipsychotic drugs, for general practitioners who have to monitor outpatient maintenance therapy or render emergency treatment to an acutely psychotic patient, and for medical students and residents in psychiatry who need clear and essential information about antipsychotic drug therapy.

Along with antipsychiatry groups, there is a growing contemporary antipsychotropic drug movement in which antipsychotic drugs are condemned in this country. A rational and scientific approach to the use of these agents will help avoid further regulatory action by federal, state and local agencies. It is believed that the incorporation into clinical practice of the fundamental principles of antipsychotic drug therapy as presented may help prevent harassment by civil liberties groups and may reduce the rise of exorbitant malpractice premiums and the constant threat of lawsuits.

We are grateful to Dr. John M. Davis for updating his table "Comparative dosages and costs" to include loxapine succinate. A special debt to Dr. Frank J. Ayd, Jr., is gladly acknowledged for permission to draw freely from his extensive publications. Finally, many thanks go to Mrs. Dottie Frazier, Miss Nancye Fightmaster and Ms. Carol Cox for their numerous hours of typing assistance in the production of this manuscript.

Contents

List of Tables

List of Figures

Clinical Handbook of Antipsychotic Drug Therapy

I

Introduction to Antipsychotic Drugs

1. HISTORICAL BACKGROUND

Few would argue that the modern pharmacologic treatment of psychosis in psychiatric medicine began with chlorpromazine (Thorazine). However, the use of chemicals to treat "madness" developed with the history of man. For the sake of brevity, only highlights in the drug treatment of psychiatric ills for 150 years prior to chlorpromazine will be examined. (Caldwell, 1978, has reviewed the history of psychopharmacology and highlighted many of the following milestones.)

Thomas Willis, the great 17th century neuroanatomist, recommended a "decoction of pimpernel with the purple flower" for the treatment of "madness." This plant contains an alkaloid with diaphoretic and diuretic properties. When light is low or it is cloudy, its flowers close and this probably enhances its medicinal appeal. In 1803, John Ford used granulated tin preparations to treat mania. Edward Sutliffe tranquilized patients with the "juice of ground ivy" and published reports of his success in 1819. Billod reported successful treatment of hallucinations with *Datura stramonium*, a plant containing anticholinergic alkaloids. Interestingly, this same plant is recognized today as a potential cause of anticholinergic delirium. Billod also treated melancholy with quinine sulfate while serving on the psychiatric service of Moreau de Tours.

3

The year 1845 is considered by many to mark the start of true psycho-pharmacology. In this year, Moreau de Tours used a drug to induce and study mental symptoms and also to treat mental disease. The drug was cannabis (marijuana) and Moreau is considered the first true psychophar-macologist. His concoction was a flavored paste of hashish mixed with black coffee and called a "Dawamsec." He published his experiences in a book, *"Du Hachisch et de l'Alienation Mentale,"* in 1845.

Chloroform and ether were tried in the therapy of psychosis 1847-1848. Effects were beneficial but, of course, transient. Chloral hydrate had its first clinical use in psychiatry, when Liebreich introduced it as a treatment for insanity in 1869. The next year, Elstun introduced it into American psy-chiatry at the Indiana Hospital for the Insane. Hyoscyamine, a belladonna alkaloid, entered psychiatry at the West Riding Pauper Lunatic Asylum in 1795. In the 1880s, cocaine was lauded as a therapy of morphine and alcohol addiction. Parke-Davis Company advertised it for these conditions and soon cocaine was widely used. Freud, in 1885, recommended subcutaneous in-jections of 0.03-0.05 mg. cocaine, insisting that it was not habit forming. Sleep therapy originated in Shanghai with sodium bromide given by mouth or by nose for 6-7 days. This began in 1897 and two years later it was used to treat mania.

The first of the phenothiazines, methylene blue, made its psychiatric debut in 1899, when Bodoni reported its sedative effect upon psychoses. Klasi introduced another sleep therapy in 1920 with "somnifen," a mixture of morphine, scopolamine and barbituric acids. His method was quite pop-ular and spread from Switzerland as far as Canada and Russia. In 1929, Bleckwenn introduced sodium amytal and in 1930 developed sodium amytal narcosis. Sen and Bose reported the root of *Rauwolfia serpentina* to be of benefit in psychosis and hypertension in 1931.

The modern chemical treatment of psychosis began with Sakel's intro-duction of insulin coma in 1933. While he was trying to determine optimal doses in some schizophrenic patients, he noted that those who fell into coma often awoke improved. In 1935, insulin coma therapy was regarded as the treatment of choice for the schizophrenias. Metrazol, intravenously as a shock therapy, was introduced the next year by Meduna. He discovered this agent while looking for a convulsive agent that would act more quickly than the one- or two-hour delay required for camphor.

Amphetamines were first used for the treatment of depressive states in 1936. They were discovered to be effective in narcolepsy the previous year. Histamine was tried as a "nonspecific desensitization" in psychosis and was introduced into the United States by Marshall and Tarwater in 1938. The first antihistamine to be tried in the therapy of psychosis was phenbenzamine in 1943. This agent's use was based on an observation that manic-depressive psychoses and asthma were somehow related. In 1943, lysergic acid diethylamide (LSD) was synthesized; it was tried in psychiatric disorders in 1947. Cade discovered the properties of lithium in 1948 and reported its successful use in mania in 1949.

The march toward chlorpromazine began in 1944 when Paul Charpentier, searching for an improved antihistamine, prepared the first amino derivation of a phenothiazine. He was then working at the Rhone-Poulenc Laboratories of the Paris drug house, Specia. Three aminophenothiazines were parent analogs of chlorpromazine: compound R.P. (Rhone-Poulenc) 3276, which was not further developed due to weak antihistaminic properties; promethazine (Phenergan), an excellent antihistamine and an isopropyl derivation of R.P. 3276; and diethazine, later used in Parkinson's disease.

During the development at the Specia laboratories, a French surgeon, Laborit, began to investigate surgical shock, which was a great therapeutic obstacle in 1945. By 1947 he had developed evidence that shock resulted from exaggerated defense reactions to stress. He postulated that, if one could control the autonomic nervous system, then shock would be controlled. Early in 1949 Laborit began to use promethazine in his surgical patients. He was surprised to find that postoperatively his patients were much calmer and more relaxed than was his prior experience. However, promethazine did not have the central autonomic blocking activity which he sought. He then tried diethazine and found that it reduced preoperative anxiety and reduced the anesthetic needs during surgery. Nonetheless, diathazine did not satisfy Laborit's needs. Working with the Paris anesthesiologist Huguenard, he urged the development of other more useful phenothiazines. In the fall of 1950, Specia undertook the specific task of finding a phenothiazine with extraordinary ability to centrally stabilize the autonomic nervous system.

Charpentier took the previously discarded compound R.P. 3276 and branched it on a chlorphenothiazine he had just developed. On December 11, 1950, he sent samples of this compound coded R.P. 4560 to Simone Courvoisier for pharmacologic testing. This drug had both sympathetic and parasympathetic blocking effects. On May 2, 1951, chlorpromazine was released for medical investigation. R.P. 3276 was actually promazine and was marketed as a weak antipsychotic drug, Sparine. Chlorpromazine is merely promazine with a chlorine atom added to one of the phenothiazine rings. The psychiatric revolution was triggered by *one* chlorine atom!

Laborit introduced chlorpromazine into every medical field that might benefit from an autonomic stabilizer, that is, every field except psychiatry. Paris psychiatrists would not touch the drug. No psychiatrist wanted to be the first to use such a drug with his patients. Their experience with new treatments in psychiatry had been so disappointing that they were unimpressed. Finally, Laborit persuaded some of his own colleagues at hospital Val-de-Grace to try the compound. Chlorpromazine was first used to treat a psychosis on January 19, 1952. The initial patient was Jacques Lh., 24 years old, suffering from his third severe "manic" attack, the others occurring in 1949 and 1951. After 20 days, he left the hospital, having received a total of 855 mg. of chlorpromazine. This case was reported to the world by Paraire on February 25, 1952, at a meeting of the Societe Medico-Psychologique in Paris. Four weeks later chlorpromazine arrived at the psychiatric hospital St. Anne. It was here that Delay and his group began using chlorpromazine. Delay, who accepted this drug with enthusiasm, evaluated its effects on behavior and developed schedules for administration. More importantly, he was the most powerful force in gaining psychiatry's acceptance of this new agent. The first study of chlorpromazine outside of France was at Padua, Italy. Early in 1953 it was first used in Switzerland. This is the same year that reserpine entered cardiology in Switzerland.

Reserpine was vaulted into Western psychiatry by the American psychiatrist, Nathan Kline. He was reading the *New York Times* one spring Sunday in 1953 and noticed that in Bombay Dr. R. A. Hakim had received an award for his paper "Indigenous Drug in the Treatment of Mental Diseases." Kline then introduced derivatives of *Rauwolfia serpentina* into the United States and successfully employed them in the treatment of psychoses. Both reserpine and chlorpromazine were available at that time in the United States and by late 1955 they were used across the entire country. Chlorpromazine was now licensed and sold virtually worldwide. Among the different trade names were Aminazine (Russia), Largactil (France) and Thorazine (United States). As drug houses began searches for new and better phenothiazines, many others began to appear.

The first chemical class of antipsychotics to differ from the phenothiazines was the butyrophenones. In 1939 Eisleb began to look for analogs of meperidine (Demerol) that could be successors to atropine and cocaine (Burger, 1976). Janssen, in Belgium, began to screen additional analogs of these compounds. In 1958, his group discovered the pronounced neuroleptic properties of haloperidol (Haldol). The term neuroleptic means "reduced neurologic tension." Since this period, literally hundreds of butyrophenones have been screened for antipsychotic properties, with 25 undergoing clinical trials. Ten are currently used as drugs in human and veterinary medicine (Janssen and van Bever, 1976).

The same year that Janssen was evaluating haloperidol, Petersen and his colleagues in Denmark were evaluating the thioxanthene analogs of chlorpromazine, promazine, and mepazine (Pacatal, no longer used). Their first compound was chlorprothixene (Taractan). This drug was administered for the first time to a psychiatric patient on November 10, 1958, at the mental hospital in Middlefart, Denmark. The Danish government subsequently approved the drug and it was marketed March 28, 1959. Thiothixene (Navane) followed and was marketed in the United States in August, 1967. By 1974 it had been used on all five continents; it is now called Navane everywhere but in Germany and Austria where it is known as Orbinamon (Ban, 1978).

Today the number of antipsychotic drugs available continues to grow. Many are available in Europe which are not used in the United States. The three chemical classes of phenothiazines, as well as the butyrophenones and thioxanthines have been noted. Two other chemical classes have recently been introduced in this country: dihydroindolone (molindone, Moban, Lidone) and a dibenzoxazepine (loxapine, Loxitane).

All known antipsychotic drugs have a number of common characteristic chemical and pharmacologic properties. Chemically they are all tertiary or, rarely, secondary amines and each contains at least one aromatic carbon ring. From a pharmacologic point of view, all produce the "neuroleptic syndrome" in man. This consists of a reduction in psychotic symptoms of hallucinations, mental confusion and delusions; reduction of psychomotor agitation, such as aggressive, assaultive or destructive behavior; inhibition of panic, fear and hostility; reduction of spontaneous movements and purposeful actions; and increased indifference towards surroundings but without impairing the sensorium or producing ataxia.

Many laboratories around the world developed animal screening procedures which would likely predict which neuroleptic compounds would have clinical antipsychotic effects in humans. One test that is often used is the antagonism of apomorphine-induced vomiting in dogs. Dogs, like humans, will vomit if given sufficient amounts of the experimental, dopamine-like agent, apomorphine. If antipsychotic drugs are administered, they will block this effect; thus, antagonism of vomiting is used as a predictor of antipsychotic activity.

There is no specific animal model of human psychosis. However, the inhibition of amphetamine-induced chewing or stereotypic motor behavior in animals correlates highly with antipsychotic efficacy in humans. When animals are given amphetamines in sufficient dose, they produce a characteristic repetitive chewing and motor syndrome. Even humans intoxicated on amphetamines will engage in repetitive motor acts. These stereotypies can be specifically blocked by all effective antipsychotic agents. Neuroleptics that are only partially effective in this test are usually not very potent antipsychotic drugs.

Side effects profiles of potential antipsychotic agents can be predicted by certain animal screening methods. Oversedation is a side effect which is potentially associated with antipsychotic drug treatment. It can be serious enough to impair intellectual and psychomotor skills. This often unwanted side effect can be assessed by determining the amount of palpebral ptosis or drooping of the eyelids in animals.

Symptoms of autonomic blockade, such as orthostatic hypotension and tachycardia, are potentially troublesome. These unwanted effects can often be predicted by determining the ability of a potential antipsychotic agent to block the effects of norepinephrine when given to an animal. Neuroleptics that are potent blockers of norepinephrine will likely cause significant autonomic blockade problems in humans.

These methods, as well as certain others, enable the pharmaceutical industry and research laboratories to screen potential compounds for usefulness as antipsychotics. However, there is a built-in flaw in this design for developing antipsychotic drugs. **Only agents which are similar to standard drugs such as chlorpromazine or haloperidol will pass this test.** Therefore, it is unlikely that novel compounds which differ dramatically in clinical antipsychotic ability or side effect profiles will be discovered by these methods. This is one of the reasons that little exciting in the search for antipsychotic agents has occurred since the 1950s.

2. MODE OF ACTION

All antipsychotic drugs share the basic property of inhibiting dopamine function in the brain. This is not to say that this sole property is responsible for antipsychotic activity. However, no presently known antipsychotic agent lacks the ability to affect substances known to act as neurotransmitters. Other important brain chemicals which act as chemical messengers are norepinephrine (NE), acetylcholine (ACh), serotonin (5-HT), and gamma-aminobutyric-acid (GABA). Many others are known to act or are suspected of acting as neurotransmitters. These chemicals transmit information from one neuron to another via a synapse or special connection between certain areas of neurons (Figure 1).

Tyrosine is an amino acid which is the precursor for dopamine. It is converted by the nerve cell body to dihydroxyphenylalanine (DOPA), which is transformed to dopamine. Dopamine is then packaged into little intracellular membrane pockets or vesicles which are stored in the presynaptic neuron. These packages are emptied across the synaptic distance (synaptic cleft) between neurons and the released dopamine activates specific receptors on the postsynaptic side. This produces electrical activity in that cell (Figure 1). Some dopamine is converted into norepinephrine, another neurotransmitter. Still other dopamine is metabolized presynaptically by an enzyme monoamine oxidase (MAO), removed from the area of the synapse

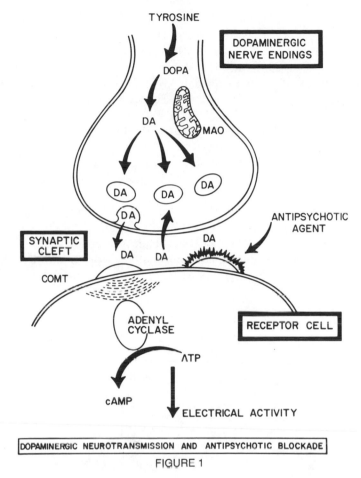

TYROSINE

DOPAMINERGIC
NERVE ENDINGS

DOPA

DA

MAO

DA DA DA

DA

ANTIPSYCHOTIC
AGENT

SYNAPTIC
CLEFT

DA

DA DA

COMT

ADENYL
CYCLASE

RECEPTOR CELL

ATP

cAMP

ELECTRICAL ACTIVITY

DOPAMINERGIC NEUROTRANSMISSION AND ANTIPSYCHOTIC BLOCKADE

FIGURE 1

and conserved by the neuron or metabolized in the synaptic cleft by the enzyme catechol-O-methyltransferase (COMT).

Dopamine-containing cells in the brain are confined to three major areas: the nigrostriatal tract, the mesolimbic pathway and the tuberoinfundibular pathway. The nigrostriatal tract begins with the substantia nigra and ascends to end upon the caudate nucleus and putamen. This is the pathway that degenerates in true Parkinson's disease. The caudate and putamen are part of the basal ganglia, a portion of the extrapyramidal system. Interference with dopamine transmission in this pathway produces the signs of parkinsonism often seen as side effects following the use of antipsychotic agents. The mesolimbic pathway is much less well known. This dopamine system projects from cells in the mesencephalon to anterior areas in the limbic brain. The limbic system is felt to be the "emotional brain" of man. Dysfunction in the limbic system is felt to account for many of the characteristic signs and symptoms of schizophrenia. These, in turn, may be related to altered dopamine activity (Stevens, 1973). The tuberoinfundibular pathway originates in the arcuate nucleus and terminates on the median eminence. This dopamine system is involved in hypothalamic control of endocrine messengers to the pituitary gland. Interference with dopamine activity in this pathway can account for many of the endocrine side effects (e.g., breast discharge) seen with antipsychotic agents (see Figure 2).

At this point in time, it cannot be conclusively claimed that the "dopamine hypothesis" explains the syndrome of schizophrenia. However, much research supports the notion that dopamine plays a unique role in inducing schizophrenic symptoms. This is further supported by the ability of dopamine-releasing agents, such as amphetamines, and dopamine precursors, such as L-DOPA, to mimic schizophrenic symptoms. All current antipsychotic drugs have only one basic pharmacologic property in common, namely an inhibitory action on dopamine transmission in the brain. The antipsy-

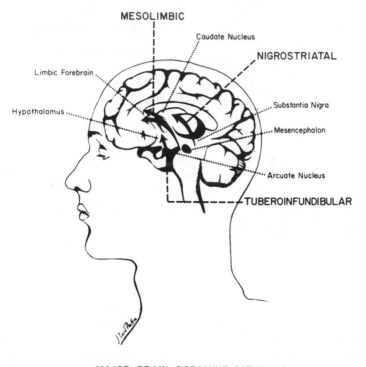

MAJOR BRAIN DOPAMINE PATHWAYS

FIGURE 2

chotic agents have other properties, such as varying ability to block acetylcholine, and these probably contribute to their antipsychotic actions, as well as accounting for differences in side effects. Nevertheless, a dopamine mechanism seems central to the disorder in schizophrenia and the ability of antipsychotic drugs to block this mechanism appears responsible for much of their antipsychotic activity. In all probability, these catecholamine systems lie in one of the limbic forebrain structures receiving a rich dopamine nerve supply (Carlsson, 1978).

3. PHARMACOKINETICS

Pharmacokinetics is the study of the time courses of absorption, distribution, metabolism and excretion of a drug in the total organism. It is not only the activity of an antipsychotic drug at its site of action in the brain that determines the intensity and duration of its desired effect, but also the amount of drug that gets there and stays there. The net effect of an antipsychotic drug depends not only upon its action on certain brain receptors but also upon the actions of the human body on the drug. The four components of pharmacokinetics must be kept in mind when treating patients with antipsychotic drugs—or any drug for that matter.

The absorption of antipsychotic drugs in the oral form can be erratic and unpredictable due to local factors in the gastrointestinal tract. For instance, enzymes in the intestinal wall often begin to metabolize antipsychotic agents before they enter the bloodstream. The use of other medications may also alter absorption. Compounds which reduce gastrointestinal motility, such as atropine, anticholinergic antidepressant agents (e.g., Elavil, Tofranil), gastric antispasmodics (e.g., Donnatal), and all belladonna alkaloids (e.g., hyoscyamine, hyosine), will increase the amount of time that the antipsychotic agent is in contact with GI wall mucosa. This, in turn, increases the likelihood of gut wall enzyme metabolism of the antipsychotic and can thereby lower plasma levels of the drug. Gastric contents can alter absorption by binding the drug and preventing uptake by the bloodstream. Certain antacids and antidiarrheal agents will commonly do this and are discussed further under Drug Interactions in Chapter V. It should be noted that antipsychotic liquid concentrates or elixirs have slightly better absorption than tablets or capsules. **The intramuscular forms of antipsychotic drugs always provide prompt absorption and bioavailability.**

Antipsychotics, when injected into skeletal muscle, are usually absorbed within 10-30 minutes (with the exception of the depot fluphenazines, Prolixin), but faster or slower absorption is possible depending upon the blood supply to the muscle site, how lipid soluble the drug is, the volume of injection, and certain other variables. If exceedingly rapid onset of action is required, the deltoid muscle is the preferred site. Blood flow through the deltoid area is at least 2-3 times greater than through a comparable size of gluteal muscle. As a general rule, intramuscular absorption is limited primarily by blood flow.

Once the antipsychotic agent is absorbed into the bloodstream, it then begins to be distributed throughout the body. All antipsychotic drugs are highly bound to protein carriers in the plasma. The percent of antipsychotic drug dose which is attached to plasma proteins varies from roughly 90-95%. Only the unbound portion of the drug is pharmacologically active. This is distributed with blood flow and passes across the blood-brain barrier into the central nervous system. Antipsychotic drugs are very soluble in fat or lipids and will concentrate at high levels in body fat and brain tissue, which is highly lipid in content. This is thought to explain the appearance of antipsychotic products in the urine of patients as much as six months following discontinuation of the drug. Apparently, they are slowly released from brain tissue and fat stores. Moreover, since these compounds are so highly protein bound, it is virtually impossible to remove antipsychotic drugs from the blood by dialysis should a patient overdose himself.

Much work has been done in the last few years in an effort to monitor plasma levels of antipsychotic agents and to find the therapeutic range of these drugs. This is analogous to monitoring lithium levels in patients. However, the results to date are not clinically practical and require highly sophisticated equipment and personnel beyond the range of community hospitals or mental health centers. These efforts are further hampered by the phenomenal number of potential metabolites for most antipsychotics. Chlorpromazine is predicted to have 168 potential metabolites, many of which have been found in humans. Since some of these compounds are also clinically active, it is presently impossible to define what is the clinically effective plasma level for chlorpromazine or other antipsychotics.

The monitoring of plasma antipsychotic drug levels has, however, given some useful information. It has been felt that many days or weeks of medication were required before behavioral characteristics of the schizophrenic syndrome showed a response to antipsychotic agents. Recently, pharmacokinetic studies have shown that intramuscular administration of mesoridazine (Serentil) at a dose of 2 mg/Kg produced favorable changes in schizophrenic pathology in 1 to 2 days. Schizophrenic patients were still quite schizophrenic 48 hours after receiving a single dose of this phenothiazine, but significant average improvement had appeared in comparison to their pre-drug mental status (Gottschalk et al., 1976). This lends some support to the use of intramuscular antipsychotic agents in initially treating acute schizophrenic patients.

The metabolism of antipsychotic drugs is confined to the liver. The majority of metabolic degradation is accomplished through sulfoxide formation, glucaronide conjugation or hydroxylation. Many other means of metabolism are potentially possible and literally hundreds of metabolites are produced from the many antipsychotic agents. Knowledge of specific metabolic products is presently not relevant to day-to-day clinical usage of these drugs.

Any substance which alters the rate of liver drug metabolizing systems will alter the rate of antipsychotic drug metabolism as well. Thus, agents such as barbiturates which speed up liver metabolism will induce drug metabolizing enzymes to be more efficient and thereby lower plasma levels of antipsychotics. This argues against using barbiturates and antipsychotic together for more than a few days. Likewise, any impairment of liver function will delay the metabolism of antipsychotic drug. Liver pathology will diminish the extent of drug metabolism in many cases. Moreover, the aging liver becomes less efficient as a metabolic organ and accounts for the lower dosages of antipsychotics necessary in elderly patients.

The elimination of antipsychotic drugs is principally through the kidneys. The ultimate aim of metabolism is to render the metabolic products of antipsychotic drugs water soluble so they may be excreted. Small portions of drug are also found in the stool due to excretion in bile. Impaired kidney function can potentially lead to accumulation of metabolic products and toxicity.

4. CLASSIFICATION AND CHEMICAL STRUCTURE

There are now five major chemical classes of antipsychotic drugs in the United States: phenothiazines, thioxanthenes, butyrophenones, dibenzoxazepines and dihydroindolones. The variations in their chemical structures are seen in Figure 3. The phenothiazine derivatives were the earliest to be developed, are the most numerous and are still the most widely used of antipsychotic drugs. There are three chemical subfamilies of phenothiazines. These are the aliphatic, piperidine and piperazine groups, which are named according to the side-chain which attaches to the phenothiazine nucleus at position 10. All effective antipsychotic phenothiazines have a molecule substituted at the 2 position. Some investigators have suggested that the phenothiazine nucleus assumes a three-dimensional shape that allows the nitrogen atom in the side-chain to swing close to the nucleus. The phenothiazine structure would then be more able to occupy the dopamine receptor. The side-chains of the long acting depot forms of fluphenazine (Prolixin) have been modified by adding long chain fatty acid esters of enanthate and decanoate. It takes longer to cleave these side-chains and further extends their duration of action.

FIGURE 3

CHEMICAL STRUCTURE OF THE
ANTIPSYCHOTIC DRUGS

Chemical Structure	Generic Name	Trade Name

A. PHENOTHIAZINES

I. Aliphatic

Promazine   Sparine

Chlorpromazine   Thorazine

Triflupromazine   Vesprin

2. Piperidine

Thioridazine   Mellaril

Mesoridazine   Serentil

FIGURE 3 (continued)

CHEMICAL STRUCTURE OF THE
ANTIPSYCHOTIC DRUGS

Chemical Structure	Generic Name	Trade Name

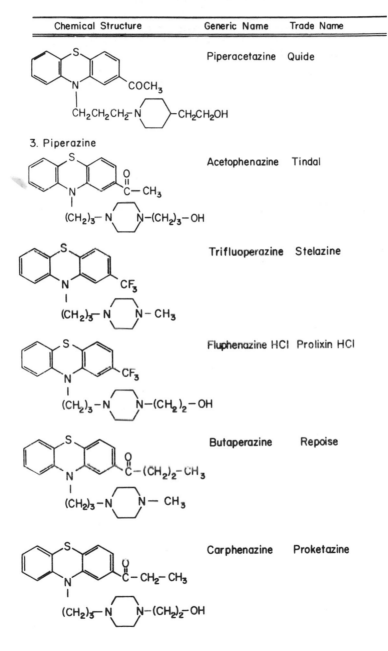

Piperacetazine   Quide

3. Piperazine

Acetophenazine   Tindal

Trifluoperazine   Stelazine

Fluphenazine HCl   Prolixin HCl

Butaperazine   Repoise

Carphenazine   Proketazine

FIGURE 3 (continued)

CHEMICAL STRUCTURE OF THE
ANTIPSYCHOTIC DRUGS

Chemical Structure	Generic Name	Trade Name

(Piperazine cont'd.)

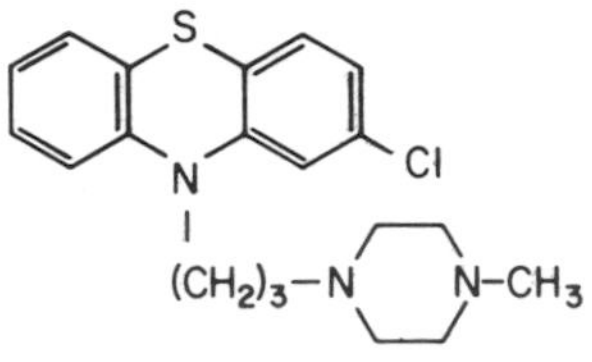

Prochlorperazine   Compazine

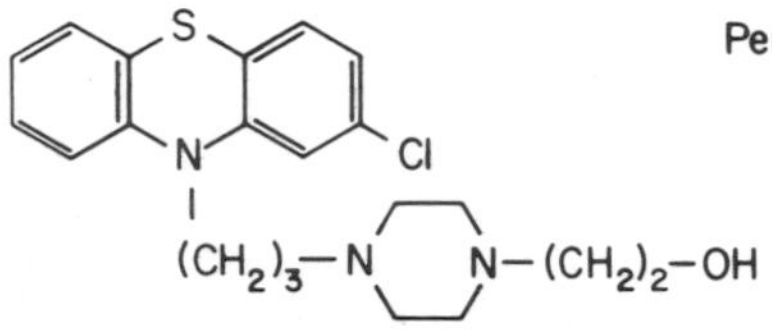

$(CH_2)_3-N$ $N-CH_3$

Perphenazine   Trilafon

$(CH_2)_3-N$ $N-(CH_2)_2-OH$

B. BUTYROPHENONES

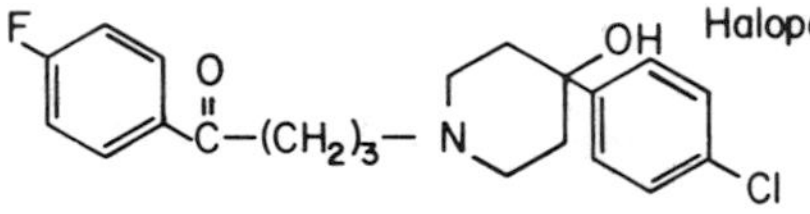

Haloperidol   Haldol

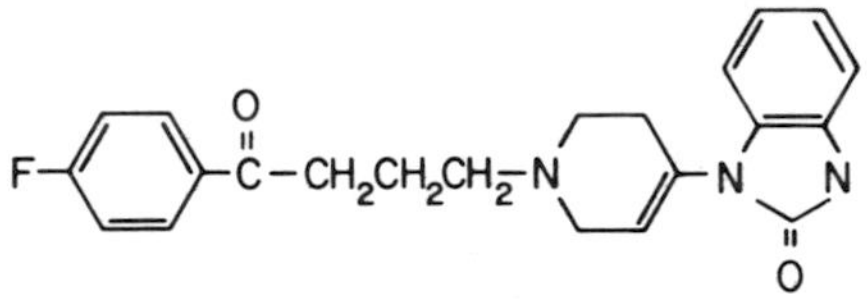

Droperidol   Inapsine

FIGURE 3 (continued)

CHEMICAL STRUCTURE OF THE
ANTIPSYCHOTIC DRUGS

Chemical Structure	Generic Name	Trade Name

C. THIOXANTHENES

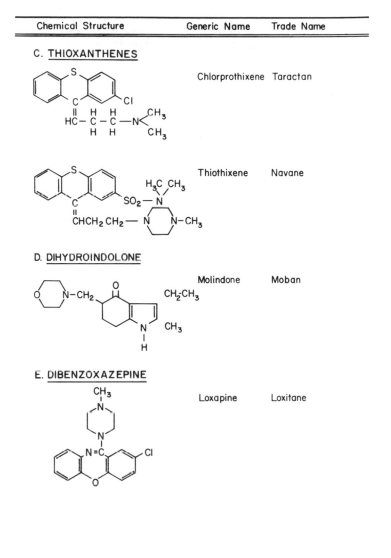

Chlorprothixene   Taractan

Thiothixene   Navane

D. DIHYDROINDOLONE

Molindone   Moban

E. DIBENZOXAZEPINE

Loxapine   Loxitane

As can be seen (Figure 3), the thioxanthenes have replaced the nitrogen with a carbon atom. This modification of the ring makes for a generally less potent group of compounds than the phenothiazines. Chlorprothixene (Taractan) is analogous to chlorpromazine, while thiothixene (Navane) is the analog of thioproperazine (Majeptil), a piperazine phenothiazine not used in the U.S. Thioxanthines seem to require a double bond between the ring carbon and their side-chain to have appreciable antipsychotic activity. However, unlike the phenothiazines, substitution at the 2 position has little effect on their biological activity.

Many structural possibilities exist for the butyrophenones. Only haloperidol and droperidol are marketed in the U.S. Virtually all other variations involve changes in the phenylpiperidine moiety which lies on the nitrogen end. However, the nitrogen can never be disturbed in the piperdine ring or the antipsychotic effect is lost.

The two newer classes of antipsychotic drugs are structurally dissimilar to the phenothiazines, thioxanthines, or butyrophenones. Loxapine is unusual in that it contains 7 members in its central ring and resembles the tricyclic antidepressants in this regard. On the other hand, molindone shares a chemical resemblance to the neurotransmitter, serotonin. Behaviorally, neither of these two agents seems to have any special advantage over the older antipsychotics.

II

Basic Principles
Of Antipsychotic
Drug Therapy

Over two decades of clinical experience with a wide variety of antipsychotic agents administered to millions of patients have established the fact that, as a group, the antipsychotics are among the safest pharmaceuticals a physician can prescribe. The incidence of serious side effects to these drugs which do not respond to treatment is quite low, in spite of the vast patient exposure to them. Nevertheless, in view of the potency of these drugs, the seriousness of the conditions they are used to treat, and their possible effects, it is important that they be prescribed as rationally and as judiciously as possible. In the following subsections, the "basic principles" or general guidelines of antipsychotic drug use, together with supporting clinical evidence, are discussed.

1. DRUG HISTORY

A comprehensive drug history should be obtained whenever possible.
The patient's past drug history is usually a reliable guide. Information

should be obtained about past drug intake, especially during recent weeks. It should include the daily dosage of the drug, when it was taken, and objective and subjective responses to medication. The patient (or his relative) should be asked: "Have you ever been on pills for your nerves?" "Which drugs do you prefer and why?" "Which drugs gave you any side effects?" "What were they?" "Which drug gave you the least side effects?"

The subjective response of the patient to past antipsychotic medication is important. Unless a patient tolerates a drug well, he is not likely to adhere to treatment. A patient who is made unbearably restless by a drug may prefer no drug. On the other hand, some patients may prefer restlessness to impairment of their sexual capacity. Therefore, the history of different side effects in the past may serve as a guide in choosing the present specific medication (Hollister, 1970). Some patients show a strong preference for certain antipsychotics based on their past experience.

It is highly important that a family drug history be included, since responsiveness to psychoactive drugs is frequently similar among blood relatives, just as certain psychotic illnesses tend to occur in families. If the patient has a blood relative who has had a favorable response to a particular antipsychotic drug, many clinicians would start the patient on the same drug. Conversely, a patient with a blood relative who has had an adverse reaction to a particular drug may react in the same manner to that drug or that class of drugs and the prescribing of these drugs should be avoided. The development of a treatment-resistant patient may be prevented through this precaution (Ayd, 1975a).

Dosage requirements are pretty much the same from one relative to the next, keeping in mind, however, that the aged generally require less medication than middle-aged or adolescent individuals. In addition, one can learn from a family drug history if the patient may be at high risk with respect to certain side effects. For example, haloperidol (Haldol) has among its pharmacologic properties the propensity to elicit extrapyramidal reactions. Therefore, before prescribing haloperidol, it would be most helpful if the physician knew that the patient is liable to be neurologically susceptible and, if so, at approximately what dose level one might anticipate a drug-induced extrapyramidal reaction.

Since many drugs tend to stay in the system for a long time after they are discontinued, there is a need to know what drug(s), if any, the individual has been taking in the immediate days or weeks before he is seen by the clinician. Necessary historical information should also include whether other drugs were taken in combination. From experience, it has been observed that most patients are taking not one, but several drugs, including over-the-counter preparations, concomitantly. It seems that this is the age of polypharmacy. Few patients on initial interview are not taking any medication.

Most patients are taking several compounds prescribed by one or more physicians. It has been noted that the average office patient is taking as many as six different drugs daily (Ayd, 1971). Thus, the patient should be questioned carefully about the specific details regarding the intake of over-the-counter preparations he may have been taking regularly—sleeping pills, hay fever pills, antacids, etc. Unless specifically asked, the patient may neglect to mention these agents. In some cases, where replies are vague, it may be useful to ask the relative to bring the contents of the patient's medicine chest for your examination.

A positive history of ingestion of drugs such as LSD or other hallucinogens, amphetamines, or alcohol may help to clarify the diagnosis and indicate the choice of treatment. Is the patient an impulsive taker of drugs or alcohol? Many physicians, especially psychiatrists, are not cognizant of the fact that many of the medications they prescribe can and do react adversely with other pharmaceuticals. The history should include a consideration of the use of other drugs for cardiac, liver, renal, gastrointestinal, dermatological, blood and other disorders.

A careful attempt must be made to elicit symptoms that later could be falsely attributed to the antipsychotic agent. It may be worthwhile to use a side-effect check list before prescribing medication. Symptoms such as dizziness, motor disturbances, dry mouth, gastrointestinal complaints, constipation, tremor, restlessness, and visual disturbances are often erroneously attributed to the antipsychotic agent, while they may be manifestations of the psychosis or other recent drug intake. Since many patients are prodigious drug consumers, a personal drug history may provide the true explanation of the patient's psychopathology. Such a history may allow the physician not only to make the clinical diagnosis, but also to select a preferable pharmacotherapy when possible.

Realistically, it is recognized that many floridly psychotic patients arrive at the admission office unable to furnish any reliable information. Their relatives are not present; often they have been transported by the police from jail to the hospital. Under such circumstances, a drug history often cannot be obtained. However, when the past history is obtained at a later date from the patient, relatives or friends, pertinent drug information should be included.

The physician should bear in mind that the patient who is seen for the first time may have a long history of drug therapy by other practitioners in private offices, clinics, or hospitals. It cannot be overemphasized that the admission physical examination should include a routine neurological examination and that all findings, positive and negative, should be recorded.

If the patient is already afflicted with a neurological disorder, the importance of these data is obvious from a medical and legal viewpoint.

2. TARGET SYMPTOMS

The target symptoms and behavior treated should be noted in the clinical record and disseminated to the entire treatment team. The effect of medication on the target symptoms and patient behavior should be recorded in the progress notes at regular intervals.

There is abundant evidence to support the conclusion that antipsychotic drugs are effective in treating psychoses and that they do not act merely by modifying the symptoms of the disorder. However, the most practical approach in assessing the therapeutic efficacy of these drugs is their action on specific symptomatic manifestations or target symptoms. Amelioration of various target symptoms should be considered a therapeutic goal and this rationale for prescribing the antipsychotic drug should be spelled out in the patient's written treatment plan (i.e., Haldol 5 mg. in a.m. and 10 mg. H.S. for hostility and agitation).

Table 1 lists alphabetically some of the target symptoms which may respond to antipsychotic drugs. It can be of assistance when developing the patient's treatment plan and establishing therapeutic goals and objectives. When recorded in the medical record, the specific signs and symptoms constitute the baseline against which change in the patient's clinical condition can then be evaluated. It is not the exception to find patients for whom antipsychotic drugs have been prescribed for months or years yet careful perusal of their medical records gives no indication as to why antipsychotics were prescribed for them or whether any symptoms were ameliorated. Small wonder that many of these patients improve or remain unchanged when antipsychotic medication is discontinued.

Schizophrenia is the most common psychiatric disorder treated with antipsychotic drugs. Klerman (1974) lists the following symptoms as characteristic of acute and chronic schizophrenic states: (1) thinking or speech disturbance; (2) catatonic motor behavior; (3) paranoid ideation and behavior; (4) hallucinations; (5) delusional thinking other than paranoid; (6) blunted or inappropriate emotion; and (7) disturbance of social behavior and interpersonal relations. He views these symptoms "target symptoms" on the basis of which patients are usually evaluated for treatment with antipsychotics.

It is important that all members of the therapeutic team, especially the nursing assistants, be made aware of each patient's target symptoms. In addition, all personnel should be trained to detect and report side effects, especially those that are truly handicapping, and to differentiate them from psychotic symptoms. Observations from the nursing staff about the effect of the antipsychotic agent on the target symptoms and about the appearance of various side effects are most valuable in regulating dosage and evaluating the efficacy of the treatment interventions. **The effects of medication on**

TABLE 1
Target Symptoms for Antipsychotic Drugs

Agitation

Aggressiveness

Anxiety

Apathy (or emotional
flattening or blunting)

Assaultiveness

Bizarre thinking or speech

Catatonic motor behavior

Combativeness

Confusion

Depressive Mood

Defective Judgment

Delusions

Delirium

Disorientation

Difficulty in relating
(poor rapport)

Deterioration of social habits

Elation

Excitement

Feelings of unroality

Flight of ideas

Guilt feelings

Grandiosity

Hallucinations

Hyperactivity

Hostility

Homicidal ideation or behavior

Irritability

Indifference to environment

Incoherency

Inappropriateness

Ideas of persecution

Insomnia

Irrelevancy

Lack of insight

Mannerisms or facial grimaces

Motor retardation

Negativism

Paranoid ideation

Poor appetite

Poor concentration

Pressure of speech

Resistiveness

Slowed speech

Social withdrawal
(seclusiveness)

Somatic concern

Suspiciousness

Suicidal tendencles

Tension

Thought disorganization

Uncommunicativeness

Uncooperativeness

Unusual thought content

Withdrawal from reality

target symptoms and patient behavior should be recorded at least weekly in progress notes of the newly admitted patient and monthly with regard to the chronic patient. The progress notes should be sufficiently detailed to enable the physician to determine what the patient's condition was at a specific time under a certain drug regimen. It should enable another physician to know what has transpired in the management of the patient and to know the patient's response to treatment in the event that this physician is required to assume the care of the patient. It should be remembered that skimpy or absent records frequently correlate with poor or indefinite care.

Target symptoms most likely to improve from the use of antipsychotic drugs include: hyperactivity, combativeness, agitation, hostility, hallucinations, irritability, negativism, acute delusions, insomnia, poor self-care and anorexia, while there is less likely to be improvement in memory, orientation, apathy, withdrawal, retardation, insight and judgment.

With the target symptoms approach, the symptoms are objectively observable pieces of behavior; nethertheless, they must be regarded within the context and in relation to the symptom complex that constitutes the disease. While antipsychotic drugs may sedate the patient, arousal to social cues is still possible. Also, they do not affect tests of cognitive function. They should be prescribed with the intent of enabling the patient to control himself and not with the intent of controlling his behavior through the drug.

As a general rule, no medication should be prescribed until as accurate as possible a diagnosis has been made and then only if the patient's symptoms are of a type known to be relieved by antipsychotics.

The aim of drug treatment should be to achieve the maximal therapeutic improvement in the patient. In some sense, one should be treating the whole patient or the underlying disease process and not a given symptom. This is particularly important when treating the depressed schizoaffective or the retarded schizophrenic patient. These patients often respond dramatically to antipsychotic drugs even though troublesome target symptoms, such as agitation or aggression, are completely absent. The goals should be for maximal cognitive reorganization and a lessening of the underlying schizophrenic process and all of its symptoms.

3. CHOICE OF DRUG

A rational approach to the selection of antipsychotic drugs is to narrow the choice.

At the present time, there are 5 major chemically different categories of antipsychotic drugs: the phenothiazines, butyrophenones, thioxanthenes, dihydroindolones and dibenzoxazepines. As can be noted from Table 2, there are about 20 antipsychotics that are available to the clinician in the United States and thus the choice may be bewildering and confusing to the neophyte. In the past, the advice has been to select a few of the antipsychotics and learn how to use them effectively.

TABLE 2
Classification of Antipsychotic Drugs and Their *PDR* Dosage Range

	Parental form available	Total daily dosage in mgs*			Estimated equivalent dose (mgs.)
		Low	Moderate	High	
PHENOTHIAZINES (Classified by side chain)					
Aliphatic					
Chlorpromazine (Thorazine)	P	to 400	401-800	801-1200	100
Trifluopromazine (Vesprin)	P	to 50	51-100	101-150	25
Piperidine					
Thioridazine (Mellaril)		to 266	267-533	534-800	100
Mesoridazine (Serentil)	P	to 133	134-267	268-400	50
Piperacetazine (Quide)		to 53	54-107	108-160	10
Piperazine					
Acetophenazine (Tindal)		to 40	41- 80	81-120	20
Carphenazine (Proketazine)		to 133	134-265	266-400	25
Prochlorperazine (Compazine)	P	to 50	51-100	101-150	15
Perphenazine (Trilafon)	P	to 21	22- 43	44- 64	10
Trifluoperazine (Stelazine)	P	to 10	11- 20	21- 30	5
Fluphenazine (Prolixin, Permitil)	P	to 7	8- 13	14- 20	2
Butaperazine (Repoise)		to 33	34- 67	68-100	10
BUTYROPHENONES					
Haloperidol (Haldol)	P	to 5	6- 10	11- 15	2
THIOXANTHENE DERIVATIVES					
Chlorprothixene (Taractan)	P	to 200	201-400	401-600	100
Thiothixene (Navane)	P	to 10	11- 20	21- 30	5
DIBENZOXAZEPINE					
Loxapine (Loxitane)	P	to 83	84-167	168-250	15
DIHYDROINDOLONE					
Molidone (Moban, Lidone)		to 75	76-150	151-255	25

*The low, moderate and high dosage categories in this table were obtained by using the maximal dosage for each antipsychotic drug as recommended in the Physicians' Desk Reference (PDR, 1978) or the manufacturer's insert and roughly dividing by three. The PDR presently states that daily doses up to 100 mg. of haloperidol may be necessary in some cases to achieve an optimal response.

A more logical approach is to select one of each of the three types of phenothiazines (aliphatic, piperidine and piperazine), one of the two thioxanthenes, and the butyrophenone (Hollister, 1970, 1973). The drugs selected should have a parenteral form available. This is important because there are many clinical situations where the parenteral form is indicated. Drugs with parenteral form are shown in Table 2. For example, it may be necessary to have an intramuscular PRN order for disruptive or violent behavior while the patient is in the process of stabilization on oral medication. If a second antipsychotic with a parenteral form has to be added, a polypharmacy situation is created with all its disadvantages, and titration with one antipsychotic to an effective dosage becomes more difficult. By choosing an antipsychotic with both an oral and parenteral form, the problem of attempting to isolate the source of side effects that may arise is avoided and the often unknown effects of medication combinations are less likely to occur.

No antipsychotic drug listed in Table 2 is any more or less effective than another in the treatment of the psychoses. Choosing five drugs on the basis of their chemical structure and availability of a parenteral form enables one to exploit the full range of pharmacological differences among the various antipsychotics. A sample choice from the array of drugs might include the following: chlorpromazine (Thorazine), an aliphatic phenothiazine; mesoridazine (Serentil), a piperidine phenothiazine; one of the low-dose, high-potency piperazine phenothiazines such as perphenazine (Trilafon), fluphenazine (Prolixin) or trifluoperazine (Stelazine); the butyrophenone, haloperidol (Haldol), and one of the thioxanthenes, thiothixene (Navane). These drugs need not be used in the order given. Obviously, many other selections are possible, although mesoridazine and haloperidol are the members of their particular chemical group that have an available parenteral form. The high-potency, low-dose thiothixene (Navane) is the more widely used and highly regarded of the two thioxanthene derivatives. The dibenzoxazepine, loxapine (Loxitane) and the dihydroindolone, molindone (Moban), two of the newer antipsychotics with different chemical structures, could be used as "back-up" antipsychotics since they presently do not have a parenteral form available. Promazine (Sparine), an aliphatic phenothiazine, is not included in the tables or discussed in the text since it has a very low efficacy as an antipsychotic, can cause a high incidence of hypotensive side effects, and is not recommended as an antipsychotic.

The physician should become thoroughly familiar with his chosen antipsychotic drugs and learn to use them well. He must know how to handle their side effects. A healthy skepticism should be maintained toward reports of the efficacy of one antipsychotic agent over others or comparisons between the injectable or long-lasting preparations and other forms of the drug.

The patient's past experience should be carefully reviewed. The readmission rate in many mental hospitals is over 75% and thus a medical record of medications and dosages prescribed, as well as of the clinical response during previous admissions, is usually available. If the patient has done well previously on a certain antipsychotic, it is unwise to change drugs or to reinstate lapsed treatment with a different drug. Patients often will relate that they have received several of the antipsychotic drugs in the past and can name the drug they feel works best for them. Rapid improvement may be lost if the patient is slowly titrated with a new drug.

The choice of drug may depend on four types of information:

(a) response to particular drug in previous illness;
(b) failure to respond to a particular drug in this or previous illness;
(c) likely tolerance of side effects (due to existing physical disease or risk of interactions with concurrent medications);
(d) need or otherwise for sedative effect. For example, an apathetic schizophrenic patient with a history of myocardial infarction could be treated with fluphenazine because this drug has less sedative action and produces fewer ECG changes than thioridazine (Blackwell, 1975).

The literature on antipsychotic drugs commonly dwells on their differential ability to produce the side effect of sedation. This requires clarification. While some antipsychotics, in high doses, may produce more sedation than others, all will reduce psychotic retardation to a significant extent. Even the apparently more "sedating" agents may improve psychomotor retardation and thus lead to normalization. Similarly, the least sedating of the drugs produce a calming of psychotic agitation and does so to an extent equal to the most sedating member of their chemical class. Indeed, all the antipsychotic compounds decrease psychomotor activity in the agitated patients, while at the same time making them more normally active. (Davis and Cole, 1975).

Oversedation is seen most frequently with the aliphatic and piperidine phenothiazines. It usually disappears after about 2 weeks, when tolerance for this reaction has developed. Clinical experience has shown that drowsiness and oversedation which develop after a patient has been on an antipsychotic drug for several weeks or months do not mean, as a rule, that the patient's dose is too high, but that he has not been taking his drug regularly—even if he pretends to have done so (Lehmann, 1975). Irregular intake of medication accounts for a loss of tolerance and increased sedation. The Forrest Urine Tests will help verify objectively whether the patient is ingesting the pills if a phenothiazine is prescribed. Such patients should be put, at least temporarily, on liquid medication and their taking of this form of medication should be carefully supervised. After two weeks of reliable drug intake—without any reduction of dosage—the symptoms of oversedation will probably disappear, as the new tolerance to the drug develops.

The belief persists that the aliphatic phenothiazines have a high initial sedative capability and they are therefore favored by many clinicians in the treatment of the excited, assaultive, hospitalized schizophrenics. This notion applied particularly to chlorpromazine, which became and still is a drug commonly used in initiating treatment in the disturbed patient. Perhaps responsible for this viewpoint are the myths that continue to exist in psychiatry (1) that hyperexcitable patients respond best to drugs such as chlorpromazine or thioridazine because they are sedating phenothiazines, and (2) that withdrawn patients respond best to an "alerting" phenothiazine such as trifluoperazine or fluphenazine. These beliefs have never been proven to be true. As far back as 1964, it was found that there was no evidence to support the view that chlorpromazine was more effective in patients requiring sedation or that the piperazine derivative, fluphenazine, was more effective in withdrawn patients in need of "activation or stimulation." In fact, NIMH studies (1964) have shown that a second order factor labeled "apathetic and retarded" predicted a differentially good response to chlorpromazine. It has been pointed out that the belief that trifluoperazine had an "alerting" or a directly stimulating effect was completely spurious and was based on its greater tendency to cause the side effect of akathisia (Hollister, 1973).

Sedation is not the most desired effect when antipsychotic drugs are used to treat the symptoms of schizophrenia. It may be better to rely on conventional sedatives, hypnotics or antianxiety drugs to manage excited states of sleeplessness. A not uncommon practice to be deplored is the use of antipsychotics, usually chlorpromazine, as a sedative for nonpsychotic patients, who may have a variety of physical complaints or illnesses. Usually small doses are prescribed. The patient thus is unnecessarily exposed to a drug which may have serious side effects. On rare occasions, tardive dyskinesia can result from the ingestion of an antipsychotic over a comparatively short period of time. More pertinent, the patient is receiving a poor sedative. Even in psychiatric disorders, the question of the sedative properties of chlorpromazine as a therapeutic side effect has to be reevaluated.

Hamill and Fontana (1975) compared the sedative properties of chlorpromazine with a placebo in newly admitted patients. During the first 5 days of treatment, the mean dosage of chlorpromazine ranged from 306.7 mg. on day 1 to 475 mg. on day 5. The results showed that the sedative properties of chlorpromazine at this dosage do not exert a calming effect on schizophrenic excitement. As many patients on chlorpromazine as on placebo showed an exacerbation of severe, agitated, aggressive or assaultive behavior. Yet many clinicians prescribe chlorpromazine within this dosage range for psychotic patients during the first 5 days of hospitalization with the expectation of sedation and control of these psychotic symptoms. They are not aware that to obtain the desired therapeutic action for florid psychotic symptoms, higher doses are necessary than the dosage range used in this study.

A recent study tested the belief that sedative antipsychotics (the aliphatic and piperidine phenothiazines) are clinically more indicated in conditions characterized by gross psychomotor excitement or hallucinations, while "activating" antipsychotics (the butyrophenone, haloperidol, and the piperazine phenothiazines) would find clinical application as more specific remedies in schizophrenics with flattening of affect and thought disorder. There was nothing to choose between chlorpromazine and haloperidol in terms of excitement or hallucinatory behavior. Neither was the sedativeness of chlorpromazine apparent in terms of sleeplessness. It seemed, rather, that haloperidol may have been more effective in reducing insomnia in schizophrenic patients. It was concluded that the "sedative" versus "activating" classification among effective antipsychotics is of dubious clinical significance (Singh and Kay, 1975). Still, the sedative effects of the high-dose, low-potency drugs continue to be cited in the literature as an advantage in drug treatment. At the same time, the sedative effect of these antipsychotics may hide the fact that the patient is receiving inadequate doses of medication for a true antipsychotic effect.

All antipsychotic drugs have some degree of alpha-adrenergic blocking which can induce clinically significant hypotension—at times to a very severe degree. Chlorpromazine and thioridazine are the most potent alpha-adrenergic blocking agents of all the antipsychotic drugs on the market. On the other hand, haloperidol is one of the least potent in terms of alpha-adrenergic blockage and, of all the antipsychotic drugs, the least likely to produce hypotension. Drugs like the piperazine phenothiazines are likewise unlikely to produce hypotension, but may not be as active as the butyrophenone in controlling the agitated or belligerent patient. Also, the potent alpha-adrenergic blockers often cannot be titrated to effective dosage levels because of cardiovascular side effects (see subsection on Cardiovascular Effects in Chapter V).

The possibility of extrapyramidal side effects produced by antipsychotic drugs is still another important consideration in choosing antipsychotic medication. The extrapyramidal effects of many antipsychotic drugs seem to parallel, to some extent, their antipsychotic potency. Milligram for milligram, the therapeutically more potent low-dose agents are far more likely to produce extrapyramidal effects but not equally more likely to produce drowsiness, depression and hypotension. A 10 mg. dose of fluphenazine will cause more drowsiness than an equal amount of chlorpromazine; therapeutic doses of chlorpromazine cause a greater degree of drowsiness or hypotension only because its antipsychotic effect is so low that it is achieved only at dose levels high enough to cause drowsiness (Jacobsen, 1971).

When the butyrophenones (i.e., haloperidol) became available, the concept of "incisive neuroleptic" was proposed by French and Belgian clinicians. They believed that the high-potency butyrophenone compound and the piperazine phenothiazines had greater specificity or efficacy particularly for paranoid and hallucinating patients—that they were more "incisive" (specific) in their ability to interrupt florid psychotic symptoms. However, careful studies have failed to substantiate these differences.

A suggested guideline for the selection of an antipsychotic drug includes the following: (1) Parenteral fluphenazine enanthate or decanoate administered on a biweekly injection schedule should be used in patients with a high possibility of noncompliance with prescribed regimens; (2) piperazine phenothiazines or haloperidol should be prescribed when sedative effects are undesirable; a piperazine phenothiazine or haloperidol should be employed for patients with cardiovascular disease or stroke. Compared to many of the other antipsychotics, these drugs produce a lesser degree of hypotension; (3) thioridazine may be the drug of first choice for patients with a high risk of developing extrapyramidal symptoms; thioridazine should be avoided if interference with ejaculation or sexual potency is of serious importance to the male patient; (4) haloperidol should be prescribed for patients who have compromised hepatic function or for patients considered to have a high risk for developing jaundice. Haloperidol has been reported to cause jaundice, but the incidence is very low and an etiological link has been difficult to establish (Byck, 1975).

A specific symptom that may be a factor in the choice of drug is visual hallucinations. This symptom occurs rather infrequently in the schizophrenic patients and there is a strong possibility that the hallucinating patient is suffering from either alcohol withdrawal or withdrawal from certain drugs, particularly barbiturate or sedative-hypnotic drugs. Patients with this symptom should not be started on phenothiazines without a definite diagnosis.

It may be the way in which the patient metabolizes oral medication that makes it difficult for him to experience an optimal therapeutic response. In some patients 90% of a 100 mg. dose of chlorpromazine may not get past the GI tract and the liver. By giving the drug parenterally, there is more drug available to target areas in the brain and therefore greater improvement. Clinical experience has shown that the most unreliable drug takers are the paranoid schizophrenics and with this type of patient it may be preferable to start with injections of fluphenazine decanoate.

Patients who are particularly sensitive to autonomic symptoms (e.g., hypotension or blurred vision due to impaired accommodation) should be treated with an antipsychotic other than an aliphatic or piperidine derivative; the same applies if undue drowsiness needs to be avoided. On the other hand, if extrapyramidal symptoms are particularly disturbing, a piperidine derivative may be indicated rather than a piperazine. If frequent intramuscular injections are required, one of the more potent antipsychotics should be used to avoid tissue infiltration with large amounts of medication. Chlorpromazine is not the preferred drug for epileptics and is unique among the phenothiazines for causing marked photosensitivity. The piperazine derivatives and haloperidol, although causing more extrapyramidal side effects, spark fewer convulsions (Lehmann, 1975).

From the above it can be seen that it may be important to anticipate possible unwanted effects in matching the drug, dosage and regimen to the patient. Certain side effects are more apt to occur in particular individuals. Acute dystonic reactions occur more often in young males and parkinsonian symptoms in elderly females. Some individuals will experience acute anticholinergic effects as dry mouth, others as constipation and some as urinary hesitancy or retention. Since thioridazine has the highest anticholinergic activity of the phenothiazines in clinical use, it may cause anticholinergic toxicity. Hypotension in the elderly may result in transient cerebral ischemia and dangerous falls, while galactorrea may be objectionable to males but more acceptable to females. In contrast, weight gain may cause great concern in women. It has been found that molindone (Moban) has a tendency to produce weight loss and therefore this drug should be considered in the treatment of the obese patient (Gardos and Cole, 1977).

During the past few years there has been an increasing tendency to use the high-potency antipsychotics (haloperidol, fluphenazine, thiothixene, perphenazine and trifluoperazine). In contrast to the low-potency drugs (chlorpromazine, thioridazine, chlorprothixene) and mid-range potency drug (mesoridazine), these drugs avoid the hypotensive and general depressant effects of low-potency drugs and minimize the tendency toward deposition in the skin, cornea, lens and tissues of pigmented metabolites with chronic administration (Shader and DiMascio, 1970). Agranulocytosis and cholestatic jaundice have been more frequently observed with chlorpromazine. The oral concentrate forms of chlorpromazine and thioridazine are remarkably bad tasting. Thioridazine is not available in a parenteral form, which limits its usefulness in agitated patients. In the past it has been prescribed extensively for elderly patients, presumably because of its low incidence of extrapyramidal side effects. This may be a questionable practice in view of possible problems with hypotensive episodes and further embarrassment of cerebrovascular perfusion. Clinicians now give less preference to these two antipsychotics, which continue to enjoy widespread popularity mainly because of historical primacy and persistent promotion (Zavodnick, 1977).

The apparent differences between various antipsychotic drugs in individual patients may be due more to idiosyncratic kinetics and the metabolism of these drugs than to any important pharmacological differences between them. The statement by Goldberg et al. (1972) is still valid: "for the clinician considering the choice of an antipsychotic drug, no system is yet available, either through empirical research or accumulated clinical experience, to enable matching of particular antipsychotics with particular schizophrenic patients in terms of their symptom profile." In other words, the formula has not yet been discovered for the "right drug for the right patient." It may well be that, at this time, the drug of choice can only be the drug best tolerated by the patient.

4. ESTIMATED EQUIVALENCY

The clinician must be aware of the estimated equivalent potency of the antipsychotic drugs.

Other than unwanted side effects, the major difference between antipsychotics is their milligram potency. Most of the aliphatic (i.e., chlorpromazine—Thorazine) and piperidine (i.e., thioridazine—Mellaril) phenothiazines are usually termed **high-dose** or **low-potency** drugs with the doses measured in hundreds of milligrams per day as compared with the piperazine phenothiazines, the more potent thioxanthenes (thiothixine—Navane), the butyrophenone (haloperidol—Haldol), the dibenzoxazepine (loxapine—Loxitane) and the dihydroindoline (molindone—Moban). The latter are considered **low-dose** or **high-potency** drugs with daily doses in the tens of milligrams. Potency should never be confused with efficacy, as despite their greater potency, low-dose drugs offer no advantage in total efficacy. High-potency antipsychotics offer a generally higher ratio between the desired antipsychotic effects and other undesired pharmacological effects such as sedation and alpha-adrenergic blocking action (Hollister, 1973).

In tables for estimated equivalent dose, all the antipsychotic drugs are compared to chlorpromazine, which is given an arbitrary value of 100. Table 3 contains estimated dosage equivalency data and conversion factors commonly used. It can be noted that 2 mg. of fluphenazine is roughly equivalent to 100 mg. of chlorpromazine. Potency is not equivalent to cost, nor does it mean that 50 times more patients will be benefited with fluphenazine than with chlorpromazine. It means that the pharmaceutical chemist used a fiftieth as much by weight in a tablet (Klerman, 1974).

In Table 4, Davis (1974) provides an empirically determined dose equivalent between different antipsychotic agents uninfluenced by drug company

TABLE 3
Estimated Equivalency of Antipsychotic Drugs

	Estimated equivalent dose (mgs.)	Conversion factor*
PHENOTHIAZINES (Classified by side chain)		
ALIPHATIC		
Chlorpromazine (Thorazine)	100	1:1
Triflupromazine (Vesprin)	25	1:4
PIPERIDINE		
Thioridazine (Mellaril)	100	1:1
Mesoridazine (Serentil)	50	1:2
Piperacetazine (Quide)	10	1:10
PIPERAZINE		
Actophenazine (Tindal)	20	1:5
Carphenazine (Proketazine)	25	1:4
Prochlorperazine (Compazine)	15	1:6
Perphenazine (Trilafon)	10	1:10
Trifluoperazine (Stelazine)	5	1:20
Fluphenazine (Prolixin, Permitil)	2	1:50
Butaperazine (Repoise)	10	1:10
BUTYROPHENONES		
Haloperidol (Haldol)	2	1:50
THIOXANTHENE DERIVATIVES		
Chlorprothixene (Taractan)	100	1:1
Thiothixene (Navane)	5	1:20
DIHYDROINDOLONE		
Molindone (Moban, Lidone)	25	1:4
DIBENZOXAZEPINES		
Loxapine (Loxitane)	15	1:6

*Estimated dosage ratio in relation to chlorpromazine. For example: A dose of 10 mg of perphenazine (Trilafon) is equivalent to 100 mg of chlorpromazine (Thorazine) since it is 10 times as potent.

promotional or medical legal decisions. His data were derived from all double-blind studies which investigated the well studied antipsychotic drugs using chlorpromazine as a standard. With some of the less well used antipsychotic drugs, where there were either no studies using chlorpromazine as a standard or very few, he calculated the rates of the drug to a more widely used antipsychotic drug whose dose potency in comparison to chlor-

TABLE 4
Dose Equivalence of Antipsychotic Drugs

Generic name (brand name)	Dose ratio equivalent to 100 mg. chlorpromazine (ratio S.E.M.*)	Oral dose† (mg/kg)	Parenteral (dose, mg/kg)
Chlorpromazine (Thorazine)	100	3.4952	1.1650
Triflupromazine (Vesprin)	28.4 ± 1.8	0.9904	0.3301
Thioridazine (Mellaril)	95.3 ± 8.2	3.3333	1.1111
Prochlorperazine (Compazine)	14.3 ± 1.7	0.5000	0.1666
Perphenazine (Trilafon)	8.9 ± 0.6	0.3100	0.1033
Fluphenazine (Prolixin)	1.2 ± 0.1	0.0419	0.0139
Trifluoperazine (Stelazine)	2.8 ± 0.4	0.0980	0.0326
Acetophenazine (Tindal)	23.5 ± 1.5	0.8190	0.2730
Carphenazine (Proketazine)	24.3 ± 2.7	0.8380	0.2793
Butaperazine (Repoise)	8.9 ± 1.1	0.3095	0.1031
Mesoridazine (Serentil)	55.3 ± 8.3	1.9333	0.6444
Piperacetazine (Quide)	10.5	0.3671	0.1223
Haloperidol (Haldol)	1.6 ± 0.4	0.0545	0.0181
Chlorprothixene (Taractan)	43.9 ± 13.9	1.5333	0.5111
Thiothixene (Navane)	5.2 ± 1.3	0.1809	0.0603

*Standard Error of the Mean.
†One-third the average daily dose in a 70 kg "person".
Reprinted with permission: John M. Davis, M.D., Dose Equivalence of the Antipsychotic Drugs. *J. Psychiatric Research*, Vol. 11, pp 65-69, © 1974, Pergamon Press Ltd.

promazine was known. Thus, in all cases he was able to calculate (directly or indirectly) an empirically determined dosage equivalent to chlorpromazine. In the first column of Table 4, there is listed the ratio of antipsychotic drugs compared to chlorpromazine given an arbitrary value of 100. The average dose of chlorpromazine per day in the double-blind studies reviewed was 734 mg. Based on the assumption of a 3 times a day dosage schedule and a 70 kg. man, the mg/kg. per dose would be approximately 3.5. If it is assumed that intramuscular chlorpromazine is 3 times as potent as oral chlorpromazine, then an average antipsychotic dose would be approximately 1.2 mg/kg. Davis further adds that there are no hard data on the equivalence of intramuscular to oral medication, so that the third column can be considered only an approximation. All the antipsychotics were found to be equally effective in these double-blind studies. Therefore, the dose equivalents listed are the mgs. of drug necessary to achieve what clinicians feel to be optimal antipsychotic effect as determined empirically from double-blind studies.

From the clinical standpoint, antipsychotic drugs administered intramuscularly are generally considered to be 3 to 4 times more potent than when given orally and doses should be adjusted accordingly. In prescribing and changing from one antipsychotic drug to another, the clinician should have some knowledge of the differences in the estimated equivalent potency. However, it is stressed that the equivalency tables are only approximate and dosing must primarily be determined by patient response. Most antipsychotics have a very high therapeutic index and seldom any life-threatening side effects.

The development of the depot fluphenazine preparations has been a major advance in the drug treatment of schizophrenia. When indicated, there are several methods of converting from oral medication to the depot phenothiazines. Grozier (1973) recommends (1) stop the previous antipsychotic; (2) start on low initial dose 0.25 ml (6.25 mg.) which is a test dose for safety; and (3) increase dose according to patient's response and the occurrence of side effects. His table compares the rough equivalency dosage of the depot phenothiazines to previous doses of an antipsychotic. Patients receiving medium or high doses of an oral antipsychotic should not immediately receive an equivalent dose of a long-acting antipsychotic. Rather, each patient's dosage should be individually titrated, since some patients will not require high doses of the depot antipsychotic (see Table 5).

A wise strategy may consist of decreasing the dose of oral medication gradually to the point of a washout period or drug holiday before starting depot phenothiazine therapy. In this way, withdrawal symptoms are not confused with reactions to the fluphenazine enanthate or decanoate. Also, this method avoids imposing fluphenazine decanoate on top of daily oral

TABLE 5

Rough Equivalency Dosage of Fluphenazine Enanthate and
Fluphenazine Decanoate Compared to Previous Doses
of an Oral Neuroleptic

Previous Dose of Oral Neuroleptic	Fluphenazine Enanthate or Fluphenazine Decanoate Dose
1. Low dosage	−0.5 to 1.5 ml (6.25 to 37.5 mg)
2. Medium dosage	−1.5 to 3 ml (37.5 to 75 mg)
3. High dosage	−3 to 4 ml (75 to 100 mg)

With permission from "The Future of Pharmacotherapy New Drug Delivery Systems." Copyright 1973, International Drug Therapy Newsletter.

medication because an extrapyramidal reaction may be generated. In an outpatient this type of side effect can be very embarrassing, particularly if the patient develops an acute dystonic reaction while he is out socially or at work. He and his family may blame the injection and refuse any more. The paranoid patient may incorporate the extrapyramidal reaction into his delusional system and believe the doctor poisoned him. Dropout data indicate that 90% of the patients who discontinue fluphenazine decanoate therapy do so during the first 3 months, generally because they get side effects which are subjectively distressing. It is for these reasons that a conservative approach is advocated—washout of the oral medication and low initial doses of depot fluphenazine (Ayd, 1976a).

Another method for converting patients to fluphenazine decanoate from all piperazine phenothiazines, haloperidol and thiothixene is one to one; that is, 1 mg. of oral trifluoperazine or haloperidol is approximately equal to 1 mg. of fluphenazine decanoate. The daily dose of the oral medication is converted to the closest dose of the injectable. For example, if a patient has been taking 20 mg. of trifluoperazine a day he would receive 1 ml (25 mg.) of fluphenazine decanoate every 2 weeks as a starting dose. The approximate guide is: 20-30 mg. of oral drug in this group converts to 1 ml of decanoate; 40 mg. converts to 1½ ml; 50-60 mg. converts to 2 ml. Ten mg. of chlorpromazine is equated approximately to 1 mg. of the decanoate (Keskiner, 1976).

Davis (1976a) offers the following method of calculating the dose of fluphenazine decanoate from the previous dose of oral medication: "Roughly speaking .67 mg. of fluphenazine enanthate (daily) is equivalent to .61 mg. of fluphenazine decanoate which is equivalent to 100 mg. of oral chlorpromazine. This evidence is based on several studies comparing the enanthate and decanoate forms and on a study by Chien and Cole (1973) that found 28.5 mg. of fluphenazine enanthate over 11 days was equivalent to 388 mg. per day of chlorpromazine. For example, if a patient has been stabilized on 200 mg. of chlorpromazine a day, computing the equivalent dose by this formula would yield 17 mg. of fluphenazine decanoate every 2 weeks."

Conversion estimates of oral antipsychotics to depot phenothiazines are very crude and empirical. For this reason it is wise to start with depot doses moderately lower than the intramuscular dose calculated by a conversion formula, remembering always that all equivalencies are "ball park" estimates and that antipsychotic dosage should be adjusted optimally for each patient.

5. DOSAGE

Adequate dosage is essential; underdosing should be avoided.

Generally speaking, any antipsychotic drug will afford satisfactory results provided it is given in sufficiently large amounts. Small doses will rarely control the symptoms of the actively psychotic patient and there is no rationale for using low dosages to avoid side effects if there is no benefit. On the other hand, after the target symptoms have been controlled, the patient should be stabilized at the lowest effective maintenance dosage.

With a new patient whose symptoms are acute, the higher the dose, the greater the likelihood of a rapid onset of therapeutic effect. An increase to the maximum dosage within 3 days to a week is recommended. Very little is gained by building up the dosage gradually unless the patient or family drug history indicates neurological susceptibility or there is a physical contraindication such as in a geriatric patient with a cardiac condition. In the chronic patient, dosage can gradually be increased, allowing 3 to 4 days between changes.

The low, moderate and high dosage categories shown in Table 2 represent a conservative range of dosages and were obtained by using the maximal dosage for each antipsychotic drug as recommended in the *Physicians' Desk Reference* (1978) and dividing by 3. Clinical experience has shown that the upper level of the high dosage range is not the absolute maximum but a guideline for the initiation of therapy. The physician should recognize that optimal dosage level may be considerably higher, that it may vary from patient to patient, and that it can be accurately determined only by careful monitoring and clinical judgment. Acutely disturbed patients may require doses above the maximum stated in Table 2 for a short period of time. However, there is one important exception to this rule. **Thioridazine should never be prescribed in amounts exceeding 800 milligrams daily.** It has been implicated in causing pigmentary retinopathy leading to blindness when given in doses above 800 mg. daily. This precaution is stressed in the *Physicians' Desk Reference* (1977) and has been repeatedly emphasized in many reports and texts on psychopharmacology. Still, during medication reviews, one continues to find occasional prescriptions where this precautionary measure is unheeded.

TABLE 6
Dosage Relationships among Antipsychotic Drugs

Drug	U.S. Trade Name	Total Daily Dosage, mg.	
		Outpatient Range	Hospital Range
PHENOTHIAZINES (Classified by side chain)			
Aliphatic:			
Chlorpromazine	Thorazine	50-100	200-1600
Trifluopromazine	Vesprin	50-150	75-200
Piperidine:			
Mesoridazine	Serentil	25-200	100-400
Thioridazine	Mellaril	50-400	200-800
Piperacetazine	Quide	10-80	40-160
Piperazine:			
Acetophenazine	Tindal	40-60	60-80
Carphenazine	Proketazine	25-100	50-400
Prochlorperazine	Compazine	15-60	30-150
Perphenazine	Trilafon	8-24	12-64
Trifluoperazine	Stelazine	4-10	6-30
Fluphenazine*	Prolixin; Permitil	1-3	2-20
Butaperazine	Repoise	5-50	25-100
BUTYROPHENONES			
Haloperidol	Haldol	2-10	4-100
THIOXANTHENE DERIVATIVES			
Chlorprothixene	Taractan	30-60	75-600
Thiothixene	Navane	6-15	10-60
DIBENZOXAZEPINE			
Loxapine	Loxitane	20-125	60-250
DIHYDROINDOLONE			
Molindone	Moban; Lidone	15-100	100-225

*Dose range for fluphenazine enanthate and decanoate are 12.5 to 100 mg. every one to three weeks. Adapted from Hollister, Leo E., *Clinical Use of Psychotherapeutic Drugs*, 1973. Courtesy of Charles C Thomas, Publisher, Springfield, Illinois.

Table 6 gives the general range of therapeutic doses for outpatients and inpatients (Hollister, 1973). **However, dosage should be adapted for the individual patient to achieve maximal benefit from the antipsychotic properties of the drug.** It is believed that since the range between a therapeutically effective dosage and a toxic overdose is very wide, it is generally safer to err in the direction of higher doses, thus avoiding inadequate dosage. Not uncommonly, clinicians will use fixed doses for long periods of time for every patient or minimal doses which fail to benefit severe symptomatology. Such routine fixed dose strategies should be avoided.

The individual metabolism of psychotropic drugs varies so markedly that it is useless to rely on body weight or even symptom severity for anything more than the crudest indication of either starting or maintenance dosage. This means that the only rational method for judging dosage in any individual is to titrate the desired therapeutic effect against the unwanted effects. This task is simplified by knowing that many side effects either follow immediately on drug administration (sedation, hypotension or anticholinergic effects) or are readily detectable (such as parkinsonian symptoms). It is therefore possible and advisable to increase dosage rapidly to obtain the desired therapeutic effect, provided careful clinical observations of side effects are made. Also, dosage can be increased until limiting side effects are observed. In general, then, one should start low but increase rapidly with regard to the ratio between therapeutic and unwanted effects. In many patients there is a "therapeutic window" in dosage below which there is no response and above which toxic effects obscure benefit (Blackwell, 1975).

When sedation seems necessary, some clinicians start the patient on chlorpromazine with a typical dosage schedule that may begin with 200 mg. on the first day. The dosage is increased to 600 or 800 mg. over the next few days. If this does not control psychotic symptomatology, the dosage is gradually increased to 1000-1500 mg. per day.

With an acutely psychotic patient in the hospital setting, a high potency drug such as haloperidol can be started at 5 mg. dose initially. Depending on the response, 1 hour later another 5 to 10 mg. may be given orally. The patient then can be placed on a dosage of 5 to 10 mg. t.i.d. and evaluated several times daily. An as-needed (PRN) order is written for 5 mg. intramuscularly or 5 to 10 mg. orally as frequently as every hour for emergency controls, in addition to regularly scheduled medication. Usually, within 2 or 3 days, an adequate maintenance dose level is achieved. If the patient is acutely agitated or floridly psychotic and will not accept oral medication, the intramuscular route can be used.

There is an increasing tendency to use predominantly the more potent, nonsedating antipsychotic agents such as haloperidol, thiothixene, perphenazine or fluphenazine because of their dose-toxicity relationship and also their low level of atropine-like side effects. The more sedating, less potent agents have several shortcomings in the upper dose range therapy. It is well-known that electrocardiographic changes are a function of the dose of thioridazine and hypotension tends to be a function of the dose of chlorpromazine. Also, patients tend to become markedly sedated, sometimes before they reach a therapeutic level. These are some of the reasons for the increasing preference of the more potent drugs when using a high dose or a rapid tranquilization method.

Patients who are refractory to standard dose medication may respond to a higher initial dose of medication. Some patients may not respond to a small dose of oral medication (i.e., 5 to 10 mg.) of one of the more potent antipsychotic drugs. But when they are given 20 to 30 mg. or even 40 mg. they will show a rapid symptom response. Dose requirements of antipsychotic drugs often vary widely in different individuals. There is no strict correlation between plasma levels of antipsychotics and their therapeutic effects. Body weight is not a good predictor of the amount of medication required. Small statured people may require very high dosage, whereas a large 200-pound male may respond to as little as 100 mg. of chlorpromazine or 2 to 5 mg. of a low-dose antipsychotic daily. There is some evidence that schizophrenic women below 50 years of age require more antipsychotic medication than schizophrenic men of comparable age (Noonan et al., 1977).

A variation of high dose therapy is used routinely by some clinicians. The younger, physically fit patient who is considered non-emergency may be started at 10 to 20 mg. per day of one of the more potent antipsychotic drugs. If there is no clinical response by the second day, the dose may be increased to 20 to 30 mg. If, by day 3, there is little evidence that any clinical response has occurred, the medication may be further increased to 40 to 60 mg. daily. If the drug used is haloperidol, the daily dosage may be increased to 80 mg. even 100 mg. to obtain a clinical response. As soon as the patient begins to show definitive improvement, the dose is stabilized and later gradually reduced to the least amount of medication that is required to prevent an exacerbation of the symptoms.

Donlon (1975), however, believes that the dose-response curve of the more potent antipsychotics plateaus in the area of 30 to 60 mg. per day. There is only a small percentage of patients who respond to doses up to 100 mg. daily. If the average patient does not respond in the dose range of 60 to 100 mg. a day of the more potent agents within a reasonable length of time, a switch to another antipsychotic is recommended.

In general, the severity and duration of symptoms may be an indication of drug dosage required. Patients with acute, florid symptomatology of a week's duration initially tend to require a higher dosage than those with an insidious illness which has developed over a number of months. Patients who exhibit dysphoria, panic or excitement also tend to require higher doses of medication for remission of symptoms.

Antipsychotics are more effective during the early stages of schizophrenia and their effectiveness diminishes the longer the schizophrenia has existed before antipsychotic therapy is instituted. Thus the more chronic the schizophrenia (and thus the more metabolically different the patient is compared to early schizophrenia), the higher the dosage of the antipsychotic must be and the more treatment-resistant the patient is likely to be.

When target symptoms fail to respond to an adequate dosage of an antipsychotic drug, patient noncompliance or inability to absorb the drug in the gastrointestinal tract should be considered. A Forrest urine test or a short course of intramuscular administration of the agent may indicate such problems and make switching to a second agent unnecessary. Usually, if little or no improvement is observed after two or three months, a trial on a different antipsychotic drug is indicated. However, a change may be warranted after a few days in a severely disturbed acute patient. Rarely, to break an episode of excitement or in other extreme situations, short-acting barbiturates may be used in addition to antipsychotic medication.

A common cause of failure with antipsychotic drug therapy is to prescribe a dosage that is too low. Often an increase in dosage in such cases results in substantial improvement and makes switching to a different antipsychotic unnecessary. Many physicians are afraid to use large doses, particularly when they do not use a specific antipsychotic agent as a prominent part of their usual clinical practice. Others may be fearful of side effects and their ability to handle them. As a result, underdosing is frequently the explanation for the persistence of florid symptoms of the psychosis, such as delusions or hallucinations.

Often low doses will reduce overt psychotic behavior and make the patient more manageable, but this should not be the goal of chemotherapy. The clinician who is content with mild or moderate improvement at low doses may prolong the patient's course of treatment and risk exacerbation of the psychotic condition. However, caution should be used in treating elderly patients. With advancing age, the patient's ability to distribute, detoxify and eliminate drugs may be reduced, thereby increasing risk of toxic effects.

Many "ultra conservative" clinicians use a slow, "stair-step" approach. Dosage is started at a low level and is slowly raised every few days to a week. Weeks or months may ensue before an effective dosage is reached and acute symptomatology is controlled. This dosage procedure not only has many disadvantages for the patient but insures an unnecessarily prolonged length of hospitalization.

Davis (1976b) reviewed 23 studies that used chlorpromazine in treating a wide variety of schizophrenic patients. The average dose of chlorpromazine was 734 mg. ± 63. Most of these studies were done on relatively sick patients who required large doses, so that the figure would be an average dose for the severely ill, hospitalized patients. This may account for the finding that the average daily dose for acute schizophrenics is about 800 mg. of chlorpromazine or its equivalent in the other antipsychotics. However, 2 to 3 weeks of drug therapy at this dosage range is necessary for chlorpromazine to exert its therapeutic effect.

Lehmann (1975) recommends that the first dose should be 50-100 mg. of chlorpromazine (or its equivalent) intramuscularly or 100-150 mg. orally. The parenterally administered drug might be expected to take effect in about 20-30 minutes, the oral administration after about 45 minutes. If the patient's symptoms have not improved after this time, either half the initial dose or the full dose may be repeated. Observation or report on the patient's condition must then be obtained after the same time interval to determine whether symptoms are adequately controlled or whether another dose of the antipsychotic needs to be administered. The pharmacological effect of the first dose or any other dose, even if it has not resulted in much symptomatic improvement, should not be allowed to dissipate before a follow-up dose is administered; this is important if a gradual accumulation of the drug effect is to be achieved. Since reduction of excitement occurs before any toxic effects become manifest, the patient's behavioral status is a good gauge of his individual dose requirements in this acute condition. After the first dose, there may be undesirable autonomic effects, particularly orthostatic hypotension, if the patient is hypersensitive to the drug, but all that is necessary for controlling such complications is to have the patient lie down.

Another common error is too-rapid changes in medication. If the physician changes the drug he is prescribing for an inpatient every 2 weeks because he is not satisfied with the therapeutic results, he might never learn the proper dose and time required to produce improvement. A good rule of thumb is not to change to another drug until the drug that was originally chosen has been given—at gradually increasing doses—over a period of 6 to 8 weeks without any noticeable improvement.

In the early stages of treating schizophrenia it is better to exceed the minimal required dose than to remain below it. Since the acute toxicity of most antipsychotics is amazingly low, there is very little risk involved in raising the dose rapidly to achieve maximum control of the most disturbing and distressing symptoms in a day or two. In certain patients, daily doses of 2,000-3,000 mg. of chlorpromazine, or its equivalent, may be required (Lehmann, 1975).

Shader and Jackson (1975) initiate treatment with a small test dose of the antipsychotic (25 to 50 mg. PO or 25 mg. IM of chlorpromazine or the equivalent dose of another antipsychotic drug). If no idiosyncratic effect develops within two hours, titrating the drug dosage into an effective antipsychotic range can begin. They believe that the usual antipsychotic dosage range for acutely ill schizophrenic patients is 300 to 1800 mg. daily of chlorpromazine or an equivalent amount of another drug. For younger patients who are acutely agitated and psychotic, they recommend that treatment begin with doses from 600 to 1200 mg. daily of chlorpromazine or equivalent. In patients over 40 or in those who have been psychotic for a long time, beginning doses of 300 to 600 mg. daily of chlorpromazine or equivalent may be more appropriate. Their general rule is to titrate the dosage until an adequate therapeutic effect is achieved or troublesome side effects are encountered.

It has been noted that the level at which antipsychotic drug therapy is instituted and the manner of its use vary widely from one psychiatric setting to another. Generally, crisis-oriented, overcrowded, public acute facilities start drug therapy in the emergency room, use intramuscular medication freely in turbulent or severely withdrawn patients and raise the dosage rapidly over 2 or 3 days to a high level—such as 1000 mg. of chlorpromazine (or its equivalent in the other antipsychotics). The dosage is reduced only after the patient is clearly much less aroused and agitated and is beginning to be quiet and even sleepy. In better staffed, more selective, private acute facilities, a drug-free evaluation period of days or even weeks may precede a rather gradual initiation of drug therapy, with levels of 300 mg. a day of chlorpromazine much more common than levels of 1000 mg. No reasonable evidence indicates which procedure leads to a better long-term remission. Under either regime, reduction of overt psychotic symptoms and a gradual cognitive reorganization are the goals of therapy (Davis and Cole, 1975). However, the ultra-conservative approach to adequate antipsychotic drug therapy practiced in many psychiatric facilities results in needless days and weeks of suffering for the psychiatric patient and enormously increases the cost of inpatient care.

Most clinicians gradually reduce the dosage of the antipsychotic drug when the patient appears maximally improved and raise the dose again if symptoms recur. A modest prophylactic increase of dosage is sometimes used when the patient is about to undergo a special stress such as returning home or starting a new job.

Rapid tranquilization may be indicated for patients who have severe psychotic symptoms. This use of antipsychotic drugs involves frequent intramuscular dosing (every 30 to 60 minutes) until improvement occurs. Emphasis is placed on the frequency of or the time interval between dosage increments. A variation of this procedure (focusing on the amount of dosage) is also gaining increasingly greater acceptance. Early large oral or intramuscular doses of drugs such as haloperidol, perphenazine, thiothixene and fluphenazine are used. The recent increase in the upper dosage limit currently approved for haloperidol to 100 mg. has fostered this approach. It is believed by many authorities that these high doses (60 to 100 mg. haloperidol per day) may place the drug in a clinically effective range that is no longer associated with the same intensity and frequency of unwanted extrapyramidal effects (Shader and Jackson, 1975). (Rapid tranquilization is fully discussed in Chapter III.)

Many physicians continue to use the same agents and dosage even when they have failed to affect the illness. The reluctance to prescribe newer drugs or to increase dosages of older ones appears to stem from a fear of possible malpractice litigation. Dosages used in the treatment of many psychiatric patients are actually homeopathic. Physicians argue that they dare not use higher dosages or prescribe new agents because too little is known about the effects of such treatment, yet the safety and efficacy of more innovative treatments have often been well established scientifically. The failure to modify treatment appropriately may account for many patients who are considered treatment failures.

In essence, the dosage of every drug must be tailored to the needs of the individual patient. Ayd (1974a) has forcibly stated: "therapists who ignore this axiom inevitably undermedicate a percentage of their patients, thereby depriving them of the chance to obtain optimal benefit and condemning them to a prolongation of suffering and disability. Not every patient needs high dose therapy. The therapist's challenge is to recognize those who do.

"Most physicians do not prescribe high doses for fear of side effects and medical-legal action against them for exceeding the dosage recommendation in the package insert. This is unjustifiable. Such doctors are protecting themselves. They are not discharging their duty to patients. High dose therapy is not without risk but, as high dose studies show, the hazards are not substantially greater than with low doses when patients are carefully selected and monitored. Furthermore, the contents of the package insert are guidelines only. **They are not a legal barrier to judicious drug therapy.** Thus, for an individual patient, it seems more rational to choose the right dosage schedule rather than the right drug."

6. SINGLE AGENT

Only one antipsychotic agent should be used at a time.

This basic principle in the use of antipsychotic drug therapy seems to require repeated emphasis. As far back as 1967, Freeman reviewed the literature with respect to the value of combinations of psychotropic drugs in various psychiatric states and discovered that the combination of two antipsychotic drugs showed no improvement over single drugs. Sheppard et al. (1969) found that when combinations of psychotropic drugs were prescribed in a large New York state mental hospital, one-third involved the use of two antipsychotics. A survey of prescription practices (Sheppard et al., (1974), disclosed that 33% of 942 psychiatrists from 4 populous states having large patient and psychiatrist populations selected some form of polypharmacy as a treatment of choice in initiating the therapy of an acute paranoid schizophrenic. Of those selecting a polypharmacy response, 79% chose a regimen consisting of two antipsychotics. After one year of ineffective chemotherapy, combinations of 3 and up to 6 potent antipsychotics were prescribed. Mason et al. (1977a), in a study of patterns of antipsychotic drug use in the four mental hospitals of a southeastern state, reported that of 1182 prescriptions written for antipsychotic drugs, 30% were for 2 antipsychotics to be administered at the same time. A survey of Veteran Administration hospitals (Mesard et al., 1976) showed that, of 17,276 psychotic patients receiving drug therapy, 26.5% had orders for 2 or more antipsychotics. Thus, it appears that we are still in the era of polypharmacy for schizophrenia and this practice still remains prevalent, even though there is no scientific evidence from well-controlled, well-designed and well-executed studies to indicate that conjoint therapy with 2 or more antipsychotics is any more efficacious than treatment with adequate doses of a single antipsychotic.

The chief result of conjoint antipsychotic drug therapy is that it leaves the physician in the position where there is uncertainty as to which antipsychotic was effective or ineffective in treating the patient. It becomes difficult for the physician to determine optimal dosage over the course of treatment and to identify the source of side effects. Medication-taking becomes more complex, increasing the risk of error on the part of outpatients and adding additional burdens on the nursing staff in inpatient facilities. Such combinations may lead to some type of drug-drug interaction that affects absorption, distribution, binding, metabolism or excretion and any one of these may negate or lessen therapeutic efficacy. They also may be responsible for tolerance and cross-tolerance, which may make the usually prescribed daily doses ineffective. Initiation of therapy with more than one antipsychotic may suggest diagnostic imprecision and haste.

Usually, the total dose of each antipsychotic in conjoint therapy is low—often so low as to justify the label of homeopathic. Compliance studies have confirmed that the more drugs a person has to take each day, the more likely it is that some doses will not be taken. The result is a patient who is underdosed. Some clinicians use antipsychotic combinations with the goal of attaining an effective level with the lower doses of each drug or fewer side effects while maintaining adequate control of symptoms. These results usually are not achieved by conjoint drug therapy. There is no firm evidence to support this type of prescribing practice and, in fact, there may be an added risk from combinations, since there may be mutually addictive effects that can produce more side effects.

Failure of the patient to respond to the first drug tried does not necessarily mean that there will be no response to other antipsychotics. However, the patient will not do better on any other member of the same subgroup. This is one of the reasons for following the suggested rational approach in selecting antipsychotic drugs (see section on Choice of Drug).

Changes from one antipsychotic to another are ordinarily accomplished by the gradual decrease of the old medication as the new agent is started at a low dose and gradually increased with careful monitoring. When it is feasible, some clinicians discontinue all antipsychotic medication for a week before starting on the different antipsychotic. The estimated dosage equivalency is taken into consideration as the new dosage is titrated upward. It should be remembered that small amounts of the first drug may be excreted slowly for several weeks to months after its discontinuation. When the physician is changing to another antipsychotic drug, the target symptoms should again be noted in the clinical record.

In attempting to explain conjoint antipsychotic therapy, Merlis et al. (1970, 1972) pointed out the belief of many physicians that the more proven a treatment, the better—therefore, the tendency to combine two proven medications. This notion gained support from successful treatment utilizing combinations of drugs in other areas of medicine. Efficacy of combined drug therapy has been demonstrated in the treatment of tuberculosis, hypertension, epilepsy and other somatic disorders. Another concept of clinical therapeutics currently still in vogue is the tendency to add a second drug to the treatment program in face of unremitting symptoms instead of increasing the initial drug of choice to maximum potential.

There is a growing appreciation of the hazards of promiscuous use of antipsychotic agents in producing tardive dyskinesia; therefore, using antipsychotics singly is becoming increasingly important. Merlis et al (1972) affirm that there is no basis in fact to justify the use of multiple psychotropic agents or support for such continued use as an effective treatment modality.

7. POLYPHARMACY

Polypharmacy should be avoided whenever possible.
Survey of drug orders for psychiatric patients shows that large numbers are still receiving simultaneously divided daily doses of one or more tranquilizers, an antiparkinson drug and a hypnotic. The result is the ingestion

of a "psychopharmacological stew" which exposes the patient to additional hazards. Many are also taking one or more other medicines for coexisting physical illnesses and a large percentage of those who are outpatients add to the mix by self-medicating with over-the-counter preparations for minor ailments or to combat side effects such as constipation.

Reliable studies have failed to show that the administration of two or more antipsychotics is more effective and safer than adequate doses of a single drug. Furthermore, there is little evidence to support the value of the co-prescription of an antipsychotic with a minor tranquilizer (the antianxiety drugs) or with an antidepressant and a minor tranquilizer. When combined drug therapy is used there is a tendency to prescribe low doses of all drugs which will not be efficacious for many patients.

Polypharmacy seldom can be considered rational or scientific and may be indicative of a serious gap in the basic knowledge and clinical use of these drugs. Most combinations are of limited usefulness, potentially dangerous and result in patients who are overmedicated or underdosed or exposed to the adverse reactions of each drug and the risk of their adverse interaction (Ayd, 1973a). It is well-known that drugs may alter each other's metabolism and as more medications are concurrently prescribed, there develops a greater possibility of toxicity, side effects and potentiation of interference with the desirable effects of any one drug. The use of polypharmacy often can result in abnormal behavioral symptoms. It is not unusual to find patients who are lethargic, asocial, disinterested or acting peculiarly. When the drugs are discontinued or the dosage reduced, these patients become talkative, alert, sociable, show a broadening of interests and many of their odd behaviors disappear. There appears to be no doubt that the patients were "drugged" and a good deal of their strange behavior was medication-induced. The geriatric patient is particularly susceptible to the effect of multiple psychotropic agents. Symptoms such as restlessness, agitation, paranoid behavior, confusion and disorientation can result, but when the medications are discontinued, there is a striking improvement. It has been shown that at least 20% of the psychogeriatric admissions are precipitated by the adverse effects of psychotropic drugs (Learoyd, 1972).

Another disadvantage of polypharmacy lies in the unnecessary burden it places on the nursing staff. The rate of medication errors grows in proportion to the number of drugs concurrently prescribed and with the frequency with which they must be given. Nurses on psychiatric wards must cope with this fact in attempting to dispense multiple drugs with accuracy. Also, studies indicate that the number of medications and age are important factors affecting the frequency of medication errors by patients on self-medication.

Hollister (1973, 1975) has described the origin and development of the myth that two antipsychotic drugs might be better than one, an idea which occurred to some pioneer psychopharmacotherapists quite early. Combination therapy was attractive in that the first two antipsychotic drugs (reserpine and chlorpromazine) had somewhat different pharmacological effects. Despite the favorable results being reported from conjoint reserpine and chlorpromazine therapy, a study (Hollister et al., 1955) indicated that patients treated with this combination were somewhat worse than those treated with chlorpromazine alone and that the prevalence of extrapyramidal reactions, such as akathisia and parkinsonism, was higher. This conclusion was apparently shared by others, for subsequently combined chlorpromazine-reserpine therapy was discarded.

Another combination that flourished during the first decade of antipsychotic drug therapy and is still frequently prescribed was the conjoint use of chlorpromazine (Thorazine) and trifluoperazine (Stelazine). It was believed that benefit would be derived from this combination since trifluoperazine had a lesser sedative effect than chlorpromazine, whereas chlorpromazine was less likely to cause extrapyramidal symptoms. However, it was found that trifluoperazine added to a stabilized maintenance dose of chlorpromazine neither reduced side effects nor increased therapeutic effectiveness (Casey et al., 1961). Also, the addition of other psychotropic drugs to maintenance programs of chlorpromazine in chronic withdrawn schizophrenics has failed to yield any further improvement.

The co-prescription of thioridazine and chlorpromazine enjoyed a degree of popularity for a different reason. These two phenothiazines are thought by many to be very effective in the management of acutely psychotic patients because of their sedative action. The maximal daily dose of thioridazine recommended is 800 mg., since higher doses raise the possibility of pigmentary retinopathy. This dosage level often fails to control the severely disturbed patient. As both drugs are strong alphaadrenergic receptor blocking agents, high doses of either or both may produce marked orthostatic hypotension. Their use of controlling agitated patients is now being replaced by substantial doses, often parenterally administered, of the low-dose antipsychotics such as haloperidol, fluphenazine or thiothixene (Sangiovanni et al., 1973; Anderson and Kuehnle, 1974).

With the advent of the long-acting esters of fluphenazine (Prolixin), a common clinical practice has arisen of administering them in combination with other antipsychotic drugs in the acute psychotic patient. However, the addition of chlorpromazine to prolixin enanthate does little to increase the enanthate's therapeutic efficacy. It should be stated that there are rare, isolated instances where large doses of single antipsychotics have failed and a combination of two antipsychotics yielded clinical improvement.

The combination of an antipsychotic agent with an antianxiety drug is rarely indicated. Even the package insert of some of the antianxiety drugs state that such a combination is generally not recommended or should be used with caution. For example, the manufacturer's insert with diazepam (Valium) states that "it should be remembered that Valium is not of value in the treatment of psychotic patients and should not be employed in lieu of appropriate treatment." Routine prescription of this combination is not advantageous in most cases. An exception is the use of diazepam for its adjunctive anticonvulsive properties in patients who are seizure-prone.

Another practice in rather widespread use is that of combining tricyclic antidepressants with antipsychotic drugs in schizophrenia. This type of combination was believed to be more effective than an antipsychotic alone in the treatment of the withdrawn, apathetic patient and that it increased alertness and thus aided in rehabilitation. Chouinard et al. (1975) found that in schizophrenic patients there was no evidence to indicate that the superiority of the amitriptyline-perphenazine combination over perphenazine alone. Amitriptyline alone was not substantially better than placebo. It can be concluded that with the exception of a combination of perphenazines and amitriptyline in schizophrenic patients with depressive features, the combination has shown no improvement over single drugs. Also, the conjoint use of antipsychotics with tricyclic antidepressants may be indicated in an agitated depression inadequately controlled by tolerable or safe doses of a tricyclic antidepressant alone. Phenothiazines added to the treatment regimen may help considerably in controlling the agitation until the antidepressant effect of the tricyclic becomes apparent. However, a combination of thioridazine with a tricyclic should be used with caution since both drugs have an adverse effect on cardiac repolarization which could be additive, possibly increasing the risk of sudden death (Hollister, 1975).

Occasionally, one finds the simultaneous administration of phenothiazines, tricyclic antidepressants and antiparkinson medication. Any two of these three may be given simultaneously but all three of them together may become dangerous or even fatal for some patients because of the synergistic effect resulting from the anticholinergic action of each one of these agents (Warnes et al., 1967). It is not recognized by many clinicians that if a tricyclic antidepressant is used with the antipsychotic drug, antiparkinson drugs usually will not be needed; the tricyclics have a similar central anticholinergic action.

Because of heavy daytime sedation, many patients have difficulty sleeping at night, for which a bedtime hypnotic may be prescribed. Incredibly, some patients are given a morning dose of dextroamphetamine or methylphenidate hydrochloride (Ritalin) to counteract the previous day's assault with sedatives.

Ayd (1973a) has posed these questions for the pharmacotherapist desirous of providing optimal benefits at the least risk and financial cost, whether prescribing for hospitalized or ambulant patients:

(1) Is a multitude of drugs necessary and in the best interest of the patient?
(2) Can the patient reasonably be expected to take multiple drugs properly, considering his circumstances, particularly when residing outside hospital and self-medicating?
(3) Is the prescribed regimen sufficiently simple for the patient to follow successfully, especially when unsupervised?
(4) Is there evidence that the patient can and will comply with prescription directions?

If the answer to each question is not affirmative, the treatment plans should be revised to ensure that the drug therapy recommended is appropriate, practical and likely to be followed. For most psychiatric patients this should be treatment with a single antipsychotic administered once daily.

Polypharmacy need not be a necessary evil. Through an educational campaign which includes periodic medication analyses and peer review, the routine use of conjoint antipsychotc prescriptions can be practically eliminated and other forms of polypharmacy markedly reduced (Diamond et al., 1976; Mason et al., 1977b).

8. DAILY ADMINISTRATION SCHEDULES

After the first week or two but especially after the patient has been stabilized on a maintenance dose, the antipsychotic drug should be administered on a once-a-day (q.d.) or at most a twice-a-day schedule.

Analysis of thousands of medication schedules of antipsychotic drugs reveal that this is the most common "basic principle" that physicians fail to incorporate in their prescribing practice (Mason, 1976). It was found that antipsychotic drugs are prescribed from three to five times a day for months and even many years. In such cases, the total daily amount to be given is administered in equally divided doses. There is no scientific basis for these practices and the use of multiple dose schedules was questioned by Tibbets as far back as 1958.

The basic principle of once-a-day medication is supported by the following well-documented facts marshalled by DiMascio (1972), concerning the antipsychotic drugs:

(1) Psychotropic drugs, in general, have a long biological half-life.
(2) The metabolism of psychotropic drugs and their excretion proceeds at a very slow rate. For example, a single dose of chlorpromazine may be detected biochemically in urine for up to 3 to 8 days and behaviorally for 8 to 24 hours.

(3) These drugs and their metabolites accumulate in various body tissues with continued drug administration until a saturation level is achieved. On cessation of the drugs, the tissues release these accumulations only slowly.

(4) The appearance of the pharmacological properties of primary clinical value in psychiatry (e.g., their antipsychotic effects) is noted later in time (days to weeks) than are the secondary properties (e.g., sedation, psychomotor inhibition) or side effects which, generally, are most prominently perceived 2 to 6 hours after administration, and tend to disappear after a few days of drug use.

Every phenothiazine, butyrophenone and thioxanthene can be and has been prescribed once or twice daily without loss of therapeutic efficacy or any significant increase in incidence or severity of side effects compared to equivalent amounts of the same drug in divided doses. Thus the common practice of initiating antipsychotic drug therapy with t.i.d. or q.i.d. doses and the continuation of this divided dose schedule as long as the patient requires medication is unnecessary for most patients. Once the optimal daily dosage is determined and the patient is stabilized, the medication may be administered either in one dose at bedtime or in two divided doses, after the evening meal and at bedtime. Usually when a b.i.d. schedule is chosen it is recommended that one-third of the dose be given in the morning and two-thirds in the evening. For most patients evening administration is preferable since most antipsychotics tend to sedate and a relatively large single dose can induce sleep. Thus, it may not be necessary to prescribe a sedative, which lessens the cost of delivery of health care and avoids possible interaction between it and the antipsychotic drug. It should be noted that the antipsychotic drugs are not good sedatives and should not be prescribed solely for this purpose.

With a single evening dose, the patient, while asleep, is unaware of pharmacologic side effects that would be annoying and subjectively distressing during the day. For this reason there is less lethargy and fewer complaints of dry mouth, blurred vision and tremor during the daytime hours. There is also less impairment of mental and physical faculties and this can make the drug more acceptable to patients, especially outpatients, and increases compliance with prescription instructions. In addition, a single evening dose for inpatients is more convenient for patients and staff than a multiple dose schedule. During the day, patients can be off the ward for therapeutic or recreational activities. When being treated with divided doses, patients must return to the ward or nursing staff will have to search for them. In the evening, most patients are on the ward and it is easier for nurses to dispense medications and to take the time to assure the patient actually swallows it. There is less risk of medication errors and a greater amount of time for nurses to take a more active role in patient care and other therapeutic duties. Outpatients who self-medicate and families or community-placement sponsors who have to supervise the patient's medication intake find a single daily dose convenient, easy to remember and economical. Patients are embarrassed by having to take drugs in the presence of others because they often have to explain why or be evasive (Ayd, 1973a).

Objections have been raised against a once-a-day dosage and the principal ones are (1) there will be an increase in side effects and (2) a single dose may be less effective than divided doses. Both of these presumptions have proven to be either false or unwarranted (DiMascio and Shader, 1969). Once daily dosages, even relatively high doses, have been given without untoward consequences to many patients with diverse physical disorders, including epilepsy and organic brain changes due to age or psychosurgery. Also, single high daily doses have been administered with other drugs patients required (anticonvulsants, hypoglycemics, cardiovascular preparations, etc.) without adverse reactions. High single bedtime doses of the more potent neuroleptics occasionally may spark an extrapyramidal reaction. However, these reactions can be treated successfully by a dosage reduction or with antiparkinson medication. The few patients who may object to taking a large number of pills at one time may be switched to the liquid concentrate.

Many studies have been carried out with a variety of antipsychotic drugs, comparing a multiple dose schedule with a q.d. or a b.i.d. schedule of administration. The latter schedule was included in the studies because certain investigators considered it beneficial to the patient to keep him under a limited degree of sedation during his waking hours, while others considered it to be of psychological value to give him a pill a second time. In each instance, it was documented that the single or b.i.d. dosage schedule of drug administration produced clinical benefit that was at least equal to—and often greater than—that produced by a multiple dose schedule.

Even when chlorpromazine was given at a dialy dose of 2000 mg., the results followed the same pattern. In a NIMH collaborative study (Prien and Cole, 1968), half of the patients received 500 mg. q.i.d.; the others received 600 mg. in the morning and 1400 mg. shortly before bedtime. There was no difference in the clinical benefit derived, but the patients on the b.i.d. schedule—with the large portion given in the evening—exhibited fewer side effects and rarely required antiparkinson drugs; 10% of the patients on the q.i.d. schedule were terminated because of side effects, while none of the b.i.d. schedule patients were terminated.

A study of compliance by chronic medical and psychiatric patients, age 20 to 65, was conducted to determine how frequency of administration affected compliance (Ayd, 1973a). The method used was a count of pills remaining in a container and tactful interrogation of patients about their medication consumption. At the end of one month the compliance of patients taking divided doses of a single drug was: q.i.d.—70% failed to take 25 to 50% of the prescribed dose; t.i.d.—60% failed to take 20 to 50% of the prescribed dose; b.i.d.—30% failed to take up to 25% of the prescribed dose; and q.d.—70% failed to take up to 20% of the prescribed dose. There was no difference between medical and psychiatric patients, nor did side effects play a major role in noncompliance. It is, therefore, evident that there is greater adherence to a once-a-day schedule than a multiple dose schedule. Many believe that a patient who is expected to take his pills regularly more than once or twice a day is almost certain to default.

Some clinicians now start their patients with a single dose given one hour before bedtime and others after the first 48 to 72 hours of treatment. In the occasional patient who reacts with restlessness or insomnia, the bulk of the daily drug dosage may be given in the morning instead of at bedtime. **Exceptions to the q.d. schedule may be the elderly and physically infirm who cannot detoxify these drugs as rapidly and require them to be given at lower daily doses in smaller units and more often.** Multiple dose administration is certainly justified in the treatment of the acutely disturbed patients until their key or target symptoms are brought under control.

Clinicians who initiate therapy with once-a-day or twice-a-day dosage follow the same dosage technique as with the more frequent schedule. Patients are usually started on fairly low doses which are rapidly increased day by day until the optimum is achieved for an individual patient. The exception may be the patient who initially needs the extra sedation and the extra control resulting from motor inhibiting properties that the antipsychotic might produce if it were taken more frequently. Such a patient can be started on a t.i.d. or q.i.d. schedule and then, when less agitated, switch over to a once- or twice a day regimen.

Patients who are switched from a multiple dose schedule to a once-a-day schedule should be physically capable of metabolizing or detoxifying the drug. Despite the decreased work load, the nursing staff may oppose the schedule changes because of the belief that patient behavior will deteriorate as a result of or because of fear that such changes would lead to staffing reductions (Callahan et al., 1975). Thus, the nursing staff must be carefully educated to potential benefits prior to any change in medication administration schedules. In this manner, the advantages of once-a-day medication scheduling can be realized without loss of staff cooperation in clinical operations.

It is difficult to change many outpatients to a once-a-day schedule after months or years on a b.i.d. or t.i.d. schedule, even though they are on a low maintenance dosage. In spite of explanations that the single pill is equal in strength to the 2 or 3 or even 4 pills they have been receiving, they will insist on a multiple dose schedule or claim that a b.i.d. schedule makes them "feel better" than "one pill." For some of these patients, it appears that a subjective sense of well-being is enhanced by a t.i.d. regimen. Therefore, when feasible, patients should be placed on a once-a-day maintenance schedule prior to their discharge from the hospital.

DiMascio (1972) has concluded that **"the single or b.i.d. dose schedule provides equal (or greater) clinical benefit to the patient than the multiple dose schedule, produces fewer side effects, results in fewer treatment terminations and reduces the need for hypnotics and antiparkinson drugs."**

9. MODES OF ADMINISTRATION

Antipsychotic agents injected intramuscularly are 3 to 4 times more potent than when given orally and dosage should be adjusted accordingly.

Administering antipsychotic agents in parenteral form (intramuscular administration) is the most reliable way to make sure that the patient is receiving adequate quantities of the drug. Surveys based on the Forrest urine tests show that an appreciable percentage of patients in mental hospitals do not ingest their oral medication as prescribed. Also, in some patients, plasma levels of the drug are nontherapeutic due to failure of drug absorption from the intestinal tract.

In the past, the general practice has been to start medication with an oral dosage form, reserving parenteral doses for disturbed, excited or hyperactive patients (Hollister, 1973). This practice developed because the intramuscular (I.M.) form of chlorpromazine (Thorazine) was highly irritating. In addition, frequent injections often resulted in sterile abcesses. The instructions for its administration as stated in the *Physicians' Desk Reference* (1978) are as follows: "Inject slowly, deep into the upper outer quadrant of buttock. Because of possible hypotensive effects, reserve parenteral administration for bedfast patients or for acute ambulatory cases and keep patient lying down for at least one-half hour after injection. If irritation is a problem, dilute injection with saline or 2% procaine; mixing with other agents in the syringe is not recommended. Subcutaneous injections is not advised. Avoid injecting undiluted Thorazine (chlorpromazine, SK&F) into vein. Intravenous route is only for severe hiccoughs and surgery." The dosage strength of the injectable chlorpromazine is 25 mg. per ml. Thus, if 100 mg. I.M. of chlorpromazine is prescribed, 4 ml. must be injected. If diluted with equal parts of saline or 2% procaine, the total amount of drug to be injected amounts to 8 ml. and this requires using two injection sites. Subcutaneous administration of chlorpromazine may cause necrosis and injection into the deltoid should be avoided (PDR, 1977). Zavodnick (1977) has stated that because the intramuscular form of chlorpromazine is bulky and so locally irritating to tissues, repeated administration verges on the sadistic. It is believed that the incidence of chlorpromazine-related hypotension reactions is far greater than reported. Thus, for intramuscular chlorpromazine administration, a small dose of 10 mg. should be used to test the patient's sensitivity. Blood pressure should then be monitored at 15-minute intervals for 90 minutes before the regular dose is given. Emergency treatment should always be available in the event of severe hypotension.

The advent of high-potency antipsychotics changed the attitude toward IM administration since the parenteral form of these drugs is comparatively well tolerated. Because of their milligram potency, effective doses are smaller in volume and the high-potency antipsychotics can be injected well within the body of any relatively large muscle. They seldom cause pain or tissue damage at the injection site. One can make a case for starting all patients on intramuscular doses over a several day period and then following with an oral dosage form (Hollister, 1973). This is one of the factors that has led to the increased use of rapid tranquilization methods. Although any of the usual sites for IM injection may be used, the high-potency antipsychotics are best injected into the deltoid and many clinicians now routinely use this site. This practice helps the patient maintain dignity and avoids embarrassment. Absorption is more rapid from the deltoid and slowest after gluteal injection. Intramuscular injections should not be made into the lower and mid-third of the upper arm. The mid-lateral thigh may be a preferred site instead of the gluteus maximus. Sciatic nerve damage is a hazard of gluteal injection if the upper outer quadrant is not used as the injection site. When repeated IM administration of any antipsychotic is prescribed, the injection site should be rotated and the site recorded following each injection. This is especially important with the use of the depot fluphenazines, since the injections may be given for many years.

As a general rule, 50% of an intramuscular dose of an antipsychotic is absorbed within 12 to 15 minutes, and within an additional 12 to 15 minutes, half of the remaining dose is absorbed. Thus, in 30 minutes from the time of the IM injection, 75% of the dose is absorbed. Although some clinicians are beginning to give the antipsychotics intravenously, this mode of administration is not F.D.A. approved for psychiatric disorders. The possible hazards of this route of administration include critical blood pressure changes and even fatal complications, particularly with the aliphatic or piperidine phenothiazines.

When fluphenazine decanote (Prolixin Decanote) or fluphenazine enanthate (Prolixin Enanthate) injections are given, the onset of action generally appears between 24 to 72 hours after injection. The effects of the drug on psychotic symptoms become significant within 48 to 96 hours. Many physicians are unaware of these facts and expect a therapeutic action within a

TABLE 7
Product Information Data—Antipsychotic Drugs*

Drug	Preparations Available			
	Tablets	Liquid	Injection	Other Forms
PHENOTHIAZINES				
Aliphatic				
Chlorpromazine (Thorazine)	Tablets: 10 mg., 25 mg., 50 mg., 100 mg., 200 mg.	Syrup: 10 mg./5 ml. Concentrate: 30 mg./ml., 100 mg./ml.	25 mg./ml.	Sustained release capsules: 30 mg., 75 mg., 100 mg., 200 mg., Suppositories: 25 mg., 100 mg.
Triflupromazine (Vesprin)	Tablets: 10 mg., 25 mg., 50 mg.	Suspension: 10 mg. per ml.	10 mg./ml. 20 mg./ml.	
Piperazine				
Acetophenazine (Tindal)	Tablets: 20 mg.			
Carphenazine (Proketazine)	Tablets: 12.5 mg., 25 mg., 50 mg.	Concentrate: 250 mg./5 ml.		
Prochlorperazine (Compazine)	Tablets: 5 mg., 10 mg., 25 mg.	Concentrate: 10 mg. per ml. Syrup: 5 mg. per 5 ml.	5 mg./ml.	Suppositories: 2½ mg., 5 mg., 25 mg. Sustained release capsules: 10 mg., 15 mg., 30 mg., 75 mg.
Perphenazine (Trilafon)	Tablets: 2 mg., 4 mg., 8 mg., 16 mg.	Concentrate: 16 mg. per 5 ml.	5 mg./ml.	
Trifluoperazine (Stelazine)	Tablets: 1 mg., 2 mg., 5 mg., 10 mg.	Concentrate: 10 mg. per ml.	2 mg./ml.	
Fluphenazine (Prolixin)	Tablets: 1 mg., 2.5 mg., 5 mg., 10 mg.	Elixir: 1 mg./2 ml.	2.5 mg./ml. Delayed release injections-fluphenazine decanoate, fluphenazine enanthate: 25 mg./ml.	

Drug	Oral	Concentrate	Injectable	Other
(Permitil)	Tablets: 0.25 mg., 2.5 mg., 5 mg., 10 mg.	Concentrate: 5 mg. per ml.		Sustained release tablets: 1 mg.
Butaperazine (Repoise)	Tablets: 5 mg., 10 mg., 25 mg.			
Piperidine				
Thioridazine (Mellaril)	Tablets: 10 mg., 25 mg., 50 mg., 100 mg., 200 mg.	Concentrate: 30 mg./ml. 100 mg./ml. Syrup: 10 mg./5 ml.		Suppositories: 25 mg., 50 mg. Sustained release capsules 30 mg., 75 mg., 150 mg., 200 mg.
Mesoridazine (Serentil)	Tablets: 10 mg., 25 mg., 50 mg., 100 mg.	Concentrate 25 mg./ml.	25 mg./ml.	
Piperacetazine (Quide)	Tablets: 10 mg., 25 mg.			
BUTYROPHENONES				
Haloperidol (Haldol)	Tablets: ½ mg., 1 mg., 2 mg., 5 mg., 10 mg.	Concentrate: 2 mg./ml.	5 mg./ml.	
THIOXANTHENES				
Thiothixene (Navane)	Capsules: 1 mg., 2 mg., 5 mg., 10 mg., 20 mg.	Concentrate: 5 mg./ml.	2 mg./ml.	
Chlorprothixene (Taractan)	Tablets: 10 mg., 25 mg., 100 mg.	Concentrate: 100 mg./5 ml.	25 mg./2 ml.	
DIBENZOXAZEPINES				
Loxapine (Loxitane)	Capsules: 10 mg., 25 mg., 50 mg.	Concentrate: 25 mg./ml.		
DIHYDROINDOLONES				
Molindone (Moban) (Lidone)	Tablets: 5 mg., 10 mg. 25 mg.			

*Extracted from the Physicians' Desk Reference (1979) and American Formulary Service (1978).

few hours when these depot antipsychotics are given to an uncooperative, severely agitated patient who must be controlled quickly. The depot flu-phenazines may be given subcutaneously as well as IM, since they are painless and do not cause local tissue reaction. A deep intramuscular injec-tion is not required.

Liquid concentrates are the next most reliable form of administration. Patients often succeed in avoiding their antipsychotic medication by pre-tending to swallow it while they are really "cheeking" it, i.e., hiding a solid pill in their cheeks or under the tongue and later getting rid of it. Liquid medication does not lend itself to this practice. It is much more expensive than the tablets or capsules and the human error in measuring out a dose can too easily result in errors. However, it is more readily and completely absorbed from the intestinal tract than the tablets or capsules. Haloperidol concentrate is especially useful when covert administration is required, for it is a colorless, tasteless and odorless solution and can be given undetected in coffee, juice or soup. Delayed-action or sustained release oral preparation (spansules) are the least reliable since their absorption is the least complete. There appears to be no indication for their use since the antipsychotic drugs have a long half-life, are highly cumulative and there is no evidence that these more expensive formulations have any advantage over standard tablet preparations. Failure of a patient to respond adequately may be less the fault of the drug than its dosage form; a brief trial of parenteral administration followed by maintenance with the liquid concentrate might be tried in patients who fail to respond to an antipsychotic table or capsule prior to switching to another drug (Hollister, 1972).

Table 7 shows the various available forms and strengths of the antipsy-chotic drugs. The clinician should have a working knowledge of this type of information about the antipsychotics commonly prescribed. It can be embarrassing when the nurse contacts the physician with the query, "Doc-tor, you prescribed 5 mg. of perphenazine (Trilafon) and we only have 4 mg. tablets on the ward. Pharmacy tells me it doesn't come in 5 mg. tablets." Again, the knowledge that chlorpromazine does not have a 150 mg. tablet available may cause the physician to prescribe either one 100 mg. tablet or one 200 mg. tablet instead of 2 tablets (one 100 mg. plus one 50 mg. tablet), thus avoiding an increase in the number of tablets to be ingested by the patient.

On many wards in psychiatric facilities, it is the custom for all patients to receive their antipsychotic drug in the concentrate for weeks, months or even years until the day of discharge. However, at the mental health center or by their private physician, the tablet or capsule form will be prescribed. This abrupt change from their accustomed form of medication often may lead to rejection of the tablets, poor patient compliance or drug discontinuation. If the concentrate is continued after discharge, the measuring out the dose of liquid medication with a dropper by the patient of a member of the family may be inaccurate and considered a nuisance. Thus, unless there is a specific reason for the continued use of the concentrate, patients should be stabilized on the tablet or capsule form of their antipsychotic agent within the first week or two of hospitalization and certainly should be weaned from the concentrate form prior to discharge.

10. ACTION TIME

An antipsychotic agent should be administered for a sufficient period of time to determine its clinical effectiveness in each individual case before a change is made to another drug.

Analyses of drug summaries of hospitalized psychiatric patients frequently show indiscriminate hopping about from one antipsychotic agent to another in short periods of time and shifts to various dosage levels for brief periods. It is unwise for the physician to switch drugs every few days. One drug should be chosen, the optimal dose found for the patient and maintained at this dose level for a sufficient time for the drug to exert its behavioral effect. As a rule, only after this procedure has failed should consideration be given to changing drugs. The length of time for a drug trial varies with different clinicians. With most, it depends upon the status of the patient. A severely agitated, acutely ill patient may be a candidate after several days of treatment at the optimal dose level, whereas a less dramatically disturbed patient may be given a longer trial, whereas a less dramatically disturbed patient may be given a longer trial, perhaps several weeks or months before the drug is changed (Davis, 1976b). Usually, when a newly admitted psychotic patient fails to improve after 6 to 8 weeks on an adequate dosage, a shift to another drug is warranted. In acute cases, the patient's management problems may be so severe that a change in drug in less than 4-6 weeks may be necessary.

There is a clinical relation between the time of response of certain symptoms to treatment and the dose of the antipsychotic the patient is receiving, and this relation can be used as a guide to a patient's individual drug requirement (Lehmann, 1975):

> Arousal symptoms (e.g., psychomotor excitement, restlessness, irritability, aggressiveness, and insomnia) are the first to be controlled—usually within 2 to 3 weeks of pharmacotherapy.
> Affective symptoms (e.g., anxiety, depression, and social withdrawal) respond next, i.e., after 2 to 5 weeks of treatment.
> Symptoms related to perceptual and cognitive functions, such as hallucinations, delusions, and thinking disorders, as a rule disappear last—in many cases only after 6 to 8 weeks of treatment.

The observation of this "timetable" of therapeutic responses to antipsychotic treatment often enables the clinician to determine whether the dose of the drug prescribed is adequate for a given patient. As an example, if the patient is still so anxious and withdrawn that he refuses to leave his room after 5 weeks, there may be a need to increase the daily dose of the antipsychotic he is receiving. On the other hand, the dose may be adequate if after 6 weeks of therapy the patient is quiet, pleasant and cooperative even though he is still hallucinating and expressing delusions and thinking disorders—symptoms that may not yield to treatment for another few weeks.

For the average patient, most of the therapeutic gains occur in the first 6 weeks of antipsychotic therapy, although further treatment gains are made during the subsequent 12 to 18 weeks. Some patients may show a rapid improvement in a single day or a few weeks but other patients may show a gradual rate of improvement over months.

It has been pointed out that improvement from antipsychotic drugs approximates the familiar learning curve. Initially, there may be a rapid change during the first few weeks, then a slowing improvement during the 6th to 12th weeks of treatment, and very slow change thereafter. Hyperactivity may disappear after a few doses of an antipsychotic while delusions and hallucinations may remain, with lessened effect, for weeks (Hollister, 1973).

Lehmann (1975) has also differentiated four stages, each to be achieved within a definite time span. Failing to do so indicates inadequate dosage or using the wrong drug. The four stages are:

(1) *Medicated cooperation*—within 1 to 5 days, the patient should no longer be in a state of motor excitement and hyperactivity should cease.
(2) *Socialization*—within 2 days to 2 months, the patient should participate in ward activities, even though his thought disorder continues.
(3) *Elimination of thought disorder*—this occurs last, often not before 1 to 6 weeks.
(4) *Maintenance period.*

The above stages are not always clearly defined. The stages through which improvement occurs—cooperation, socialization, elimination of thought disorder—are somewhat available. Some patients improve dramatically over a few days while others improve gradually over a few months. A lag may occur in time between the decrease in overt psychotic decompensation and cognitive improvement.

Klein and Davis (1969) used the term "resolving phase" to distinguish the period between acute psychotic symptomatology and the eventual residual state. It is characterized by fearful demoralization with a trend toward maladaptive social or self-isolating behavior. The patient's self-esteem is impaired and often there may be vacillation between massive denial of difficulty and feeling overwhelmed by interpersonal, social and economic tasks. The "phase" is of varying length. During this stage of illness, the residual pattern of social effectiveness or ineffectiveness starts to emerge. They believe that it is during this period that adequate maintenance dose levels should be established.

The acute schizophrenic who fails to respond to adequate dosage may require the administration of a different antipsychotic drug. The length of time before this change is made varies. Some clinicians switch after several days or 2 to 3 weeks, others 30 days, and still others 40 days. Sometimes it is obvious within a few days that the medication and the patient are not made for each other because of particular severe side effects, although the most common side effects, sedation and extrapyramidal symptoms, do not usually make a shift to another drug necessary. The therapeutic decision should probably rest on the patient's level of improvement. If the patient is much better, the dose can be decreased. If the patient is still very psychotic, an antiparkinson drug can be added and the dosage of the antipsychotic drug raised if clinically necessary. If only a partial response is obtained and limiting side effects are encountered as the dose is increased before the desired therapeutic end point is reached, a switch to an antipsychotic of a different chemical class may be indicated.

Ayd (1974a) believes that a patient should be treated with a single antipsychotic, the dosage of which should be increased steadily over a 3-month period until therapeutic benefit occurs or undesirable side effects intervene. If a patient does not react to maximally tolerated doses with substantial improvement within 3 months, he should be categorized as refractory to the compound and treated with another antipsychotic. For many types of schizophrenics, Klein and Davis (1969) advocate a period of 6 weeks on adequate dosage. If the patient does not respond within this period, the question of misdiagnosis is considered after checking to insure that the patient is actually ingesting the prescribed medication.

The action time may be quite different when a rapid titration technique (or rapid tranquilization procedure) is used in the acute schizophrenic. Donlon and tupin (1974) have observed that excitement and the behavioral manifestations are among the first to be reduced in the symptom picture, normally within a matter of hours or a day or two. This is followed by the remission of the more bizarre thought content and perceptual distortions. The last remnants to abate are the cognitive disorganization and perhaps some of the delusions. When patients are discharged after an average of 1 week of hospitalization, they are no longer psychotic but some psychotic residuals are still present. Thus, the gross psychotic symptoms may respond rapidly to treatment but evidence of emotional brittleness and cognitive disorganization usually remain for days to weeks and in some cases indefinitely. They feel that the healing process requires a matter of weeks before the patient returns to a prepsychotic cognitive state. Anderson (1976) disagrees with the above only in the area of some of the time frames. In his experience with rapid titration, the cognitive disorder, the delusional activity and the hallucinatory process in 50% of his patients went away as rapidly as the agitation—within hours. These, incidentally, were the patients who had a good social support system.

Chronic patients may require 12 to 24 weeks at an adequate dosage before a different medication is indicated. Some clinicians use the rule of thumb of keeping the chronic patient on the same drug 1 month for every year of illness.

11. MAINTENANCE THERAPY

After the patient's mental condition has been stabilized for a period, the antipsychotic medication should be reduced to the lowest effective maintenance dosage.

Skillful dosage adjustment is essential after the acute psychotic symptomatology has subsided. Too low a dosage may precipitate a recrudescence of symptoms while too high a dosage may establish a pattern of overmedication that can persist for years. After the main target symptoms have been controlled, patients should be placed on maintenance doses as low as possible to still retain therapeutic gains. The dosage should be reduced gradually to avoid relapse.

The most common error in maintenance therapy is to reduce the dosage too quickly. It is not unusual for the clinician in the mental health center or outpatient clinic to reduce the dosage by as much as 50% during the patient's first clinic visit following discharge and continue this rapid reduction upon subsequent visits. This type of prescribing practice often contributes to readmission rates as high as 50 to 80% in many mental hospitals. Some physicians are not fully aware of the need for a continued large dose of an antipsychotic to maintain a good remission in many chronic schizophrenic patients. It is most discouraging for the hospital staff to see, almost daily, schizophrenic patients who had achieved a remission within the hospital under intensive antipsychotic drug therapy regress and relapse following discharge because family physicians or community psychiatrists had prematurely reduced the maintenance dosage. Often the community physician will switch the patient to another antipsychotic and frequently at a lower dosage instead of an equivalent dose. The multiple readmission of so many patients caused by the faulty practice of drug reduction or drug substitution outside the hospital has become known as the drug dosage "Merry-Go-Round" (Forrest et al., 1964).

There are few, if any, occasions on which it would be appropriate or safe to reduce or discontinue medication at the time of discharge. At this moment the patient is about to be subjected once more to the environmental and social stresses that may have precipitated the illness. Ideally, each patient should be allowed to self-medicate for several days before discharge and not be expected to graduate from complete dependence to total independence overnight. If this were done routinely, subsequent compliance would be much enhanced. Many hospitals have such self-medication programs.

Forrest and his associates (1964) found that the tendency to reduce medication below an effective maintenance level may be due to (1) the emphasis in the literature of minimal doses rather than the importance of optimal dosage; (2) an exaggerated fear of side effects or permanent damage from the continued use of antipsychotic drugs at effective dosage levels; (3) the expense of the drugs which may result in pressure on the patient, his family or the treating physician to reduce maintenance medication. It is important to realize that relapse as a consequence of drug discontinuation is frequently a slow process. Especially in the case of gradual reduction, the former target symptoms may not reappear for several months. This may be one of the reasons why community physicians treating former chronic psychotics in private practice, mental hygiene clinics, community mental health centers, outpatient clinics, VA offices, etc., often do not recognize the causal relationship between reduced drug dose and incipient relapse. The subsiding of some side effects, such as dryness of mouth, muscular rigidity or dyskinetic phenomena, may produce in the patient a temporary euphoria, which tricks the therapist into believing that the patient who "feels better" is improving. Weeks later, when the patient becomes tense, sleepless, withdrawn or delusional, all sorts of dynamic explanations may be advanced and the usual interval of several months between drug reduction and full relapse is sufficient to obscure the true causal relationship.

Upon discharge, the patient's drug history should be provided to the aftercare physician to facilitate any required change in drug or dosage. The patient on maintenance dosage in the community must be carefully monitored through frequent clinic visits. Some patients require an increase in dosage for a month or two following discharge to enable them to cope with various community stresses. The clinicians should be prepared to raise the dosage at the earliest signs of decompensation. Most patients after rapid tranquilization are discharged at a fairly high dosage and, as yet, have not been stabilized at the lowest effective maintenance level. Usually, it is unwise to reduce their dosage for 2-3 months post-discharge. Once acute psychotic symptoms are controlled and the patient's condition is stabilized (usually 4 to 12 weeks), the daily dose of medication may be gradually reduced. The necessary reductions should be made over long intervals (at least 3 months) because the effect of the higher dose may take such a long time to wear off (Morgan and Cheadle, 1974).

Maintenance dosage, like all other aspects of antipsychotic drug therapy, must be individualized. The physician must consider the matter of drug adjustment of mental patients not only in lowering the high dosage but also in terms of increasing dosage, since there may be many instances when an increased dose might prevent full relapse. Detre and Jarecki (1971) believe that, in most instances, a maintenance dosage of 12 to 16 mg. of perphenazine (Trilafon), 8 to 12 mg. of trifluoperazine (Stelazine) or 6 to 8 mg. of fluphenazine (Prolixin) daily affords sufficient protection against relapse. In some cases, however, somewhat higher maintenance doses are preferable. The great majority of clinicians are in sharp disagreement with setting maximal maintenance dosages for most patients.

The minimal dose at which the patient functions at his highest level is preferred to any arbitrarily imposed maintenance dose such as one-third or one-fourth of the peak dosage. Doses of 300 to 600 mg. of chlorpromazine or the equivalent in the other antipsychotics may be an adequate maintenance level for most patients; however, some clinicians claim to maintain patients on doses of 50 to 100 mg. chlorpromazine or the equivalent. Lehmann (1975) recommends that after the patient is symptom free, one should aim at maintaining him in remission with daily doses of 100-200 mg. of chlorpromazine or its equivalent. He believes that some patients may be successfully protected against recurrences of their illness with as little as 50 mg. of chlorpromazine 2 or 3 times a week, although these patients are in the minority. Other clinicians have reported that often antipsychotic medication may be tapered over a period of weeks to a dosage range of 75 to 400 mg. a day of chlorpromazine or equivalent. However, the reduction of a patient's maintenance dose to a fraction of the original by many physicians may result in nothing more than a placebo effect.

Higher maintenance dosage levels are indicated in patients whose premorbid functioning has not been restored or has always been poor. If the patient is free of acute symptoms but shows some impairment in social functioning, it may be useful to increase the medication and, if this helps, to continue increasing it every 2 to 3 months until the patient either stops improving or develops unmanageable side effects (Detre and Jarecki, 1971). The fact that the patient has been on maintenance medication for a long period of time (many years) should not become a factor in the discontinuance of medication, except for the development of a disabling side effect.

While no particular antipsychotic can prevent relapse better than others, many clinicians tend to avoid using the sedating phenothiazines such as chlorpromazine or thioridazine as maintenance medications. The high potency antipsychotics may be preferred since they are effective at lower dose levels, and are less likely to make the patient feel drowsy, impair his reaction time or otherwise interfere with his normal daytime functioning. The patient's subjective reaction to the drug helps to determine its long-term effect. Patients taking the more sedating phenothiazines are more likely to complain about the way the drug makes them feel and are more likely to stop taking the drug.

Hollister (1970) has stated that another problem with low-potency drugs is that if treatment is continued over a long period (and for many patients, it may be for life), choosing these drugs commits one to a course that will eventually lead to the administration of kilograms of drugs. He has noted that it is not known whether it is preferable to give 20 mg. daily of a foreign molecule rather than 200 mg., since the harmful effects of drugs or chemicals in the environment are not appreciated for decades after their introduction. It therefore seems prudent to reduce the total body burden as much as possible. Hollister recalls that several years elapsed before it was recognized that lenticular deposits were a dose-related effect of chlorpromazine. Consequently, consideration should be given to only short-term rather than long-term use of the low-potency drugs, substituting whenever possible high-potency drugs for chronic treatment.

Switching the patient to the less soporific antipsychotics can best be accomplished during the "resolving phase." Ideally one should add the new medication, observe, and then decrease the old, thus changing only one medication at a time. One can easily attribute untoward changes in clinical condition to the specific change in management. Difficulties rarely occur if one adds the new medication while decreasing the old. The routine use of conjoint antipsychotics is only of value in this switching phase.

Abrupt changing to another antipsychotic, even though equivalent doses are prescribed, may be fraught with danger. Gardos (1974) investigated interchangeability of effective antipsychotic agents in a clinical setting. Sixty formerly hospitalized schizophrenics were randomly assigned to one of three drug groups: (1) thiothixene, (2) chlorpromazine, or (3) continued doctor's choice medication (control group). The first two groups were abruptly switched from the previous medication to equivalent doses of chlorpromazine or thiothixene. During the two-year study period, 16 patients (44%) of the switched group (combined chlorpromazine and thiothixene group) underwent clinical deterioration to an extent that required termination from the study. In contrast, only two patients (12%) of the control group relapsed during the same period. Relapses were equal in number during the first and second 6 months of the study and the significant difference in relapse rates was attributable to the change in antipsychotic medication. Gardos believes that his findings imply that antipsychotic drugs are not inter-changeable and that the clinician should be wary of switching drugs in a stabilized chronic schizophrenic since a relapse may result from the change.

Burgoyne (1976) however, found that upsetting long-standing medication rituals had little effect on the attendance of stabilized, chronic schizophrenic patients as a group and medication changes were tolerated by such a group. He reported that the clinician should exercise judgement in changing med-ication but it certainly appears safe to do so. Patients often look upon med-ication reviews as evidence of therapist's enthusiasm and interest and as cause for new hope. Therapists who make no changes in medication routines because of patient fragility should reconsider this policy to be sure they are not rationalizing their own wishes to keep their interaction with patients unmolested and unbothersome.

It should be remembered that, after the substitution of a new drug, the patient is responding not only to increasing doses of that drug but also to the continuing effect of the previous drug for a potential period of several months. If the old drug was, in fact, more effective than the new one, the change will eventually result in delayed deterioration. The longer the delay before relapse, the more difficult it becomes to realize, in retrospect, what has happened. The patient can have remained as well as before for some months, apparently from taking the new drug, but actually because of the continuing effect of the old one. Once a patient has been initiated on an-tipsychotic therapy and some therapeutic response has been achieved, the therapist must be persistent and flexible to assure that the patient is receiving the rational, safe and effective treatment to which he is morally and legally entitled. This means that the therapist must continue to prescribe the same effective dose of the antipsychotic for at least 3 to 6 months to preclude relapse in those patients whom he has reasons to believe faithfully ingest the medication. Then the therapist should gradually reduce the antipsychotic dosage while carefully monitoring the patient for early warning signs of impending relapse. If the latter is detected and is occurring despite faithful consumption of the antipsychotic, prompt dosage increase usually will fore-stall relapse (Ayd, 1976b).

In the resolving phase, schizoaffective patients may develop low spirits and generalized unhappiness associated with depressive signs such as inertia, apathy, loss of appetite and loss of sexual interest, even after a phase of apparent normality. Insomnia is not uncommon. This phase of illness re-sponds very well to the addition of antidepressant medication of the imi-pramine type (Klein and Davis, 1969).

The depot phenothiazines represent an opportunity for progress in main-tenance therapy for certain psychiatric patients. Already some fluphenazine decanoate clinics have been established and found to be practical and effective. Patients at these clinics receive an injection of the drug from a nurse or trained paramedical personnel. When necessary and feasible, a visiting nurse from the clinic goes to the patient's home to give the injection. If the patient is fully compensated on a maintenance injection of fluphenazine decanoate every 2 weeks, the clinician may lengthen the time interval to every 3 weeks for several visits. If the patient's condition remains stabilized, the interval may be lengthened to an injection every 4 weeks. Later, consideration may be given to reducing the amount of each dose. This type of program has the potential of preventing further periods of hospitalization in many patients who have had repeated readmissions.

The importance of maintenance medication cannot be overemphasized. Maintenance medication may not protect the patient against every manifestation of his illness. Even if his initial symptoms have improved and he continues to take antipsychotics as prescribed, he may remain socially awkward or somewhat uncomfortable and, at intervals, have a mild exacerbation of the cognitive disorder. These episodes do not usually progress further and can be regarded as subclinical relapses, in the sense that the patient would exhibit psychotic symptoms at this time were he not taking medication. With these reservations, patients who continue to take the prescribed dose of an antipsychotic following remission of their first or second episode of schizophrenic illness rarely relapse severely enough to require hospitalization (Detre and Jarecki, 1971).

It has been pointed out by some clinicians that many untreated patients experience but a single episode of schizophrenic illness during their lifetime, which may cast some doubt on the favorable results reported of maintenance treatment. Nevertheless, many patients, whose illnesses had recurred repeatedly for many years and who recover once they are given antipsychotics, remain well as long as they take them, relapse each time they stop taking them, and remit again as soon as antipsychotic treatment is reinstated. Some of these patients have few or no symptoms when on medication, while others function only marginally. The important thing is that they do not relapse again irrespective of the level of their integration.

Patients on long-term maintenance therapy must be checked periodically for cardiovascular, liver and other complications. Two important complications are ocular changes and tardive dyskinesia. Drug holidays should be considered for the patients who will be taking the medication indefinitely. Maintenance use of antipsychotics should reflect active consideration of the patient as a person receiving treatment, not as an individual receiving chemical care. Patient records should show thoughtful changes in dosage within reasonable time frames, consideration of intermittent administration and attentiveness to the symptoms of illness and undesired actions of the medications.

Hansell and Willis (1977), in their continuing study of 575 schizophrenic patients treated in a mental health center for many years, found the average daily maintenance dose equal to 2-5 mg. of fluphenazine; the average daily dose during a psychotic episode was equal to 30-60 mg. of fluphenazine. They ascertain the lowest effective dose and propose arrangements for a long-term pattern of continuous or semicontinuous use of medication. Patients are counseled that their disease is likely lifelong, that it may involve altered brain biology and that it is often modifiable with chemical and social regulation. Their counseling focuses on analogies to diabetes, on fluctuations in the course of the illness due to adaptational challenges, and on self-regulation of medication within a prescribed range. They tell patients that lifelong care for their condition, if done with precision, does not result in an increase of sickness but in an increase of health function. Patients are also informed that if their condition later warrants a less continuous mode of care, the approach can be shifted on the basis of strategic observations.

Hansell and Willis (1977) "try to teach schizophrenic patients to be more effective managers of their adaptational episodes. During such crises most of the patients increase the dose of medication that is usually effective in controlling their symptoms; this increase averages a doubling or tripling of their ordinary dose and lasts from several weeks to several months." They "encourage patients: to watch their sleeping-waking and resting-working rhythm as markers of the completeness of their regulation; to get rest, food, water and relaxation during the period of challenge, remembering that the problem-solving effort may extend over many weeks; to name their helpers and to keep in regular reporting contact with them." They estimate more than 400 of the 575 patients in their study group are systematically increasing and decreasing their own doses successfully.

If a patient wants to stop taking medication when well clinically or voices an intention to assess the consequences of stopping medication, Hansell and Willis encourage him or her to do so, but only under close supervision. Patients are instructed in a method for looking for the earliest signs of deregulation, i.e., the symptom cluster of disturbance of the sleeping-waking cycle, floating effects (sadness, panic, suspicion, perplexity), difficulty concentrating, preoccupation with a narrow range of thought, and loss of pleasure in social contacts. They report that in the past 2 years 38 of their 575 patients have assessed the effects of stopping medication; 36 patients experienced a return of the early-warning symptom cluster of frank psychosis and returned to the use of medication.

Cohen (1975) has averred that the antipsychotics are not utilized to the full extent of their potential. Dosage schedules during maintenance are not flexible enough: Some patients are overdosed; others are undermedicated. The early identification of side effects remains to be learned. Even with the drugs available, better results could be obtained by using the antipsychotics more skillfully and thoughtfully.

It has been stated that there is an art of maintenance antipsychotic therapy in which some clinicians are more skilled than others. This accounts for the divergent results reported by different clinicians whose technique of therapy and willingness to take legitimate risks vary. Some, for example, simply dispense antipsychotics with little attention to the individual needs of the patient, to the frequency of administration, or to the hazards of polypharmacy. Others tailor the therapy to the individual needs of the patient, administer the total daily dose once each evening and carefully monitor the patient to achieve optimal results with minimal risks. The latter clinicians are the most successful.

12. AS NEEDED (PRN) ORDERS

As needed (PRN) orders for antipsychotic drugs are rarely indicated after the first 2 or 3 weeks or after stabilization on an effective dosage.

A PRN order for an antipsychotic agent is frequently used to control acutely disturbed behavior or other psychotic symptoms. The need for such use usually indicates that the patient has not yet been titrated to a clinically effective dosage. One exception might be the PRN usage of chlorpromazine for the treatment of flashback due to LSD, even though the patient is generally stabilized for his anxiety on a successful dosage.

A PRN order for the chronic mental patient is usually written because of the possible occurrence of outbursts of sudden disruptive behavior. Logically, it would call for the parenteral administration of the antipsychotic drug to bring the patient rapidly under control. In an in-depth study of PRN orders (Mason and DeWolfe, 1974), it was found that only 45% of the PRN orders called for intramuscular administration. It was also significant that in 52% of the patients, the PRN orders were written for an antipsychotic agent differing from the drugs prescribed in the daily regimen. This prescribing practice violates two of the basic principles in the use of antipsychotic agents, namely (1) that one antipsychotic agent should be used at a time, and (2) polypharmacy should be avoided whenever possible (Mason, 1973).

In this study, about 77% of the patients were on a daily medication schedule of an antipsychotic drug that had a parenteral form available. It would appear that the rational prescription practice should be to use the parenteral form of these drugs in clinical situations calling for a PRN order. Such a practice would be of help in titrating to an effective dosage of one drug and polypharmacy could have been avoided. When the physician turned to a different antipsychotic agent for the PRN order, it usually was chlorpromazine (87%). Perhaps the physician felt more comfortable for this purpose with the phenothiazine drug that is the oldest and most commonly used. However, it may reflect a lack of knowledge or an inability to use the high-potency or newer antipsychotic agents.

It is believed that the high degree of correlation between the large percentage of patients receiving daily medication within a conservative dosage range and the many PRN orders indicates that some of these patients had not yet stabilized on a clinically effective maintenance dosage. This conclusion is reinforced by the fact that agitation is the most frequently cited reason for writing a PRN order; yet this target symptom usually responds to adequate doses of an antipsychotic agent.

In many instances, once a PRN order is written, there is an almost automatic continuation of the status quo in regard to the patient's drug regimen, with the same orders rewritten every month. This seems to be the practice as long as the patient causes no problems. Over half of the patients with a PRN order are on open wards, indicating that they have achieved a level of social competence and are able to attend and participate in their activity program without nursing staff supervision.

It is a recognized fact that during the early phase of drug therapy a PRN order may be necessary for a short time as the dosage is raised to a high level for rapid onset of therapeutic effect or when the form of the antipsychotic agent is changed (i.e., parenteral to oral form) or when attempting to stabilize the patient at the lowest effective dose. Also, there are some agitated, refractory and volatile patients whose response to medication is minimal and who thus may require a PRN order for extended periods. Otherwise, the PRN order, continued month after month, may indicate that the patient is not yet receiving an adequate dosage or that the order is no longer necessary and is serving as a "security blanket" for the staff. Thus, PRN orders should receive special attention when orders are rewritten and during the periodic critical review of the patient's drug regimen.

13. RAPID URINE COLOR TESTING (THE FORREST URINE TESTS)

A Forrest urine test should be routinely and periodically performed with the urine of most patients on phenothiazine medications and constitutes an essential element in the management of patients for whom this class of antipsychotics is prescribed.

The Forrest Tests are valid, simple, inexpensive methods to determine qualitatively (and semi-quantitatively) whether patients are actually taking their phenothiazine medication. Spot checks as well as systematic testing of mental hospital populations have shown that from 5 to 15% of patients in well-staffed hospitals successfully "cheeked" their drugs (Forrest et al., 1958; Pollack, 1958). Blackwell (1973) reported on 6 studies whereby the Forrest test was used as a method of detection and found a range of 5 to 30% of inpatients who were drug defaulters. With outpatients, the number of defaulters rose as high as 44%. Irwin et al. (1971) showed that 32% of open ward patients and 63% of patients on hospital leave did not take their prescribed phenothiazines.

At a Veterans Administration mental hospital, it was found that 62% of the readmissions had failed to adhere to their prescribed medication regimen, according to the Forrest urine tests (Mason et al., 1963). Most of these patients had been receiving aftercare at a mental hygiene clinic and none of the clinic workers—psychiatrists, psychologists, or social workers—was aware that the patients were defaulting on their drug intake. Surveys indicate that generally 25 to 30% of all outpatients, psychotic and nonpsychotic, fail to comply with medication schedules. With schizophrenics, the proportion is even higher. Park and Lipman (1964) showed that while verbal reports suggested a deviation among only 15% of outpatients, a pill count revealed that 51% were defaulting. It is well known that hospitalized patients will spit out, hide, regurgitate and discard their medication. Interrogating the patient about his tablet-taking habits is at best embarrassing and at worst unreliable. Many schizophrenic inpatients are especially noted for the length they will go to "cheek" medicine and deny defaulting (Neve, 1958; Wilcox et al., 1965).

In view of the above, it is difficult to understand why clinicians at psychiatric inpatient facilities and community mental health centers, as well as in private practice (many at teaching centers which take pride in their quality of care), fail to utilize the Forrest tests in the management of patients on phenothiazine drugs; yet very few hospitals or outpatient clinics employ the tests as a routine procedure. The findings and conclusions of dozens of elaborate, costly, time-consuming clinical research studies (many double-blind) involving the phenothiazines, using various rating scale instruments and complex statistical analyses are suspect or erroneous due to failure to check drug compliance objectively.

The urine tests for phenothiazines were developed by Drs. Fred and Irene Forrest, a husband and wife team of psychiatrist and biochemist, who devised a series of ferric chloride color reactions that have become the standard test for the phenothiazines (Forrest et al., 1958, 1960, 1961, 1966, 1972). These tests have become known by their name and their validity has been independently corroborated (Pollack, 1958; Caffey et al., 1963). The testing of the patient's urine is the simplest and most convenient means of drug detection, especially since the urine is the major source of excretion for the phenothiazines. It can easily be done as an office procedure using standard, readily obtainable laboratory equipment. At the hospital where these tests were developed,* a nursing assistant on each ward performed these tests routinely for many years. Virtually no false negatives have been encountered with these tests (Forrest et al., 1961, 1966). False positive reactions can occur but are uncommon. A few substances produce false positives, including the urine of phenylketonurics and high doses of amino salicylic acid (PAS), estrogen therapy and liver failure may also interfere. The long-acting injectable fluphenazine preparations in the form of the decanoate or enanthate, whereby 25 mg. doses are given at two or more week intervals, cannot be detected by these tests. The test most frequently used, the "F.P.N." or Universal Test, can detect and measure the intake of a wide variety of the phenothiazines drugs.

Almost any urine specimen in the high and medium dosage ranges of the phenothiazine drugs, i.e., the doses usually prescribed in hospital psychiatry, may be used. Equal volumes (1 ml.) of urine test reagent are measured into a test tube by means of 2 graduated rubber-tipped medicine droppers, 1 for urine and 1 for the brown reagent bottle, the latter being mounted in a plastic screw top as a permanent, tight-closing stopper. The color produced in the test tube is promptly compared with the colors on a color chart which is placed against a light surface away from a window. Urines may be stored for several weeks, refrigerated with a few drops of toluene as preservative, without appreciable loss of drug.

The Forrest Tests should be available in all hospital laboratories, clinics and physicians' offices and should be an integral part of the routine procedure in managing patients on phenothiazine medication or whenever toxic ingestion of such a drug is suspected. Most outpatients who have improved with phenothiazines do not relapse with adequate medication levels. Hence, the objective criteria offered by the Forrest Test to evaluate drug intake are essential to the professional personnel dealing with the increasing number of patients on maintenance therapy in the community and can be the fundamental factor in preventing relapse.

The failure of patients to adhere to their medication results in an enormous economic waste amounting to hundreds of thousands of dollars annually. Cupboards stacked with unused tablets of various phenothiazines accumulated over the years pose a potential hazard to health (Hare and Wilcox, 1967; Gardiner, 1968). It is not unusual for relatives to bring shopping bags of unused medication when returning the relapsed patient to the hospital. The routine use of the Forrest test can go a long way in preventing this

---

*Veterans Administration Hospital, Brockton, Mass.

state of affairs and in ameliorating the "revolving door syndrome" of mental hospitals.

14. ANTIPARKINSON MEDICATION

As a general rule, an antiparkinson drug should be added only when drug induced extrapyramidal side effects appear. When an antiparkinson drug is prescribed, it should be discontinued after 3 months and then reinstated only in those patients whose extrapyramidal symptoms return. Antiparkinson drugs should never be used routinely.

The commonest drug combination in psychiatry is the use of an antipsychotic with an antiparkinson drug. It has been estimated that 30 to 50% of patients on antipsychotic medication receive antiparkinson drugs. During a 2-year period at the Massachusetts Mental Health Center, all hospitalized patients who were placed on pharmacotherapy were seen weekly and all side effects were recorded. It was found that 62% of 555 patients admitted into the hospital were placed on antipsychotics and that 30% of these were also given antiparkinson drugs. Of the latter group, 59% received an antiparkinson agent after a side effect had been observed—but 38% of them were started on an antiparkinson drug at the same time they initially received the antipsychotic drug (DiMascio, 1972). Mason et al. (1977a) found that 41.5% of the patients in the 4 mental hospitals of a southeastern state had an antiparkinson drug order. Antiparkinson drug use more than tripled between 1960 and 1974. In a study of the prescribing practices in 42 Veterans Administration hospitals, data regarding 3,860 patients revealed that 34% of the patients were receiving antiparkinson drugs and that 52% of these patients had been taking them for longer than 6 months (Schroeder et al., 1977).

The incidence of drug-induced extrapyramidal symptoms has been reported to vary from 4% to 50%, depending upon the antipsychotic employed, the dosage, the criteria used for reporting symptoms and the diligence of the clinical investigators (DiMascio and Demirgian, 1970). Lehman (1975) found that extrapyramidal symptoms usually occur in approximately 30% of patients who receive aliphatic or piperidine phenothiazines and in more than 50% of those who receive other antipsychotics.

The prophylactic use of antiparkinson drugs has an element of controversy. Soon after the introduction of the first antipsychotics, reserpine (Serpasil) and chlorpromazine (Thorazine), it was recognized that these compounds could provoke in neurologically susceptible individuals diverse extrapyramidal reactions, depending on the dose and route of administration. It was also quickly learned that these drug-induced neurological reactions often could be modified or abolished by adequate doses of antiparkinson drugs without even a temporary reduction in the dose of the responsible antipsychotic. Consequently, many physicians prescribing antipsychotics began to co-administer an antiparkinson agent prophylactically, especially when the antipsychotic was known to cause a high incidence of extrapyramidal responses, the starting dose was high, the drug was administered parenterally, or there was a family history of antipsychotic-induced or naturally occurring extrapyramidal reactions, and continued to do so as long as the patient received an antipsychotic. This became standard practice, particularly in public mental hospitals, so that it was not unusual in such institutions for many antipsychotic-treated patients to be on long-term antiparkinson medication. This was also true for a large percentage of outpatients on antipsychotic therapy.

The low-potency drugs such as thioridazine and chlorpromazine are less likely to produce extrapyramidal involvement than the other antipsychotics. However, antiparkinson drugs may be just as frequently prescribed with them. Often, once an antiparkinson drug is used, the order will be renewed as long as the patient is on antipsychotic medication. Occasionally, medication analyses reveal instances where the antipsychotic medication has been discontinued years before but the patient is still receiving an antiparkinson drug.

One of the first points of controversy surrounding drug-induced extrapyramidal side effects was the exact relationship of the neurological disorder to the therapeutic efficacy of the antipsychotic drugs. Many clinicians simply considered extrapyramidal side effects as an undesirable adverse effect and attempted to utilize those medications which produced a minimal amount of neurological disturbance but remained equally efficacious in their antipsychotic effect. Other clinicians were proponents of the theory that the neurological disorder was indicative of therapeutic effectiveness and used extrapyramidal side effects as a clinical measurement of either an adequate therapeutic response or as an indicator of appropriate blood levels. Clinical studies have since indicated that the antipsychotic efficacy of a drug is not significantly related to the degree of extrapyramidal side effects produced as an untoward effect and that the psychotic symptomatology can be alleviated without the production of this type of side effects (Coleman and Hayes, 1975).

Pecknold et al. (1971) delineated 3 patterns of prescription of antiparkinson drugs in psychiatric patients: (1) pertinent—prescription upon development of extrapyramidal symptoms; (2) prophylactic—prescription along with high dosage antipsychotic therapy; and (3) precautionary—prescription with all antipsychotic medication. On the basis of their observations, they concluded that precautionary and prophylactic antiparkinson therapy should not be a routine indication.

Patients have been studied who had been on antiparkinson agents concomitant with antipsychotic medication for over 3 months and were then abruptly withdrawn from the antiparkinson medication (Orlov et al., 1971). It was found that fewer than 10% had a recurrence of symptoms requiring the restarting of the antiparkinson medication. Therefore, the common practice of sustained administration of antiparkinson medication was found to be unwarranted and most patients who have been treated with antiparkinson medication for over 3 months can continue on the same regimen of antipsychotic medication without the antiparkinson drug and have no remission or exacerbation of symptoms. The few patients requiring antiparkinson medication demonstrated extrapyramidal symptoms within 2 to 4 weeks of drug withdrawal and it was concluded that 90% of the patients had been receiving antiparkinson medication unnecessarily.

DiMascio (1971) has stated that (a) antiparkinson drugs are being used "with undue frequency"; (b) most patients who have been treated with antiparkinson medication can continue on the same regimen of antipsychotic medication without the antiparkinson drug and have no exacerbation of extrapyramidal symptoms; and (c) the concomitant prescription of antipsychotics and antiparkinson compounds actually increases certain types of side effects such as lethargy, dizziness, gastric irritation, and blurred vision. DiMascio also claims that while the prophylactic use of antiparkinson drugs may or may not lessen the intensity of extrapyramidal reactions, "the evidence does not substantiate the clinician's hope that they will prevent them."

An assessment of the duration of antiparkinson administration and the frequency of extrapyramidal symptom recurrence after withdrawal of the antiparkinson agent disclosed that, of the patients who had been on these drugs less than 1 month, two-thirds developed side effects necessitating reintroduction of an antiparkinson compound, but, of those who had been taking an antiparkinson drug for more than 3 months, only 3 to 6% required readministration of the antiparkinson agent. All patients needing the represcription of an antiparkinson drug had a resurgence of extrapyramidal symptoms within 3 weeks after it had been stopped (DiMascio and Demirgian, 1970).

Ayd (1974b) found that only 30% of patients treated with antipsychotics will develop extrapyramidal symptoms and since there is no way to predict with any certainty which 30% will develop these reactions, there is no reason to give antiparkinson drugs to the 70% who will not have them. Some clinicians believe that prophylactic drugs are warranted in at-risk patients such as outpatients on antipsychotics that produce a high incidence of extrapyramidal symptoms but that, on the psychiatric wards, staff members are experienced in handling extrapyramidal symptoms so prophylactic antiparkinson medication is unnecessary. Paranoid patients who would refuse antipsychotic drugs if an extrapyramidal side effect developed are often included in the at-risk group.

There are other facets in the use of antiparkinson drugs which must be taken into consideration. The addition of benztropine to haloperidol reverses the course of some of the therapeutic changes. The nontherapeutic interaction is slective, involving what may be called "social avoidance behavior" (inwardness, poor social and emotional interactions) but not the cognitive integrative dysfunctions. It has been suggested that antipsychotic effects on social avoidance behavior in schizophrenics may be mediated through a cholinergic system which is blocked by antiparkinson drugs. Caution is therefore advised in use of antiparkinsonism agents with antipsychotics (Singh and Smith, 1973). Also, in a comparison study of haloperidol and chlorpromazine, it was found that benztropine had the effect of diminishing the therapeutic response to both antipsychotics (Singh and Kay, 1975). However, haloperidol proved less susceptible to this effect. It has been shown that the concomitant administration of trihexyphenidyl (Artane) with chlorpromazine results in lowering of plasma chlorpromazine level—another reason why antiparkinson agents (anticholinergics) such as Trihexyphenidyl (Artane), benztropine mesylate (Cogentin) and diphenhydramine (Benadryl) should not be used prophylactically with chlorpromazine in anticipation of parkinsonian reactions to the drug. The anticholinergics probably exert their antiparkinsonian effects at least partly by reducing the level of chlorpromazine in the plasma. In some patients this may be more logically and economically achieved by reducing the dose of chlorpromazine, and thus also avoiding the problem of having to cope with the undesirable adverse effects of anticholinergics (Rivera-Calimlim, 1976). The outpatient on antipsychotic and antiparkinson agents may be ingesting other anticholinergic drugs such as atropine and scopolomine in over-the-counter medications. This may precipitate the anticholinergic syndrome.

Many clinicians withhold antiparkinson drugs in all patients except those who are "high risk" or cannot be followed very closely. Others will start only outpatients with an antiparkinson agent, especially if it felt that the patient might not be able to recognize extrapyramidal symptoms. However, if there is a reliable family member who has been informed about extrapyramidal symptoms, therapy will be started with just the antipsychotic. Also pertinent is the fact that antiparkinson drugs such as trihexyphenidyl and biperiden seem to have a euphorizing mood-elevating effect in many patients taking antipsychotic medication (Jellinek, 1977). This effect may account for the significant resistance encountered when attempting to discontinue antiparkinson medication even in patients no longer on antipsychotic drugs.

The question arises as to whether antiparkinson drugs should be given prophylactically to all patients receiving depot phenothiazines. Like all the phenothiazines of the piperazine group, the butyrophenones and thiothixenes, the depot phenothiazines cause a relatively high incidence of extrapyramidal reactions. This question is important since (1) there is a steady increase in the use of depot phenothiazines in clinical practice; (2) these drugs are used extensively as maintenance medication for chronic patients who are either hospitalized or in the community, or have a history of drug-defaulting, relapses and readmissions; and (3) a fear exists among clinicians that the injection of a depot phenothiazine may cause unmanageable extrapyramidal side effects that would persist until the drug is excreted from the body, a process that might take weeks. This fear often leads to the prophylactic use of antiparkinson medication with the belief that it is essential to protect the patient from an industrial accident or from embarrassment in community life should an extrapyramidal reaction to the antipsychotic drug suddenly occur.

Bakke (1973) after 2½ years of experience with fluphenazine enanthate and decanoate, found that the frequency of extrapyramidal side effects was clearly dependent on whether the maintenance dosage was individualized and whether a gradually increasing dosage schedule was used (see Table 8 for his dose schedules). If side effects occurred, the dosage was reduced by postponing the next injection by 1-2 weeks, then giving an actual dose some 25-50% lower than before. Dosage reductions were continued until an absence of side effects was achieved without leading to relapse. A more rapid progression than in the table—e.g., beginning with 0.5 ml (12.5 mg,)—led to unreasonably frequent and moderate-to-strong neurological side effects. He found prophylactic antiparkinson medication to be "inappropriate."

Ayd's analysis (1975b) of available data on the extrapyramidal reactions caused by the depot phenothiazines led him to conclude that neither the enanthate nor the decanoate induce a higher incidence of any type of extrapyramidal reactions that the potent oral antipsychotics, as commonly believed. He found that the incidence of neurologic reactions due to decanoate is somewhat less than that of the enanthate. He also noted that the response of the extrapyramidal reactions due to the depot antipsychotics is as prompt and satisfactory as for similar reactions due to the oral antipsychotics when treated with the antiparkinson agents. More importantly, he concluded that antiparkinson drugs should be prescribed only to treat emergent extrapyramidal symptoms since the prophylactic administration of an antiparkinson agent neither prevents nor modifies these symptoms.

TABLE 8

Dose Schedules of Fluphenazine Enanthate and Decanoate I.M.

A			B	
Day	ml.		Day	ml.
1	0.1		1	0.1
3	0.1		3	0.1
5	0.2		5	0.5
12	0.5	or	19	0.75
26*	0.75			

*Thereafter dosage according to clinical judgment, every 14th day, with lower dosages being given for fluphenazine decanoate than for the enanthate. For patients over 60 years of age, half the above dosage should be given.

From Bakke, 1973.

Other therapists prescribe trihexyphenidyl or one of the other antiparkinson agents routinely on initiating depot phenothiazine. After the patient has adapted to the antipsychotic, the antiparkinson agent is gradually withdrawn if no side effects are observed. The customary dosage of trihexyphenidyl may be as low as 2 mg. twice a day. It has been observed that it usually does not completely suppress akathisia or the more frightening dystonias. However, some clinicians (e.g., Owens, 1978) feel that it makes readily available to the patient a means of easily controlling the extrapyramidal side effects by merely increasing the dosage. Although there is the occasional abuse of trihexyphenidyl, it is believed that on countless occasions it has preserved an all too tenuous relationship between patients and the mental health professionals at the outpatient clinic.

Some clinicians give the patient or a family member a supply of an antiparkinson agent with instructions for oral self-medication as needed if side effects occur. Frequently, very small doses of the antiparkinson drug suffice and usually these are only needed for the first few days after injection of a depot phenothiazine such as fluphenazine decanoate. There are other therapists who routinely prescribe the antiparkinson drug prophylactically for 4 to 5 days after an injection and thus the patient does not receive the antiparkinson drug during the rest of the 2- to 3-week interval between injections. It is much easier to discontinue the drug entirely after 3 to 4 months of such a regimen than if the patient had been taking the antiparkinson drug daily for several months.

In 1975, Groves and Mandel, after an extensive review of the literature on the long-acting phenothiazine, advised that antiparkinson drugs be prescribed only as indicated by the development of extrapyramidal reactions.

Tolerance to extrapyramidal effects (even the acute dystonias) of the long-acting drugs does not develop after a few months of therapy as it may with medications taken orally. Therefore, patients should be monitored for such symptoms throughout the treatment period with long-acting drugs.

A recent study (Johnson, 1978) clearly demonstrated that almost half the patients who experienced morbidity while on the depot fluphenazines did not require anticholinergic drugs. (Morbidity was recorded as present if the patient, a relative or a member of the clinical team reported that the patient was experiencing a discomfort or a disability that limited a physical or social function.) When antiparkinson drugs were prescribed, the need for these drugs was often limited. It was suggested that, when morbidity develops within the first 3 months of treatment, antiparkinson drugs should be prescribed and continued until the end of the 4th month, unless the resolution of symptoms is almost immediate. However, after this interval antiparkinson drugs need be used only for the duration of morbidity. Again, the risk of a return of morbidity following discontinuance of antiparkinson drugs was small (<10%).

Rifkin and his associates (1978) are in disagreement with the consensus described in the foregoing pages. They believe that the relevant literature is not conclusive, that most studies were not done in a double-blind fashion using a control group, and that many studies also lacked a clear definition of extrapyramidal symptoms or, if symptoms were defined, excluded the subtle adverse extrapyramidal symptoms or the behavioral manifestations of akinesia. They believe that the main difficulty lies with extrapyramidal symptoms that mimic psychopathology. Akathisia can appear to be psychomotor agitation, commonly part of the clinical picture in many illnesses for which antipsychotics are used. Akinesia, which they defined as decreased spontaneity, at its most extreme is manifested as markedly diminished speech, gestures and, at times, almost all movement. Less severe akinesia may be seen only as diminished social activity or interest in work and they averred that this symptom is generally ignored or easily confused with "depression, demoralization or residual schizophrenia."

After a controlled study of procyclidine withdrawal in patients of an aftercare clinic, using a broader definition of akinesia, Rifkin et al. (1978) found that no patient taking procyclidine experienced extrapyramidal symptoms, whereas 54% (20 of 37) of those receiving placebo did. Furthermore, their experience does not bear out the usual belief that the addition of any antiparkinson drugs adds to the anticholinergic side effects in patients receiving antipsychotics. They believe the data that antiparkinson drugs lower the blood level of antipsychotics, thus interfering with the clinical effect, are, as yet, meagre and unconvincing.

In summary, however, it is not considered advisable to administer antiparkinson drugs prophylactically. In outpatient clinics, a clear explanation of how to recognize extrapyramidal side effects should be given to the patient and his family. A supply of an antiparkinson agent should be furnished with specific instructions as to dosage and when to call the clinician should a side effect occur. There are a few possible indications for prophylactic use of the antiparkinson drugs, namely patients receiving high initial doses of the long-acting antipsychotics without supervision, patients with a previous history of susceptibility to extrapyramidal involvement or with a family history of neurologic side effects to antipsychotic drugs, and the older female patient (Grozier, 1973). Finally, all patients on antipsychotic drugs, whether acute or chronic, inpatient or outpatient, must be carefully scrutinized at regular and frequent intervals for the subtle manifestations of extrapyramidal side effects which may indicate the need of an antiparkinson drug. If long-term use of an antiparkinson drug proves to be necessary, the drug should be titrated slowly to the lowest effective dosage.

15. MEGADOSES

The use of megadoses should be considered in selected schizophrenic patients.

When doses within the usual range of the 5 chosen antipsychotic agents have failed in chronic patients and in some nonchronic treatment-resistant patients, the selective use of very high dosages or megadoses may prove effective.

The National Institute of Mental Health (NIMH) sponsored two multi-hospital collaborative studies on high dose phenothiazine therapy (Prien and Cole, 1968; Prien et al., 1969, 1970). In one study the effectiveness of large doses of chlorpromazine was tested by comparing a dose regimen of 2000 mg. per day of chlorpromazine with a dose regimen of 300 mg. per day, a placebo, and physician's choice (consisting of whatever medication or dose the hospital chose to administer). In the second study, a large dose regimen of trifluoperazine (80 mg. daily) was compared with a low dose regimen (15 mg. daily) and a placebo. These studies of 24 weeks' duration were double-blind and involved several hundred chronic schizophrenics. The results have been summarized as follows:

(1) Some chronic schizophrenics are responsive to high dose therapy. The most likely candidate for this treatment is a young (under 40), physically healthy individual who has been ill less than 10 years, who manifests at least a moderate degree of affective reaction, who has florid symptoms such as conceptual, delusional, and perceptual disturbance, who has been partially responsive to the usual ther-

apeutic dose of an antipsychotic, and whose clinical condition has been stable with little variation in dosage for 3 to 6 months. Before shifting to another drug, such a patient should be treated with gradually increasing doses to the limit of his tolerance. He should be kept on the highest tolerated dose for 3 to 6 months before being judged unresponsive. In the high dose chlorpromazine study most high dose patients reached a plateau of improvement by 4 months.

(2) High dose therapy carries a high risk of side effects that are especially frequent and severe in patients over 40. Even with the carefully selected patients (under 40 years and hospitalized less than 10 years) used in the high dose chlorpromazine study, approximately half of them had at least one moderate-to-severe side effect during treatment. Ten percent had side effects serious enough to warrant withdrawal from the study. However, the fact that 45% of the younger, short-stay patients showing improvement had no moderate-to-severe side effects indicates that high doses are both safe and clinically effective. Any patient treated with high doses must be monitored carefully. Dosage should be reduced at the earliest sign of a serious side effect, especially persistent dyskinesia (Ayd, 1971).

(3) High doses of trifluoperazine (a piperazine) were most effective with short-term patients who had been receiving a piperazine phenothiazine, whereas patients who had been taking non-piperazine phenothiazines showed relatively little improvement. Similarly, high doses of chlorpromazine (a non-piperazine) were found most effective with short-term patients who had been prescribed a non-piperazine phenothiazine. Thus, there was the implication that if the patient was not responding to less than substantial doses of his current medication, a trial on high doses of the same drug may be warranted before shifting to another antipsychotic.

(4) A chronic schizophrenic refractory to high doses of a phenothiazine for 6 months should receive consideration for treatment with another antipsychotic, preferably a non-phenothiazine.

The oral form of fluphenazine (fluphenazine hydrochloride) has been used in the dosage range of 700 to 1200 mg. daily on 14 chronic schizophrenic patients refractory to other treatment (Polvan et al., 1969). Six of the 14 patients showed marked improvement and three showed some improvement. Itil et al. (1970) reported on the treatment of resistant schizophrenics with extremely high doses of fluphenazine. Patients were started on relatively high doses of fluphenazine, 50 mg. daily, and then the dosage was increased weekly to 100, 200, 400, 600 and finally 800 mg. daily by the sixth week of the treatment. The patients were maintained on 800 mg. for 4 weeks and then the dosage was gradually decreased to 30 mg. over a period of 6 weeks and maintained at this level for another 4 weeks, after which it was cut down to 20 mg. daily. Six out of 22 patients showed marked improvement with high dosage and 3 patients showed marked improvement with low dosage treatment. Extrapyramidal side effects were seen with both dosages but more frequently with the low dosage. Rifkin et al. (1971) used massive doses of fluphenazine (300 to 1200 mg. daily) and found that both chronic and acute treatment-resistant schizophrenics had good to excellent responses. In a later study, Quitkin and his associates (1975) found that a "standard dose" (30 mg. daily) of fluphenazine produced greater improvement than megadoses (1200 mg. daily) in non-chronic treatment-refractory patients. Their data indicated that some apparently refractory schizophrenics will have good remissions only after being treated for 3 months with aggressive antipsychotic regimens (i.e. fluphenazine, 30 mg. daily) and that the community practice of short-term hospitalization (1 to 3 weeks) followed by the usual small dosage aftercare pharmacotherapy may seriously undertreat such patients.

The use of high dosage piperacetazine (Quide) with doses of 160 to 400 mg./day strongly suggests that piperacetazine is therapeutic at such high doses and that psychotic symptoms resistant to standard dose piperacetazine may respond to high dose therapy without increasing the risk of liver, blood, or renal toxicity (Donlon and Rada, 1974). The judicious administration of high dose piperacetazine to patients refractory to standard doses may greatly expand its overall therapeutic potential as an antipsychotic agent and it can accelerate the reintegration process in some acutely ill schizophrenic patients. Accelerated reintegration means reduced emotional trauma, shortened hospital stay, and earlier exposure to psychotherapeutic and rehabilitative community programs.

A study by Wysenbeek et al. (1974) provided no support for the contention that very high doses of trifluoperazine (600 mg.) are more effective than doses of 60 mg. per day (it should be noted that the dosage of 60 mg. of trifluoperazine exceeds the recommended maximal level in the *Physicians' Desk Reference*). In a double-blind trial of 6 months duration, McClelland and his co-workers (1976) found no significant difference between a very high dosage of fluphenazine decanoate (250 mg. weekly) and a standard dose of 12.5 mg. weekly in chronic schizophrenic patients. Until recently, haloperidol doses up to 100 mg. daily were in the megadose range. The former maximal conservative daily dosage of 15 mg. has now been raised to 100 mg. in *Physicians' Desk Reference* in view of many reports of its clinical efficacy and safety in doses above 15 mg. daily. Interestingly, megadoses of potent antipsychotics such as haloperidol or fluphenazine have not caused a significantly higher incidence of extrapyramidal reactions than low dose therapy. It has been observed that extrapyramidal side effects with fluphenazine are more common in dosages below 100 mg. per day and tend to disappear with higher dosages.

Davis and Cole (1975) have stated that a significant number of patients who do not receive maximal benefit from the usual doses may respond to double or quadruple this amount. Ketai (1976), in discussing high dosage drug therapy with treatment-resistant psychotic patients, stated his belief that many patients in our state institutions and community mental health centers have nothing to lose, but much to gain, by receiving aggressive pharmacologic treatment. It appears that the piperazine group of phenothiazines, haloperidol, and thiothixene are the best tolerated drugs in high dosages for long periods. Extrapyramidal problems are the most common side effects with these drugs and can usually be effectively controlled with appropriate agents such as trihexyphenidyl and benzotropine.

Within safe medical limits, the dosage of these antipsychotic agents should be gradually increased until the desired effect is achieved. Complete blood counts should be done periodically, although they may not necessarily forewarn of an impending drug-induced agranulocytosis. Careful observation, including checking for signs of infection, should be mandatory. If an agranulocytosis is to develop, it is more likely to occur within the first 8 weeks of treatment. It is also wise to have baseline and periodic liver function tests performed, as well as E.K.G.'s.

Persistent or tardive dyskinesia may be an increased risk, particularly with high dosages of piperazines and haloperidol. However, fear of that possible development should not prohibit high dosage treatment of an otherwise chronically psychotic person. In addition, it should be stated that no concrete correlation has been found between the development of tardive dyskinesia and megadoses or the duration of time on antipsychotic medication. Nevertheless, proper observations and interventions are indicated. A trial of from 3 to 6 months of the same antipsychotic drug, with increasing dosages, may be necessary before deciding to switch to another.

Willingness to experiment with many different antipsychotic agents in high dosages is necessary if a determined effort is going to be made to establish effective pharmacotherapy for severely and chronically psychotic patients. Not every patient needs high dose therapy. However, the studies discussed help to identify the clinical characteristics of the candidate for such therapy. Megadose therapy is not without risk but the hazards are not substantially greater than with low doses when the patients are carefully selected and monitored.

16. DRUG HOLIDAYS

Drug holidays may be considered for patients on stable maintenance doses of antipsychotic agents.

For the great majority of patients on stabilized maintenance doses, withdrawal of drugs 1 or 2 days a week may be feasible and beneficial to both patient and staff. Very few patients require high doses for prolonged periods. The antipsychotic drugs and their metabolites accumulate in various body tissues with continued drug administration. Thus, the elimination of medication for 1 or 2 days a week for 2-4 months will result in no significant difference in clinical efficacy for most of the chronic, long-term patients on stable maintenance doses.

After the introduction of antipsychotic drugs, Good et al. (1959) reported these conclusions:

(1) Chlorpromazine can be withdrawn from chronic schizophrenic patients for at least 10-12 weeks without any noticeable regression in behavior or intellectual function.
(2) Withdrawal of chlorpromazine for periods of 3 months or longer results in marked regression in some schizophrenics. Typically such regression is characterized by the return of hallucinations, delusions, incoherence, and confusion which constituted the patient's symptomatology prior to successful treatment with chlorpromazine.
(3) There is no relationship between duration of previous chlorpromazine treatment and tendency to regress when chlorpromazine is withdrawn.
(4) Resumption of chlorpromazine after 3 months without it produces the same effects as continuous treatment, suggesting that periodic short-term withdrawal of chlorpromazine is a feasible treatment program for chronic schizophrenics.

Since then, a number of clinical studies have reported on the feasibility and efficacy of drug administration schedules in which drug-free periods are tested. Some investigators have used a 1-day-a-week drug-free period, a weekend drug-free period, the administration of drug only on alternate days, administration during alternate weeks and even during alternate months. In each study the total daily dose remained the same, but was administered less frequently. Elimination of medication for 1 or 2 days per week resulted in no statistically significant difference in clinical efficacy from that noted with the administration on a daily basis. If the medication was withheld for longer periods of time, deterioration of clinical status and even relapse began to show up after a few months.

Ayd (1966), who coined the term "drug holiday" for intermittent drug-free schedules, initiated a "Never-On-Sunday" policy for his chronically ill patients on maintenance antipsychotic therapy. On Sundays these patients did not take medication. He found that this proved practical and safe, since only rarely did a patient feel the need to take some, but not all, of the usual daily dose of the medication. Later some of these patients had the drug-free interval increased to Saturday and Sunday or to Friday, Saturday and

Sunday. Others were better maintained by 2 days on and 1 or 2 days off drugs. Another group was maintained successfully on a program of 3 weeks on and 1 week off drugs. Occasionally, a patient had to resume medication earlier than planned because of reaction to some moderately severe personal or environmental stress. The most suitable patients for drug holidays have been found to be those on maintenance medication whose clinical condition has been stable and who have not required any variation in dosage for 3 to 6 months minimum (Diamond and Marks, 1960; Greenberg and Roth, 1966).

The evidence clearly indicates that for the great majority of patients, once a tissue saturation level is reached (i.e., after 2-3 weeks of daily drug administration), there is no loss in clinical efficacy if the medication is not given on a daily basis (DiMascio, 1972). Those few patients who clinically cannot tolerate any drug-free periods must obviously remain on daily drug administration, but it is only by trying such drug-free schedules that a physician can determine in whom various schedules may or may not be successfully employed. Drug holidays result in the reduced use of drugs and reduced nursing time involved; more importantly, the use of drug-free periods gives the patient's body the opportunity to rid itself somewhat of these drugs and/or their metabolites that have accumulated in the tissues and that in time show up in a variety of body organs (eyes, skin, heart muscles, etc.). Also, drug holidays may result in freedom from some of the drug side effects that may interfere with social, occupational and recreational activities.

In a V.A. collaborative study, Caffey et al. (1964) evaluated a schedule in which medication was administered only 3 days a week. In this double-blind study of 348 chronic schizophrenics, one group received antipsychotic drugs daily, another only on Monday, Wednesday and Friday with drug-free days in between, while a third group received a placebo every Monday, Wednesday and Friday with drug-free days in between. At the end of 16 weeks, 5% of the patients on continuous treatment had relapsed, compared to 15% on intermittent treatment and 45% on no medication.

In a later study (Prien et al., 1973a), 375 patients were assigned on a double-blind random basis to one for 5 groups: (1) patients continued to receive their pre-study medication; (2) drugs were given Monday through Friday, with a drug holiday on Saturday and Sunday; (3) drugs were given on Monday, Tuesday, Wednesday, Friday and Sunday, and placebos were given on Thursday and Saturday; (4) drugs were given Monday through Thursday, and a placebo was given on Friday through Sunday; (5) drugs were given Monday, Wednesday, Friday and Sunday. In the four intermittent schedules there was no increase in the daily dose to compensate for the omission of 2 or 3 days' medication; hence, the patient's weekly dose was reduced by 29% to 43% below his pre-study level. After 16 weeks, relapse had occurred in 1% of the patients continued on the daily schedule, in 6% on the first conventional 5-day schedule, in 8% on the second 5-day schedule, in 7% on the first 4-day schedule, and in 6% on the other 4-day schedule. The results of the V.A. studies demonstrated that the large majority of chronic schizophrenics on stabilized doses of antipsychotic drugs can have their medication withdrawn for 2 or 3 days per week without significant deleterious effects. However, it does not mean that intermittent schedules should be used indiscriminately.

To institute a drug holiday program which meets with the least resistance and creates a minimum of anxiety in the nursing staff, a gradual introduction is recommended. The initial step is to withhold medication for 1 day per week for 1 month and then go back to the daily drug regimen for a month. A weekday such as Wednesday instead of Saturday or Sunday should be chosen since there is a full staff complement during weekdays in contrast to the minimal coverage on weekends and thus the staff feels quite secure with this innovation. After twice alternating months on this type of 2-month schedule, the drug holiday is increased to 2 days during each week every other month. By this time, staff anxiety and fears will be allayed and both the patients and staff will be ready for a drug-free weekend (Saturday and Sunday) program every other month. Later the period of drug-free weekends can be expanded to 2 months. Finally, some patients can be placed on drug-free weekends throughout the year.

In addition to the benefits of a drug holiday program already mentioned, the patient has less need to bother continually with medication and thus may develop the feeling that he is not completely dependent on drugs, as well as possibly feeling he is improving. For the nursing and medical staff there is reduced workload on the drug holidays (weekends) when fewer personnel are on duty and therefore more time is available for recreational and other therapeutic activities. Furthermore, drug holidays used in a systematic way can encourage and enable physicians to assess the needs of patients for their medication.

Although intermittent drug withdrawal is feasible, it must be tempered with concern for patient and staff. Patients who have required recent dosage adjustments and whose clinical condition is not stable are not ideal candidates for a drug withdrawal program. Also, caution should be observed with young patients who have been hospitalized under 10 years. Intermittent drug withdrawal should be initiated only when the clinician is satisfied that the patient will not benefit from upward adjustment or change in medication. Special care should be taken to familiarize the staff with intermittent schedules to be employed on the ward. A staff faced with a program of decreased medication for many patients may be apprehensive. It has been shown that staff attitudes can be a crucial factor in the success or failure of any treatment program. Personnel should know that the risk of relapse following short-term drug withdrawal is small. In addition, it should be pointed out that when relapses do occur, they are usually gradual rather than abrupt and are easily handled in the early states by returning the patient to a daily medication schedule.

The drug holiday program has not gained the wide acceptance it deserves. A recent survey study of 42 Veterans Administration hospitals compared the prescriptions of 3,860 patients from 257 wards with the drug holiday recommendation in "Guidelines for Antipsychotic Drug Use" (Prien and Caffey, 1975). The specific V.A. guideline for drug holidays was as follows: "For patients on stabilized maintenance doses for 6 months or more, withdrawal of drug 2 to 3 days a week is feasible and could be beneficial to both patient and staff and should be tried." It was found that drug holidays were not often used; 74% of the hospitals reported less than 5% of their patients on this type of scheduling.

Yet this program has many advantages when compared to uninterrupted drug administration. Long-term uninterrupted antipsychotic medication may contribute to institutionalization by reducing drive, initiative and planning ability in the chronic patient. Also, drugs are expensive and considerable staff time is spent in preparing and dispensing medication. Drug holidays allow the patient to engage in weekend visits and other activities without the inconvenience of medication. It helps the physician to avoid heavy reliance on drugs to the exclusion of psychosocial and rehabilitive therapies. Drug holidays also provide a means of limiting the total amount of medication administered over a long period of time.

The risk of relapse during the suggested drug holiday program is very slight and can be further minimized by careful monitoring of the patient. If possible, patients should have the experience with intermittent drug therapy prior to discharge since many patients, once out in the community, will strongly resist and refuse to accept any change in their medication regimen.

When an intermittent program is tried with outpatients, the visits to the physician or clinic should continue to be regularly scheduled, perhaps more frequently. When feasible, the family of the patient should be informed about the program and requested to report any behavioral change or early signs of decompensation so that the former daily medication schedule can be promptly reinstituted. Also, reassurance can be given that relapse will be easily prevented. A successful period of drug holidays should precede the trial period off medication for patients in remission from their first psychotic episode. Finally, Carpenter (1978) recommends a trial of 4 to 6 weeks without maintenance medication in the belief that this will expose mose cases of "covert dyskinesia," which may possibly represent a subgroup of early tardive dyskinesias potentially reversible with drug cessation.

17. DRUG DEVIATION

The physician and the rest of the mental health team must be aware of the many factors that may cause the patient to discontinue maintenance medication and must take action to prevent or control these factors.

The most important single cause of the return of psychotic symptoms, relapse and readmission to a psychiatric facility is still the failure of the patient to take the antipsychotic drug or in the dosage prescribed. Hollister (1973) found that the number of patients who do not take their medication or reduce the dose increases rapidly in the first few months following return to the community, reaching as high as 40%. While the need for long-term treatment may well be recognized by the physician, it is frequently not recognized or accepted by the patient. Consequent failure to take the medication has given rise to the term "drug defaulter."

Obviously, there is a wide variety of reasons why patients default. The patient's daily drug schedule may be responsible for failure of the patient to adhere to this medication schedule. It is the usual practice in mental hospitals for a member of the nursing staff to administer medication on a t.i.d. or q.i.d. schedule up until the day of discharge. At this time, the patient is assumed to have reached, overnight, the level of mature responsibility for taking his drugs. To prepare the patient for this responsibility, many hospitals have developed self-medication programs whereby the patient is given a prescription, fills it at the hospital pharmacy and is given the opportunity to take his medicine on his own initiative.

Often patients do not take their medications because they are given too complicated a drug regimen to follow after discharge. A simple but very important rule is to reduce the pill-taking to a once-a-day schedule, preferably at bedtime. A person feels "less sick" if he takes only one pill a day. The patient who is expected to take his medicine regularly more than once or twice a day is almost certain to default. A strategy to combat drug forgetting is "habit tailoring," which links the taking of medication to a routine procedure such as brushing teeth.

Embarrassment is often a factor when the patient is supposed to take his drugs in situations other than the privacy of his home. It is particularly true when the patient is at work and thinks his co-workers are aware of his situation. Taking pills on the job leaves the patient open to questioning and may involve uncomfortable explanations or evasions. The same situation prevails during social occasions. Also, the necessity for medication may be interpreted by him as a reflection of his inferiority and is a daily comparison which constantly undermines his feeling of adequacy. The result is frequent forgetfulness in taking the medication. This not only decreases the appropriate drug level but disrupts the medical pattern, which engenders more "forgetting" other times. The missed doses usually do not affect the patient's functioning immediately and thus may delude him into believing that perhaps he doesn't really need the drug (Brophy, 1969).

The side effects of the antipsychotics play a prominent part in the creation of a negative attitude in outpatients toward maintenance medication. Irwin et al. (1971) found that significantly more chronic ambulatory patients for whom thioridazine had been prescribed (55%) were not taking minimal amounts of their medication as compared to patients on chlorpromazine (15%). Impotence is one of the main reasons male patients will avoid taking medication and, because of the relationship of thioridazine to this side effect, this drug is least likely to be taken. It appears that psychiatric patients placed on antipsychotics, especially chronic schizophrenics, are not usually asked about their sex lives. Amdur (1976) has commented that the experience at a university aftercare program indicated a high incidence of sexual dysfunction in men taking thioridazine. In practice, therefore, they no longer prescribe thioridazine to male patients. It is important that clinicians be aware of sexual dysfunction in males due to antipsychotics and of the reversibility of this side effect, so that patients will be questioned about their sexual functioning. If impotence is occurring, reassurance can be given and a switch to another antipsychotic can be promptly made. This action, along with weekly contacts with the patient, will indicate whether or not the dysfunction has been alleviated.

Drug reluctance on the part of patients has been found to be significantly associated with extrapyramidal side effects, most notably a subtle akathisia (Van Putten, 1974). A dysphoric response to antipsychotic drugs has also been associated with extrapyramidal involvement (for full description of extrapyramidal symptoms and their treatment, see Chapter 5 on Side Effects of Antipsychotic Drugs and Their Management). Hostile, paranoid schizophrenics were found to be most intolerant of any extrapyramidal side effects. Dysphoric responders complained bitterly about the drug and were strongly "drug reluctant." Akinesia also is a poorly recognized drug-induced extrapyramidal behavioral side effect which is common in patients receiving antipsychotic drugs and can be the only manifestation of extrapyramidal involvement. It has been recommended that once it is established that maintenance on an antipsychotic drug is necessary, every effort should be made to avoid the development of even mild extrapyramidal involvement. Such involvement can be unbearable and lead to outright drug reluctance or self-prescribed reduction of dosage. Hansell and Willis (1977) encourage their outpatients to discuss side effects fully, including the subtler forms of akathisia. More than two-thirds of their group of 575 outpatients experienced some side effects, most of which were manageable with persistent attention. Twenty-two percent of their group are taking antiparkinson agents for control of motor side effects and 46% have done so occasionally. It pays to ask the question, "How does the medication agree with you?"

Presently, many patients are discharged quickly from the hospital once their acute symptoms subside. Some patients may develop a depression a few weeks or months later and stop taking their medication. This type of post-psychotic depression must be differentiated from neurologic side effects such as akinesia. The patient has early awakening, morning retardation, self-reproachfulness and a depressed mood. The depressions often remit spontaneously along with other extrapyramidal side effects. Prompt differential diagnosis may be accomplished by giving an antiparkinson drug intravenously. If the depressive symptoms are in reality extrapyramidal effects, they will subside, often within a half-hour. If the depression is not drug induced, the antiparkinson drug is of no benefit. Then the depression may be considered a natural concomitant of the illness course and may require treatment with antidepressants. Increasing the dosage of the antipsychotic can make the depression worse. Physicians should be especially alert for depression in patients treated with the depot fluphenazines.

Van Putten et al. (1978) also has called attention to a group of hard-core drug refusers who experience a "resurgence of a florid psychosis characterized by grandiosity and relative absence of such dysphoric affects as anxiety and depression." This group of chronic schizophrenics had a history of numerous readmissions and discharges and symptoms that responded to antipsychotics. It appeared that they never became reconciled to the need for antipsychotic drug therapy and could not tolerate the drug-induced increase in reality contact. When they were switched to fluphenazine decanoate, very few returned with any regularity for their bimonthly injections. It seems that some schizophrenics may prefer an "ego-syntonic grandiose psychosis" to a relative drug-induced normality. A gratifying relationship with a skilled clinician appeared to be the only approach in keeping these patients on maintenance medication.

Drug intake may be altered by the patient who is troubled by some side effects such as daytime drowsiness or an unusually large weight gain. Cognizance, however, must be taken that when some schizophrenic patients in the community complain about the side effects of the antipsychotic drug, especially those that are vague or not well documented, the effects may be spurious. The complaint may be related to the patient's unwillingness to take his medication. For example, the patient may claim that he is allergic to his medicine. He may display a post-drug rash that on close inspection does not exist. Also, patients who are resistant or indifferent to treatment are an especially high-risk category. The clinician must take the time to deal with their resistance by developing a good relationship with these patients even though they may be considered poor treatment prospects. In many community mental health centers and outpatient clinics, the patient is not seen by a physician but by a psychologist, psychiatric social worker, nurse or some other mental health worker. Therefore, it behooves not only the physician but all members of the mental health team to become very knowledgeable about possible side effects. An available checklist of physical symptoms, specifically including side effects, may be helpful. This type of quick review by systems would not be dissimilar to that taken by a nurse or clinician during an office visit for a physical disorder. Along the same vein, checking the weight and taking the patient's blood pressure may contribute to a positive attitude toward keeping clinic appointments. The questioning of the patient must be tactful and skillful to avoid suggestibility. Alert observations during a clinic visit may disclose some signs of extrapyramidal involvement. Failure of the physician to respect the patient's objective complaints is one of the common causes of patients' refusing to take their medication and dropping out of treatment.

The patient's family plays a vital role in determining whether the patient will continue to take his medication and keep his clinic appointments. It is important that the physician, besides establishing a good rapport with the patient, strive to develop a good relationship with relatives and to create family-physician rapport. Relatives can be a help or a hindrance to successful antipsychotic therapy. If they are to be a help, every effort should be made to include them in the therapeutic team by indoctrinating them about what they can realistically expect drugs to do for the patient and what they can do to help the patient, especially by making sure that he takes his medicine exactly as prescribed (Ayd, 1970).

The family should be told clearly of the possibility of recurrence when the drug intake is altered. The family, as well as the patient, should be informed about side effects and be cautioned about possible drowsiness and interference with skilled movements. Many patients have a recurrent pattern to their psychosis which can be detected in the incipient stages. Such patterns are unusual expenditures, unusual loquacity, insomnia, instability and secual preoccupation may signify the recurrence of psychosis. The family should be made aware of these symptoms based upon the history of the individual case and should be advised to contact the therapist at the first appearance of symptomatic behavior. If a good relationship exists with the family, they may recognize failure to take medication as a sign of impending difficulty and bring the patient quickly to the psychiatrist to avoid a relapse. Sometimes a nurse through home visits can be helpful in fostering this type of relationship.

Family members are often opposed to the "doping" of a relative in remission and making them take his maintenance treatment seriously often presents more of a problem than the original treatment of the psychosis. It should be remembered that when some patients have no symptoms, neither the patient nor his family consider him sick. This may account, at least partially, for the fact that a substantial number of patients apparently adjust dosage in accordance to their self-identified needs and that this is in the direction of scaling the dosage downward. Large numbers of these patients do not feel free to inform their therapists of the change (McClellan and Cowan, 1970). Open-ended, nonthreatening, nonjudgemental questions (e.g., "You don't seem to be doing quite as well as we hoped; are you having any difficulties with the medication, or is there something that I didn't explain?") can be effective in elicited nonadherence (Francis, et al., 1969). A substantial amount of education focused on the patient's role in self-regulation of medications within a prescribed range may result in improvement in the safety, precision and reliability of drug intake.

Clinic staffs must remember that, after a patient discontinues his medication, it may take many months or perhaps a year before a relapse occurs. This increases the chances that the patient and relatives will have lost contact with the psychiatrist or any member of the treatment facility, which complicates the situation. Traditionally, psychotherapists have been reluctant to maintain active communication with the relatives of their patients. Psychiatrists treating schizophrenic patients cannot afford the luxury of noncommunication with relatives. **Failure to involve the patient's family in the treatment program often results in the patient's not taking medication regularly or discontinuing medication with resultant relapse and hospitalization.**

Many patients do not give reliable information regarding their drug intake. Some may allege that they are taking their medication when, in fact, they have stopped. It has been found that clinic staff cannot determine with any degree of accuracy which patients are failing to adhere to their medication schedule unless the patient shows a recrudescence of symptoms signifying relapse. To objectively determine whether the patient is taking a phenothiazine drug and the dose prescribed, the Forrest urine tests, a simple office procedure, should be made a routine part of every clinic visit, just as a urine test for sugar is standard practice in diabetic clinics. Many outpatients are still on chlorpromazine and thioridazine and the Forrest urine tests give their most accurate semi-qualitative determinations with these phenothiazines. Particular indications for the tests are a patient who (a) is paranoid, or (b) complains of having to take too many tablets but is persuaded to remain on the same regimen, or (c) is relapsing unaccountably, or (d) is receiving a drug or a dosage which is not having the expected therapeutic results, or (e) has a history of relapses and hospital readmissions. (See section of Forrest Urine Tests). Compliance can sometimes be improved by switching to liquid medication.

Detre and Jarecki (1971) have pointed out that psychological factors may cause the patient to discontinue his medication against medical advice. There may be a denial of illness, which is usually reflected in such statements as, "I feel well, so why should I take medication," or "if I continue medication it proves that I'm still sick." In some cases, the patient may feel that the use of drugs diminishes his image in his own eyes or those of his family; he may be trying to prove that he is no longer (or perhaps never was) ill or a weakling. He may resent taking medicine and may look upon it as a crutch. Wishful or magical thinking and indignation over his disability may also be reasons for patient's desire to terminate his drug intake. Continued treatment may serve to remind him of the cloud under which he feels he must live. It may mean to him that decompensation is possible at any time or that he is incurable. Some patients manipulate their medication regimen as a psychological means through which they can express certain feelings to their physician. Sometimes the patient simply cannot believe that a pill can help prevent a breakdown. Others, noticing their discomfort when they withdraw, become concerned they will become addicted to the drug in spite of their physician's assurance that the medication does not lead to craving or other signs typical of sedative, opiate or alcohol addiction. Patients who discontinue medication and are at the point of relapse are often extremely negative about resuming medication or getting back into psychiatric treatment of any kind. Rehospitalization is almost always necessary.

The development of rapport between the patient and his physician, with a positive attitude on the part of the physician, may lead to a more conscientious attitude toward taking medication regularly. The patient needs to be cautioned that he must continue medication even though he feels well. If the patient does not cooperate, the physician should explore the reasons with the patient. He should be concerned with both the psychological and social aspects of the giving of medication. **In fact, it is believed that any physician who uses long-term antipsychotic therapy should spend as much effort on the non-drug factors of the total care of the patient as he does on selecting the dosage and monitoring the drug regimen.** Default may be the patient's way of controlling or defeating other people. It may also indicate the patient's lack of knowledge regarding how to comply with the physician's instructions (Jobe, 1976).

An important determinant may be the patient's perception of the physician's interest in him as a person. However, at many community mental health centers, the psychiatrist may be responsible for 200-300 patients in addition to other duties and does not have the time to develop a therapeutic relationship with these patients. Thus, the mental health workers of the center must be trained and relied upon to develop the patient-therapist rapport.

The patient should be taught to recognize the signs of incipient trouble early enough to take appropriate countermeasures while he still has enough insight to do so. These countermeasures may include increasing his drug intake until he can reach his physician. He must be instructed how important it is to seek consultation early in the course of a relapse and whenever he changes his residence to contact a local physician to whom he can turn for treatment (Astrachan and Detre, 1968). Most importantly, the patient must be taught about the risks inherent in abrupt, unsupervised drug withdrawal and to understand and accept the necessity of taking drugs for as long as recommended. The clinician must talk to patients and let them know that he is flexible in his thinking and open to hear any kind of problem that may arise in regard to their medication. Patients often ask about decreasing or stopping medication and these requests must be consistently discouraged. The social and often the occupational cost of a relapse into a psychosis is too high a risk.

Education of patients about the need to take medication for a long time and perhaps indefinitely in order to stay well should start in the hospital and should continue as long as the patient needs the antipsychotic. It should be emphasized to him that there are hundreds of thousands of people with physical illnesses who must take medicine for the rest of their lives. Some examples which might be mentioned are the people who require continued treatment for diabetes, epilepsy, high blood pressure, pernicious anemia, and many heart and kidney diseases.

Often, the blanket warning of total abstinence from alcohol may produce a drug defaulter (Marshall, 1971). Many chronic patients can find companionship only in a bar or tavern. Their community placement may consist of a boarding house, hotel room or a large personal care home which engenders feelings of loneliness and social isolation. Their sole source of recreation may be a visit to a tavern where they can find some sociability and relief from boredom. In spite of the firm admonition that alcohol and their medication do not mix, they start drinking and soon discontinue taking their medication. It may take several months, but the ultimate result is the return of the psychotic symptoms and rehospitalization. Some patients repeat this pattern time and again.

Patients should be advised about the use of alcohol and their medication regimen on an individual basis. It may be advisable to counsel certain patients that they may have one drink or two beers if they must rather than none at all. When patients are told they cannot have a drink while on medication and a holiday or a birthday or a celebration of one sort or another comes around, they take the drink and not the medication. Drug compliance can be greatly influenced by the restrictions placed on an outpatient. The re-education with respect to recreational outlets in the community is important for many chronic patients.

Despite all efforts, there are many chronic patients in the "revolving door" group who will not take their medication as prescribed each time they are released from the hospital. To assure that these unreliable and uncooperative drug takers receive their medication, they can be treated with the long-acting depot injectable forms of fluphenazine. If, however, a patient is known to be reliable in taking oral medication, then there is no reason to change his treatment regimen to intramuscular injections. However, when it is considered unlikely that a particular patient is going to take his tablets conscientiously outside the hospital, it is advisable to stabilize him on a program of depot fluphenazine injections before discharge.

The cost of medication may represent a heavy financial burden to the patient and his family if they cannot obtain the drug free or at low cost at the clinic. The monthly drug bill may exceed $50 since psychopharmaceuticals are expensive and, in these inflationary times, other expenditures (i.e., food, clothing and shelter) must receive a higher priority. This economic factor is responsible for many patients ceasing to take their medication and it is essential that a continuous supply of drugs be made available to these patients.

Perhaps the main factor governing the intake of antipsychotic medications appears to be direct patient supervision. In foster homes, mini-homes and convalescent homes where the sponsor assumes some responsibility in making certain that the patient takes his medication, the readmission rate drops to 5 to 15%. Patients living alone are much more likely to default; schizophrenic patients living with a spouse or relatives are twice as likely to take medication as those living in isolation (Parkes et al., 1962).

To reduce the likelihood of drug deviation, Blackwell (1973) has recommended that the minimum number of different medications be prescribed; the minimum frequency of daily dosage be used; relatives, friends or social workers become involved in the supervision of medication; the possible side effects that may occur be carefully explained; regular follow-ups be instituted in prolonged therapy; and information be given regarding the possible consequences of drug defaulting.

His suggestions for identifying the drug deviator consist of (1) tactful questioning, if possible by a person well-known by and concerned with the patient and (2) use of available tests in a nonthreatening manner. Patients found to deviate should not be confronted in an accusatory manner but the suggestion may be made that they appear to be unusually forgetful. At this time, inquiry may reveal evidence of impending relapse or elicit complaints of side effects. Such measures are helpful in obtaining compliance as has been found in lithium clinics where close attention to blood levels seems to be interpreted by the patient as an additional expression of interest and concern rather than an attempt to expose drug deviation.

18. DRUG DISCONTINUATION

Maintenance antipsychotic medication will be required indefinitely for most schizophrenic patients and is essential if relapse is to be avoided.

There are conflicting views in psychiatry as to how long antipsychotic drugs should be continued. In an effort to find an answer to this problem, many drug discontinuation studies have been conducted. An early study (Caffey et al., 1964) found 45% of hospitalized chronic schizophrenics relapsed within 16 weeks when taken off medication and placed on placebo in contrast to a 5% relapse rate for the patients who remained on drug therapy. In addition, the "non-relapsed" patients on placebo showed significantly more thinking disorganization and agitated depression than the medicated patients at the end of 16 weeks.

Prien and Klett (1972), in their review of the drug discontinuation literature, found that (1) indiscriminate withdrawal of antipsychotic medication for long periods of time carries a high risk of relapse. Most studies indicated that 40% or more of the patients taken off medication relapse within 6 months. They concluded that the probability of relapse appears too high to recommend long-term drug withdrawal as a general treatment policy for chronic schizophrenics. Discontinuation was most feasible with patients who had been hospitalized for long periods and were already receiving low doses of antipsychotic medication. The risk of relapse with these patients is relatively low.

Various studies show that discontinuation of antipsychotic drug therapy may lead to relapse in 73 to 95.5% of patients within a year, in 51 to 75% of patients in 6 months and in approximately 25% of patients within 4 weeks (Ban, 1974). In a review of 24 controlled studies on the use of maintenance antipsychotic drugs, Davis (1975) observed that 698 out of 1068 patients who received placebo relapsed (65%), in contrast with 639 patients out of 2127 who received maintenance antipsychotics (30%). Thus, the percent of relapse in the drug-treated groups was less than half that observed in the control group. Objective determinations of drug intake were usually not done and in all probability would have revealed that many of the "drug-treated" group who relapsed had not complied with their drug regimen. Lehman (1975) noted that relapse rates vary widely according to different studies—from 7 to 33% in a year follow-up of patients on maintenance medication and from 20 to 70% of patients not on treatment.

Perhaps the best long-range study to determine the ability of maintenance drug to forestall relapse was carried out by Hogarty and his associates (1973, 1974, 1975, 1976), using patients at 3 different clinics. They reported that by the end of one year, 67.5% of patients placed on placebos relapsed but only 30.9% of the "drug-assigned" patients had relapsed. By the end of 2 years, 80% of the placebo patients but only 48% of the patients on an antipsychotic drug had relapsed. Interestingly, 30% of the patients did well on a placebo for a period of 10 months and then suddenly relapsed without warning. The differences in relapse rate between drug and placebo were remarkably consistent at each clinic. Hogarty et al. also noted that "in all probability the true relapse rate on active medication was lower to some unknown extent than 48%, particularly in light of the fact that some drug-assigned patients were not taking medication as prescribed at the time of relapse." They felt that the relapse rate of those on active drug therapy would have been lower—20% or less—if all patients on the drug had taken it regularly.

Sex had a strong influence on the relapse rates for men and women. While drug was superior to placebo for both men and women, nevertheless, after 2 years, 63% of the male schizophrenic patients assigned to drug had relapsed but only 37% of the female patients. At the same time, nearly identical numbers of men and women relapsed on placebo (82% and 80%, respectively). It may well be that women have a greater tendency to adhere to their medication schedules, resulting in fewer relapses.

Hansell and Willis (1977) found that not taking medication was highly correlated with a return of symptoms and with rehospitalization in their large group of outpatients. It often required 3-6 months or longer for such exacerbations to occur. Drug holidays lasting several days to several weeks usually did not actually foreshadow longer-term consequences.

The reports of Hogarty and his associates (1976) further suggest that the need for prophylactic antipsychotics continues to exist throughout the third and 4th years after discharge. They found that nearly one-third of the successfully maintained patients appeared "too ill" clinically to risk drug discontinuation. For those thought to be suitable candidates, two thirds relapsed following withdrawal. It appeared to them that the need for maintenance chemotherapy may be indefinite and that the physician who fails to maintain schizophrenic outpatient medication for an extended period of time runs the enormous risk of inviting relapse. Finally, it appears that in studies carried out in a variety of settings—in private, state or V.A. hospitals, in inpatient and outpatient facilities—more patients relapsed with placebo than with antipsychotics. It is very unusual to find such agreement in psychiatry.

However, it should be noted that some patients do not relapse even if their drugs are discontinued and there is general agreement that a subgroup of schizophrenic patients should not be treated with maintenance medication. There is, as yet, no way of telling who the patients are who will remain well and not relapse when medication is stopped. The clinician has to make a decision whether to embark on a maintenance regime of possibly indefinite duration or to take the risk of letting the patient have another breakdown. When the patient's past history reveals that discontinuance or reduction of antipsychotic drugs in the past was followed by clinical relapse, it is safe to assume that this patient has already been tested without medication with negative results and therefore should remain on maintenance therapy indefinitely. In the United States, there is a 50% chance for readmission within 2 years; in fact, 70% of all state and county hospital admissions for schizophrenia are readmissions. Thus, it would appear that the majority of chronic schizophrenics have already had a test period without antipsychotic drugs. However, Gardos and Cole (1976) stress "that every chronic schizophrenic outpatient maintained on antipsychotic medication should have the benefit of an adequate trial without drugs."

In the hospital, it is relatively easy to discontinue antipsychotic medication in the chronic patient. Nursing staff can be trained to detect early signs of relapse and, if behavior deteriorates, medication can be represcribed. A sounder drug treatment program for the chronic schizophrenic who has reached a "steady state" of functioning and whose condition has not changed for months or years consists of a gradual decrease of drug dosage. The dosage is reduced by 20-25% and continued at this reduced dose to determine whether it is sufficient to stabilize the mental condition. Those patients who show an intensification of their symptoms within a short time—sometimes within days—should resume their former antipsychotic regimen immediately. However, if there is no change in the mental status after 3 months, the dose can be further decreased in 20-25% decrements until the minimal dose that brings about the greatest improvement has been found.

A number of patients may temporarily improve when the antipsychotic medication is stopped. They may become more alert and more cooperative and show increased participation in activity programs. This apparent improvement is due to the disappearance of an undiagnosed mild akinesia. However, after 2 to 4 weeks without medication, many of these temporarily improved chronic schizophrenics will relapse and manifest their former psychotic symptoms. These patients need continued pharmacotherapy.

Careful review of clinical records will reveal some chronic schizophrenics who have received substantial doses of several antipsychotics over the years and whose psychotic symptoms have remained essentially unchanged since admission. These patients are receiving antipsychotic drugs needlessly since they have not responded to the drugs. They may be candidates for having their medication gradually phased out. The observation has been made that patients who need relatively high doses of antipsychotic drugs to maintain improvement have a greater frequency of relapse and thus are not good candidates for drug discontinuation.

It has been advocated that since some patients, whether acute or chronic, do not regress or relapse when the drug is discontinued and since there is presently no method to identify these individuals, it seems reasonable to treat them for 6 months to a year and then discontinue medication. If regression or relapse takes place, the physician can resume the drug on an indefinite maintenance basis. Such a treatment program is feasible when a good doctor-patient relationship exists and the patient's aftercare program provides for reasonably frequent visits. Under thee circumstances, it is possible for the physician to detect the early signs of a relapse that may occur and antipsychotic medication in adequate dosage can be initiated quickly to abort the relapse. It must be remembered that antipsychotic drugs are excreted from the body slowly and therefore relapse may not occur until weeks or months after drug discontinuation. Thus, in most instances, medication can be reinstituted before frank relapse occurs.

Many authorities seem to "hedge" on the question of whether the "one episode" patient should continue with maintenance medication indefinitely. A common recommendation is that this type of patient should *probably not* be treated with long-term medication. Leff and Wing (1971) state that there are patients who are likely to remain well for at least a year without any drug treatment. These are patients with acute onset whose clinical state included symptoms of "endogenous" depression and who had a good personality before the onset of the illness. They conclude that *it might be considered justifiable* to withhold maintenance treatment from such patients.

Other clinicians feel that the patient who has had one schizophrenic episode and seems to have outgrown the environmental events that led to the episode, with no other clinical indications that he is at risk for relapse, should probably not be treated with long-term maintenance medication. Also, for the first episode "reactive" schizophrenic patients short-term maintenance treatment should be given to ensure that the patients have made a solid recovery from the first episode but to avoid long-term maintenance. Factors such as acute episode, youth, rapid onset and good premorbid history further describe this patient. Hogarty and his associates' findings (1976) are contrary to these views. Unequivocally, their studies show that the characteristics of patients who survive drug discontinuation after 2 or 3 years of successful maintenance are not able to be clearly definied. They have stated that "whoever they are, they are certainly not patients that allegedly do not require phenothiazine treatment (e.g., acute, non-paranoid, young, first episode, rapid onset or good premorbid history)."

The consequences of drug discontinuation in a patient who has responded well after his first psychotic break must be weighed carefully. Another attack of schizophrenia can be a major catastrophe and may ruin the patient's chances in his chosen occupation. Family disruption may result in divorce and the patient may acquire the reputation among his relatives and friends of having unpredictable "crazy" spells. Yet patients who have responded to antipsychotics and have remained relatively asymptomatic represent the clinical dilemma of whether to continue or discontinue maintenance drug therapy after a prolonged period of successful outpatient treatment.

It has been the experience of Lehman (1975) that it is best to continue maintenance treatment after the first schizophrenic attack for at least 2 or 3 years, after the second attack for 5 years, and after 3 or more relapses indefinitely, possibly for the patient's lifetime. Zavodnick (1977) recommends that treatment should be continued for 6 months after a first schizophrenic episode and, after 2 or more episodes, probably indefinitely. Rifkin et al. (1976) consider it best to provide the acute schizophrenic who has remitted with a prophylactic drug for at least a year. At any rate, a trial on intermittent drug therapy prior to the discontinuation of the antipsychotic seems to be a wise course of action, even for the first-episode patient on maintenance medication.

It has been found that patients who have been hospitalized for a long period of time (i.e., over 15 years) and are on relatively low doses of antipsychotic drugs (i.e., the equivalent of 300 mg. or less chlorpromazine) have a relapse rate of 15% compared to a 33 to 60% rate in other subgroups. These long-stay hospitalized patients on low doses of antipsychotic medication would seem to be particularly good candidates for drug discontinuation trials. On the geriatric and semi-infirm wards in mental hospitals, in nursing and convalescent homes, and in extended care facilities, there are thousands of elderly patients who have been receiving very small, usually homeopathic doses of antipsychotic medication for many years. Their history often discloses that at some time in the past they displayed some aggressive or uncooperative behavior which resulted in an antipsychotic drug order. The medication of many of these patients can be gradually phased out and there would be no resultant behavioral changes. If disruptive symptoms recurred, small doses of maintenance medication could be promptly reinstituted. However, to allay anxiety of the nursing staff it is best to first place them on a drug holiday program for a period before drug discontinuation. There is some reason to suspect that most geriatric patients, whether with good prognosis or very poor prognosis, may fare at least as well if not better without maintenance drug therapy.

The concept of risk/benefit ratio, which often governs clinical decisions, can be utilized in solving the clinical dilemma of whether to continue or discontinue maintenance drug therapy after a prolonged period of successful outpatient treatment. The possibility that tardive dyskinesia may develop eventually makes it necessary to weigh the drug's benefit against relapse. The social and other consequences of relapse must be evaluated for each patient; social workers, psychologists, nurses and even the patient can be consulted on what the consequences of relapse might be as part of the decision-making process.

The outpatient on maintenance medication must be carefully monitored for early warning signs of impending relapse as the dosage is slowly and gradually reduced to the lowest effective maintenance level. If the patient required a maintenance dosage of more than 300 mg. chlorpromazine daily to prevent relapse, a drug holiday regimen may be considered with progressive increase in the duration of the drug holiday.

19. CHRONIC AND TREATMENT-RESISTANT PATIENTS

Do not forsake the chronic and treatment-resistant patient.

In most psychiatric facilities, there is a sizeable group of chronic psychotic patients who are considered treatment-resistant. It has been estimated that there are, in and out of hospitals, at least one million patients who have responded partially or not at all to the antipsychotics prescribed for them. The great majority of these patients are chronic schizophrenics. A review of their drug histories usually indicates that they had a trial on small to moderate doses of many antipsychotics, often with conjoint antipsychotics prescribed (2 or more), for varying periods of time and with no significant improvement. Others had received a trial with only 2 or 3 of the oldest antipsychotics as they became available. Most have shown no change from their medication or dosage for many months or years. No change in therapeutic approach has been tried for years. No attempt has ever been made to treat them with higher than the usually recommended dosage. They have never received the benefit of a trial with the newer antipsychotics, with dosage alteration, with a short trial on parenteral administration, or with new formulations of old antipsychotics such as the long-acting injectables. Although forsaken, these patients represent a formidable challenge to the therapeutic skills of the psychiatrist.

Clinicians have noted that patients who fail to respond to one phenothiazine occasionally show a good response to another phenothiazine or to an antipsychotic with a different chemical structure. Studies have shown that some of the chronic schizophrenics may respond to the newer antipsychotics, such as loxapine (Loxitane), molindone (Moban, Lidone) or mesoridazine (Serentil).

It can be noted in the section on the Forrest Urine Tests that some patients are considered treatment-resistant when, in reality, they do not ingest their total daily dosage. If phenothiazines are prescribed, the Forrest Urine Tests usually will detect these patients. Those patients who fail to adhere to their maintenance medication can be treated effectively with the long-acting injectable antipsychotics, fluphenazine enanthate or decanoate.

Polypharmacy with low doses of each antipsychotic contributes to the number of drug-resistant patients and many chronic schizophrenics will respond to higher doses of an antipsychotic (see sections on Polypharmacy and Megadoses). Gardos and Cole (1973), in a review of clinical dose-response studies, concluded that high doses or megadoses (1000-2000 mg. of chlorpromazine or the equivalent in other antipsychotics) ofter are indicated for some treatment-resistant schizophrenics who are under 40 years of age with less than 10 years of hospitalization. Treatment with lower doses may be optimal for apathetic or depressed schizophrenics who are not floridly psychotic. Duration of the schizophrenic illness and length of hospitalization may be the key factors in determining whether high doses of antipsychotic medication will be effective.

Some patients are fast metabolizers who destroy the antipsychotic drug so rapidly that they receive ineffective brain levels unless they are given very high doses. Others are slow metabolizers who may have unusually high brain levels that may be toxic even when they receive standard doses. Thus, some phenothiazine-resistant patients may be fast metabolizers who would respond if ultra high doses were used (Davis, 1976b).

It has been shown that chlorpromazine and other antipsychotics may be metabolized in the gut wall. Other patients may show an inadequate therapeutic response because of poor absorption from the intestinal tract. To bypass poor absorption or inefficient metabolism, fluphenazine decanoate has been administered to antipsychotic-resistant patients and has achieved good results in many of these patients. Some patients may respond to a few days of parenteral administration of an antipsychotic followed by a return to oral medication (i.e., haloperidol 5 mg. t.i.d. for 2-4 days followed by oral dosage).

An aggressive trial with the piperazine group of phenothiazines, haloperidol or thiothixene has been advicated since they are well tolerated in high doses for long periods. A trial of from 3 to 6 months of the antipsychotic drug, with increasing doses, may be necessary before deciding to switch to another. The more florid the psychotic symptomatology, the more likely the patient will respond to proper dosages of antipsychotic medication, provided there is no detactable brain disease. Also, clinical response seems to be particularly likely when major affective components are evident (Ketai, 1976).

Rapid tranquilization methods have been used successfully in the treatment of acute psychotic patients with the diagnosis of schizophrenia or mania. However, consideration should be given to a trial of one of these rapid titration methods for the chronic patient who still presents florid symptoms of conceptual disorganization, hallucinations, delusions and disorientation. (For details of rapid tranquilization methods, see Chapter III). Some refractory patients respond dramatically when a tricyclic antidepressant is added. The addition of an antiparkinson drug may negate the therapeutic efficacy of the antipsychotic and result in an apparent treatment-resistant patient. Discontinuation of the antiparkinson drug may produce a higher plasma level of the antipsychotic and patient improvement. Occasionally, a trial on a small dose may result in a therapeutic response for the patient who has been resistant for a long period on a substantial dosage.

Ayd (1974a), after a review of the literature and calling upon his extensive research and clinical experience, has formulated a set of guidelines for rational psychopharmacotherapy with antipsychotics. It is his belief that, if followed, these rules would radically change the way the majority of chronic schizophrenics are treated today and would offer many of them the hope that because of adequate antipsychotic therapy they no longer would be prisoners of their psychosis. The guidelines are:

(1) A neuroleptic should not be prescribed until as accurate a psychiatric diagnosis as possible has been made and the patient has symptoms known to be relieved by such medication.

(2) When possible, the choice of a neuroleptic should be determined by the patient's family history. If a blood relative has responded optimally to a particular neuroleptic, the patient should first be treated with this drug. If blood relatives did not respond to a particular neuroleptic the patient should not be treated with that neuroleptic but with another neuroleptic.

(3) A patient should be treated with a single neuroleptic, the dosage of which should be increased steadily over a 3-month period until therapeutic benefit occurs or undesirable side effects intervene.

(4) If a patient does not react to maximally tolerated doses with substantial improvement within 3 months, he should be categorized as refractory to the compound and treated with another neuroleptic.

(5) A patient refractory to a piperidine or aliphatic phenothiazine should be treated with either a piperazine phenothiazine, haloperidol, thiothixene, or molindone but not with chlorprothixene.

(6) A patient refractory to a piperazine phenothiazine should be treated with either haloperidol, thiothixene, or a molindone but not with a piperidine or aliphatic phenothiazine or with chlorprothixene.

(7) A patient refractory to haloperidol should be treated with either a piperazine phenothiazine, thiothixene, or molindone but not with a piperidine or aliphatic phenothiazine or with chlorprothixene.

(8) A patient refractory to chlorprothixene should be treated with either a piperazine phenothiazine, haloperidol, thiothixene, or molindone but not with a piperidine or aliphatic phenothiazine.

(9) A patient refractory to thiothixene should be treated with either

a piperazine phenothiazine, haloperidol, or thiothixene but not with chlorprothixene or with a piperidine or aliphatic phenothiazine.

(10) Before a patient who seems to be refractory to a neuroleptic is switched to another drug, he should be evaluated clinically to determine if he is truly a candidate for neuroleptic therapy or if his lack of response is due to failure to ingest or absorb the medication. The latter may be checked either by a Forrest Urine Test or, better still if feasible, by a short course of parenteral administration of the neuroleptic.

During the early days of antipsychotic drug therapy in the 1950s, small doses of chlorpromazine were added to large doses of reserpine, especially in patients who were resistant to reserpine alone. A major concern about reserpine was its role in causing serious depression and numerous cholinergic side effects. Newer phenothiazines were introduced which were reported to be more rapid and more effective as antipsychotics. Thus, the use of reserpine in psychiatry diminished after 1960.

Recently reserpine, 0.75-6 mg./day, was added to various antipsychotic medication of 27 refractory patients (Bacher and Lewis, 1978). Reserpine was started at a low dose which was increased but discontinued or reduced at the first appearance of unusual discomfort or side effects. There was slight to marked improvement in mood, affect and social interaction and a decrease in somatic concern, hallucinations and withdrawal in 12 patients. Reality orientation and ability to cope with life situations improved. After 8 months, there was no evidence of increased depression in this group of patients. Refractory patients to the therapy, who were receiving relatively small doses of reserpine, rejected the combination after a few days to two weeks because of tiredness, sluggishness, depression and other uncomfortable somatic feelings. These patients tended to be younger, less compliant and more aggressive about discontinuing the medication. It is cautioned that objective, controlled, long-range studies are necessary before this combination is utilized to any extent.

20. PSYCHOTROPIC DRUG SUMMARY

The use of a psychotropic drug summary form is vital for the treatment of the mental patient.

A psychotropic drug summary form is a necessary tool for the appropriate administration of antipsychotic agents. Such a form has been devised to obtain essential data during the course of a research study into the use of the antipsychotic drugs. In chronological sequence, this form lists the name of the drug, the daily dose schedule, the total daily dosage and the number

TABLE 9

Psychotropic Drug Summary

Name: John Doe   Date of birth: 4-21-49   Diagnosis: Schizophrenic Reaction, Chr. Paranoid Type.   Admission Date: 7-20-73

DRUG*	DAILY DOSE SCHEDULE	TOTAL DAILY DOSE	DATES FROM	DATES TO	TOTAL NO. DAYS	PROGRESS NOTES (Include target symptoms, response to therapy, reason for drug changes: describe side effects, their treatment and response.)
Thorazine	100 mg. t.i.d.	300 mg.	1/10/74	1/16/74	6	1-10-74—Patient is still hostile, suspicious, incooperative and delusional; states God is controlling his mind.
Thorazine	100 mg. a.m. 200 mg. noon & h.s.	500 mg.	1/17/74	2/6/74	20	
Thorazine	200 mg. a.m. 400 mg. h.s.	600 mg.	2/7/74	2/21/74	14	2/15/74—More cooperative to ward routine but still suspicious and delusional.
Haldol	5 mg. h.s.	5 mg.	2/22/74	3/1/74	7	2/21/74—Condition unchanged; will try Haldol.
Thorazine	200 mg. b.i.d.	400 mg.	2/22/74	3/1/74	7	
Haldol	5 mg. t.i.d.	15 mg.	3/2/74	3/8/74	6	3/5/74—Patient is cooperative, no longer hostile and suspicious, still delusional.
Haldol	5 mg. a.m., 10 mg. noon & r.s.	25 mg.	3/9/74	3/15/74	6	3/10/74—Patient drooling and restless. Artane 3 mg. t.i.d. prescribed.
Haldol	10 mg. a.m., 10 mg. noon, 20 mg. h.s.	40 mg.	3/31/74	4/20/74	14	3/30/74—Still can elicit delusions but there is lessened affect. Participates fully in activity program.
Haldol	10 mg. 4:00 P.M. 20 mg. h.s.	30 mg.	4/21/74	5/6/74	21	4/20/74—Denies delusions; in good remission; medication will be tapered down to a maintenance dose. Extrapyramidal symptoms controlled by Artane.
Haldol	10 mg. 4:00 P.M. 20 mg. h.s.	30 mg.	4/21/74	5/6/74	14	

*Trade name used—a customary practice by physicians.

of days the patient has been on a particular drug schedule (Mason, 1975).

An attempt was made to cull from the clinical record, target symptoms, response to medication, side effects and their treatment and any other pertinent data usually included in progress notes. Many hours were spent poring over hospital charts attempting to decipher illegibly written orders, trying to figure out the responses to various psychotropic medication schedules or the reasons for the numerous changes in dosage or drugs. It soon became apparent that a psychotropic drug summary would enable the physician to quickly review the patient's drug history and would disclose which drugs or combination of drugs had been tried, at what dosage, for what length of time and whether there was any resultant improvement. A brief sample of a psychotropic drug summary is reproduced in Table 9.

Drug summaries reveal the occasions where the psychotropic drugs are overused, underused or used incorrectly. They show where the prescribing practices of various staff physicians have failed to incorporate the latest scientific findings and the drugs were not used in the most effective and economical manner. For example, one summary revealed a situation where a specific combination of two antipsychotic drugs was prescribed on 3 different occasions in the same dosage at intervals of several days by three different physicians, even though the progress notes culled from the clinical record showed that this particular drug combination always had been ineffective in ameliorating the patient's symptoms.

Copies of the summary should follow the patient as his status changes (i.e., from inpatient to outpatient). This practice should eliminate the many instances where readmitted patient is placed on a new drug even though perusal of the clinical records would reveal that there had been an excellent response to a different drug during the patient's previous hospitalization.

The psychotropic drug summary or a similar form (Levenson and Dunbar, 1977) can be used as a teaching tool since it highlights the manner whereby the antipsychotic drugs are used inappropriately. An educational campaign can then be instituted to teach physicians the basic principles in the use of the antipsychotic agents and thus help develop their professional skill and expertise in this important aspect of psychiatric treatment (Mason, 1973). Inquiry can be made why a particular therapeutic regimen was prescribed and what the clinician's reasons were for the frequent and often multiple changes that take place in the course of a patient's management. The form forces the clinician to identify the target symptoms, to indicate the efficacy of drug(s) prescribed, to indicate the reason for drug changes, and to note any side effects.

It is not feasible to develop drug summaries for the many long-term patients in mental hospitals or outpatient clinics who have been receiving psychotropic drugs for years—even decades. However, it is recommended that a drug summary be started for each new and currently for each old patient in psychiatric clinics, services or hospitals. With minimal assistance or training by the physician, it can be easily maintained by a clerk with the help of a psychiatric nurse or some other mental health professional. The problem-oriented record will not supplant this type of summary. In addition to improving the quality of care by making data easily retrievable, the form is suitable for various medical audit functions, for large-scale studies of therapeutic efficacy, and for the surveillance of adverse effects.

It is generally acknowledged that the antipsychotic agents are the most powerful treatment available for the psychoses. Thus, an up-to-date psychotropic drug summary could well be one of the most essential and valuable documents in the medical records of the mental patients.

21. DRUG REGIMEN REVIEW

The past and present drug regimen of each psychotic patient should be critically reviewed once a year at a minimum.

A high proportion of hospitalized schizophrenic patients have been maintained uninterruptedly on antipsychotics for many years—even more than a decade—without change in the dosage or specific drug. Many of these patients have never been given the opportunity to show further clinical improvement with a different dosage or the newer drugs. They may have stabilized at a new level of functioning that does not require as much medication. A periodic review will enable the physician to discover these cases and enable him to make appropriate changes in the drug regimen.

Also, review of patients' medical records frequently shows that the mental status of many chronic patients is unchanged even after years on antipsychotic therapy. The patients' target symptoms are still present and it would appear that the antipsychotic drug may be safely discontinued.

In most mental hospitals, the physician must reevaluate the drug regimen and rewrite the drug orders every month. Since the workload is heavy, orders are routinely continued month after month unless the patient is causing a "problem" and the nurse suggests that a change in medication may be indicated. Commonly, the drug regimen is not reviewed in the light of the objectives of the patients' treatment plan since the physician is not present during the reevaluation of the treatment plan conducted by the other members of the treatment team who have different professional orientations. Thus a semi-annual or at least an annual formal review of each patient's drug treatment by the physician is essential in maintaining quality patient care.

The physician must find (or take) the time to review the patients' charts.

In the psychiatric facilities of some states such a review of each inpatient's and outpatient's drug treatment plan is mandatory. The results of these reviews and new treatment recommendations should be recorded in the patient's clinical record. At some centers, a specific form is devised which must be completed after the review. This type of review gives the physician an opportunity to evaluate his prescribing habits, especially from the standpoint of the accepted basic principles in the use of antipsychotic agents (Mason, 1973). An up-to-date drug summary can expedite these reviews and eliminate the alternative of thumbing through a clinical folder several inches thick. If available, the clinical pharmacist should be involved in the therapy review. At the time of the drug review, the neurological status should be reevaluated, especially if the patient is on long-term drug therapy.

During the review, the clinician should seek objective evidence that the drug is needed and is producing real benefits. Especially with outpatients, the physician must be keenly aware of developing medical symptoms, since many chronic mentally ill patients do not receive ongoing medical care. A workable dosage evaluation program could result in less risk of toxicity for the patient and reduced medication costs for the hospital.

III

Rapid Tranquilization Methods

1. AN OVERVIEW

"Rapid neuroleptization," "crash" tranquilization, rapid "digitalization," "rapid titration," "crisis psychopharmacologic techniques," or "rapid psychotolysis" are terms used for rapid tranquilization methods with antipsychotic agents. During the past decade, there have been comparatively few reports on this subject but its use is becoming increasingly important in the treatment of psychotic patients, especially those in states of excitement or manifesting agitation, assaultiveness, hyperactivity or other acutely psychotic symptoms.

In the days before the advent of antipsychotic agents, extremely excited and disruptive patients could exhaust themselves and die. If this were prevented with cold packs, seclusion, or warm baths, the patient could remain severely psychotic for a long time. The violent, delusional patient often directed his aggression against persons and property and was a possible source of serious injury or death to other patients and personnel.

The care and treatment of combative, hyperactive, destructive and hostile

109

patients is still one of the difficult problems in hospital psychiatry. Such traditional methods and devices as restraints, seclusion, maximum security rooms and wards, courses of electroconvulsive therapy and heavy sedation may be used but have limitations and may actually do more harm than good by inflicting physical injury and interfering with continuity of therapy. Use of large numbers of aides is feasible for brief periods but not practical for longer courses of therapy. These problems are compounded in open wards and general hospital situations by lack of such control as is afforded by the locked ward. Even on a locked ward, these patients are not always amenable to verbal communication from the staff, nor are they able to control their own actions. They are frightening to the staff and to themselves. Therefore, since their violent behavior is disruptive to ward procedures and often dangerous to themselves and others, control of such behavior in these patients is the first order of treatment. This should be done as quickly, safely and humanely as possible (Fann and Linton, 1972).

Since the advent of psychotropic drugs, state mental hospitals have dramatically reduced their population and much of the psychiatric care has been shifted to satellite mental health centers. However, most of these centers are understaffed and ill-equipped to handle extreme psychiatric emergencies such as agitated, assaultive, acutely psychotic patients who are a danger to themselves and others. These patients are often taken to the state mental hospital where generally they are secluded for several hours to several days or more, and usually administered inadequate doses of IM or oral antipsychotic drugs every 4 hours. Under these conditions, many are not adequately controlled and remain agitated, assaultive, hostile and manic to the point of exhaustion, or they are managed by sedative control. Incomplete and/or sedative control requires 2 to 3 days or more of treatment with constant medical monitoring and nursing care, which results in overburdening all available facilities. The failure of this traditional method may be related to non-innovative investigation concerning the best method to control a highly disturbed patient. The fear of adverse reactions expressed by some physicians generally results in inadequate dosage and drawn-out intervals of titrating antipsychotic medication to effective levels.

Prolonged exposure to severe psychotic symptoms may decrease the patient's chance for an early and relatively complete recovery. He may experience accumulating, irreparable ego damage and an almost irreparable "social damage" to his relations with members of the treatment team. Often it may be impossible to give such patients oral medication. Consequently, it is important that the disturbed behavior of the severely ill psychotic patient be controlled as soon as possible—preferably within 24 hours of his being admitted to the hospital. Rapid tranquilization may offer an effective tool in the management of these patients.

The physician can acquire a fundamental knowledge of the methods of rapid tranquilization through an overview from the chronological standpoint. This type of review reflects the increasing experience of clinicians and investigators with the antipsychotic drugs and their side effects, especially as the newer high potency drugs with parenteral forms become available and widely used. Furthermore, it is hoped that the overview of detailed reports by many of the leading clinical psychiatrists will reassure the physician who is hesitant to use parenteral medication or exceed the suggested maximal dosage (mentioned in the manufacturer's insert) for short periods and will encourage him to incorporate this treatment procedure in his therapeutic armamentarium. A word of caution—in some of the comparison studies on rapid tranquilization, equivalent doses of the antipsychotics were not used and it is suggested that Table 3 be consulted before accepting the validity of comparative efficacy and side effects. Some of the early methods of rapid tranquilization are no longer used, nor are they recommended. They are included to furnish a fuller historical background to this procedure.

Kinross-Wright (1955) reported on intensive chlorpromazine (Thorazine) treatment of schizophrenia. The patient received 200 mg. on the first day. On the second day he was given 400 mg. Thereafter the dose was increased by 400 mg. daily until the therapeutic level was reached. For the first few days, half the total daily dose was given intramuscularly. In very disturbed patients, the whole amount was given by injection until tablets were accepted. Medication was usually given in 4 divided doses throughout the day. The therapeutic level was reached when the patient began to communicate, to become socially responsive, and to show an improved quality of affect. This level varied from 800 to 3600 mg. per day, with a mean of 2400 mg. Improvement was usually rapid at this dosage, which was maintained for 1 to 2 weeks. Chlorpromazine was then decreased by 400 mg. daily until a maintenance level of 200-400 mg. was reached. At this point the patient was discharged to the outpatient clinic, while dosage was "tapered off" over a period of weeks or months.

The plan of treatment was tailored to meet individual needs. The period of intensive treatment occupied about 3 or 4 weeks, and the length of hospital stay in Kinross-Wright's series of 108 schizophrenics averaged slightly less than 1 month. The treatment was easily administered and was not reported to be unpleasant. Complications were rarely severe.

This report illustrates the "loading doses" of phenothiazines often used during the first decade of antipsychotic drug therapy. It was exemplified by Mountain (1963), who reported on his principles and method of "crash tranquilization" as follows: "(1) Give the largest dose of chlorpromazine that can be tolerated rather than the smallest dose possible to make the symptoms barely tolerable. (2) Give the medication in full dose as soon as it can be estimated. This can only be done by trial." As soon as the patient was admitted, he was given chlorpromazine 50 mg. p.o. Serious idiosyncratic drug reactions (very rare) were looked for. Chlorpromazine, 50-100 mg., was then given each hour unless (a) the patient was asleep; (b) the symptoms were much diminished; (c) serious side effects occurred. Hypotension was not an indication to stop medication unless serious signs and symptoms developed. In Mountain's study, after 3 or 4 doses were given, the hourly dose could be doubled. After 4 or 5 more doses, it was possible to estimate the dosage indicated for the first day, so that medication could be given q.i.d. instead of q. 1 hour.

If oral medication was refused, intramuscular chlorpromazine, 50-100 mg., was given in its place. Usually, after a few injections, the oral route was elected by the patient. Gavage was used in exceptional cases. The dosage might be increased from 2400 mg. to 3500 mg. on the second day and within a week the daily dose could be 5000 mg. At this stage much sleepiness was seen and accepted. Although the patient was still expected to attend group activities, less involvement was demanded of him.

After the symptoms had been controlled for several days, medication was gradually withdrawn, but care was taken to prevent re-emergence of florid symptoms. After several weeks, the patient was completely off medication or on maintenance dosage. Chlorpromazine was the drug discussed in his report because Mountain had several years' experience with it and found it most effective and without an unacceptable level of side effects. However, he felt that the other antipsychotic drugs could be just as acceptable and much depended on the experience of the physician.

This concept, developed at the Fort Logan Mental Health Center in Denver, was further expanded there and in 1971 Polak and Laycob reported on 3 years' experience with a "rapid tranquilization" approach to the treatment of acute psychosis which was integrated with "intensive social-system intervention centered on the patient's real-life setting." With this method, they were able to effectively treat the majority of acutely psychotic patients in less than 7 days of hospitalization. Their revised technique was described as follows: "The patient is given a test dose of 25 to 50 mg. of chlorpromazine orally and is observed for 1 hour for side effects, especially hypotensive reactions. If no major side effects are observed, chlorpromazine is prescribed in amounts ranging from 50 mg. to 200 mg. orally every hour for 6 to 8 hours, depending on the patient's weight and the degree of psychotic disturbance." The elixir or IM administration (at one-third of the oral dose) was prescribed for patients who showed reluctance or refused to take the tablet form. Their objective was to reach "a stage of initial control of psychotic behavior within the first 6 hours of treatment." Thus dosage adjustments were made during this period on the patient's response. The initial daily dose was obtained "by extrapolating from the amount of medication required to reach the tranquilizing end points in the first 6 to 8 hours." For example, if the patient required 600 mg. of chlorpromazine during the first 6 hours, they started him on roughly two-thirds of his 24-hour rate of 2400 mg., specifically, 1600 mg. of chlorpromazine daily in divided doses. Also, there was always a p.r.n. order for 100 mg. of chlorpromazine every 2 hours to be given for agitation or the return of the target symptoms of the psychosis. Each morning, the previous day's supplemental medication was added to the daily dose and adjustments were made throughout the day if necessary.

In their experience, "most mistaken judgements about chlorpromazine are made because of a lack of understanding about the shift of side effects on the third day. In the first two days, adequately tranquilized patients may sleep a good deal in the daytime and they often sleep well at night for the first time in many weeks. However, on the third day a rapid decrease in drowsiness usually takes place without a decrease in medication level." Dryness of the mouth and symptoms of postural hypotension also tended to lessen after the third day. They believe it is a common error to reduce the dosage as a result of the patient's complaints about side effects on the very day the same side effects would attenuate or disappear.

As the patient improved, the daily dosage was reduced by one-third after the third day and a further reduction was made 2 days later. Typically, a patient may have been on a 2400 mg. dosage of chlorpromazine during the first or second day, would have this reduced to 1800 mg. on the fourth day, decreased again to 1200 mg. on the sixth day, discharged during the seventh day on a dosage of 800 mg. with a further reduction to 600 mg. one week after discharge.

They observed that this type of dosage regimen usually prevented the development of serious side effects. Blood pressure was taken before each dose and if the systolic blood pressure fell below the 80-90 range, medication was withheld. Severe hypotension resulting in termination of treatment was rare and parkinsonism did not make a frequent appearance. However, antiparkinson agents were routinely prescribed if the maintenance dosage was higher than 1000 mg. of chlorpromazine after 7 days or if an appreciable degree of parkinsonism occurred.

They further reported that when adequate medication had been given, the patient's psychotic behavior could be observed to be strikingly diminished or attenuated. The specific target symptoms to be controlled by rapid tranquilization were unique for each patient. Hallucinations, delusional behavior, states of extreme anxiety or panic, and other target symptomatology of the psychotic state sharply attenuated or disappeared. Although they used chlorpromazine in their report, they found the other "major tranquilizers" to be equally effective.

Brauzer and Goldstein (1968) compared the effects of intramuscular thiothixene (Navane) and trifluoperazine (Stelazine) in psychotic patients in a double-blind fashion. Each cc of medication contained 2 mg. of thiothixene or trifluoperazine. The maximum length of treatment for any one patient was 72 hours and no patient received more than 20 mg. of medication per day. The patient's blood pressure and pulse were determined prior to each injection and again at 30 to 60 minute intervals after the injection. The sites of injection were alternated and no more than 3 cc (6 mg.) of drug was given at any one site. The medication was administered in divided doses with a maximum of 5 cc at any one time.

The results indicated that thiothixene was as effective as trifluoperazine on a milligram-per-milligram basis in the treatment of recently admitted psychotic patients. Auditory hallucinations, agitation and ideas of persecution were the most favorably affected target symptoms. Side effects occurred in 10 of the 18 patients receiving thiothixene and 13 of the 18 patients receiving trifluoperazine. The most commonly occurring side effect was drowsiness, followed by extrapyramidal side effects. The latter were readily controlled with the use of benztropine mesylate (Cogentin) in doses of 1 to 4 mg. daily. The patients did not exhibit symptomatic hypotension or compensatory tachycardias.

Feldman and his associates (1969) reported on the use of parenteral haloperidol (Haldol) in controlling patient behavior during acute psychotic episodes. Their method consisted of injecting haloperidol intramuscularly, 5 mg. 3 times a day, generally for a maximum of 3 days. The patients were then treated with oral (tablet) haloperidol. Their choice of antipsychotic to be administered was based on the fact that the chlorpromazine parenterally may be painful at the site of injection; the possibility of resulting systemic complications such as severe hypotension and oversedation was also considered.

They found that 3 days of parenteral administration of haloperidol resulted in significant improvement in all symptom areas such as affect, social behavior, motor behavior, perception and ideation. Side effects were mainly controlled extrapyramidal symptoms. Haloperidol appeared to produce a true reduction in symptom severity instead of masking symptomatology by sedation. The lack of orthostatic hypotension and torticollis was particularly gratifying to them.

In 1969 Nilson described his procedure to ensure that new admissions received prompt and intensive psychiatric treatment. Drug treatment began immediately with chlorprothixene (Taractan) administered intramuscularly in doses of 25 to 75 mg. four times a day or as needed for sleep. He found that the drug had a very useful sedative effect because it produced a sound sleep from which the patient could be readily awakened without feeling sluggish. The patient was kept asleep for 3 to 6 days and awakened for meals, baths and nursing procedures. The physician visited regularly while the patient was awake to let him know how his treatment was progressing and how his family was faring, and to give him other reality-oriented information.

For very psychotic and aggressive patients, sleep was often induced with chlorpromazine instead of chlorprothixene; it also produced sound sleep for several days, but left the patient still sedated while awake. Sometimes, to induce sleep in a very excited or frightened patient, the sedative effect of either drug was increased with rapid-acting barbiturates, such as 125 to 250 mg. of sodium amytal injected intramuscularly. After the patient was asleep, it was usually possible to discontinue using barbiturates, but if not, he received 100 to 200 mg. of phenobarbital every 8 hours.

In most cases, however, Nilson found that the initial treatment with chlorprothixene was effective. By the fourth day the patient usually developed a tolerance to the side effects and it lost most of its sedative effect. By that time he usually was past the state of acute distress and could be placed on oral medication. In another 24 hours, the patient was completely alert, bored with the clinical environment and ready to see his psychotherapist to begin working on his problems. The patient was then transferred to a readjustment area, which was intensively programmed to reinforce the expectation of the patient's being responsible, independent and self-motivated. He had regular interviews with his psychotherapist, who was the same physician who admitted him and conducted the intensive treatment phase. Patients treated with this method by staff psychiatrists usually were released in 3 weeks.

Klein and Davis (1969) found a regimen of 100 mg. chlorpromazine t.i.d. intramuscularly to be effective for the manic, excited or schizophrenic patient. Out of caution and concern for the rare massive orthostatic hypotensive response to intramuscular chlorpromazine, they advised that a test dose of 25 mg. I.M. be given initially. They further stated that the intramuscular medication should be injected deeply into the buttocks. "Intramuscular chlorpromazine is an irritant and will produce a fairly marked inflammation upon repeated use. However, most patients can withstand 5 or 7 days of intramuscular medication, and the value of quick control of a psychosis far exceeds the drawback of a tender buttocks. Actual abscess formation was never observed. To mitigate the distress of intramuscularly injections, the chlorpromazine may be diluted with saline, as recommended by the manufacturer. However, 100 mg. are 4 cc and diluted with saline equally would result in an 8 cc injection" (Klein and Davis, 1969).

This regimen also consisted of starting liquid oral chlorpromazine medication concommitant with the intramuscular injections, building to a level of approximately 1500 to 2000 mg. daily. When the intramuscular medication was discontinued, the patient was receiving 1500 to 2000 mg. daily of chlorpromazine. In the period immediately after discontinuance of intramuscular medication, the patient was closely observed for exacerbation. This was an indication for either increasing the oral dose or reinstating intramuscular medication.

The effectiveness of parenteral administration of haloperidol as compared to that of perphenazine (Trilafon) in acutely psychotic patients was tested (Fitzgerald, 1969). Haloperidol and perphenazine were supplied in identically appearing 1 ml. capsules, each containing 5 mg. of drug. Intramuscular injections were administered every 8 hours as required for a period of 48 hours. The mean total of haloperidol administered was 25.7 mg.; the mean total dose of perphenazine was 27.6 mg.

Improvement occurred in 90% of the patients receiving perphenazine and in over 95% of those receiving haloperidol. On the basis of global improvement and reduction in target symptom severity, it appeared that haloperidol and perphenazine were equally effective. Psychomotor agitation, hostility and overactivity, which frequently cause problems in patient management, were reduced markedly. Blood pressure, pulse and respiratory rate, on the average, showed no clinically significant changes after injections in either drug group. No unexpected adverse experiences were observed.

The management of severely disturbed soldiers in Vietnam posed special problems. Continuous sleep induced with chlorpromazine for 24 to 48 hours proved particularly effective and efficient and represented another demonstration of the use of a rapid tranquilization techniqe (Bloch, 1970).

As other new antipsychotic drugs with a parenteral form became available, their efficacy continued to be compared to chlorpromazine in the rapid control of acute target symptoms of the psychotic patient. In a double-blind study to measure the differential response to parenteral chlorpromazine and mesoridazine (Serentil) in psychotic patients, male and female patients were randomly assigned to 1 of 2 therapies and treated in a double-blind fashion for 3 days (Brauzer and Goldstein, 1970). Drugs were supplied in 1 cc ampules, each cc containing either 25 mg. chlorpromazine or mesoridazine. The maximum duration of treatment for any patient was 3 days and no patient received more than 225 mg. (9 cc) per day. Medication was given in divided doses, the injection sites were alternated, and no more than 3 cc (75 mg.) was administered to any one site at any one time. Blood pressure and pulse were determined in a standing position prior to and 30 minutes after each injection. The most frequently occurring side effects were drowsiness, soreness at injection site and hypotension. These occurred in both treatment groups with relatively similar frequency and intensity.

The results of the overall global evaluations indicated that, in the treatment of newly admitted psychotic patients, mesoridazine was at least as effective as chlorpromazine on a milligram-per-milligram basis when administered by the parenteral route. However, mesoridazine was significantly more effective in controlling the target symptoms of indifference to environment and conceptual disorganization.

In 1971, Oldham and Bott of London described their three years of experience (1964-1967) in the management of excitement in a general hospital psychiatric ward. They utilized haloperidol since it appeared to have advantages over other major tranquilizers and hypnotics in its relative safety and effectiveness in controlling excitement; its main disadvantage was the production of dystonia. Their regimen was as follows: Patient was kept in bed continuously or allowed to sit in a chair beside the bed. Every patient was examined daily by a doctor and the following routine observations were recorded: hours of sleep; blood pressure, morning and evening; fluid intake and output; daily ward urine analysis, temperature, pulse and respiration morning and evening; weekly blood examination for Hb % and WBC." An initial injection of 10 to 30 mg. haloperidol was given with dosage dependent upon the weight, age and sex. Patients also received a daily I.M. dose of 10 mg. procyclidine (Kemadrin).*

Later doses of halperidol were equal to the initial level or increased until "tranquility" developed. the majority of patients received a daily dosage range of 20-39 mg. haloperidol daily. The time needed to control excitement varied from 3 to never more than 17 days. A therapeutic objective was attainment of 8 hours sleep nightly and, if necessary, nitrazepam (megadon—a hypnotic not available in the U.S.) was used.

Routinely, antiparkinson drugs were prescribed for all patients. Dystonic side effects occurred infrequently and were usually mild. Treatment was discontinued in one patient who developed dystonia associated with hypotension. A drop in the systolic blood pressure of over 20 mm. Hg. or to below 100 mm. Hg. was considered significant and this factor occassionally determined the discontinuation of treatment.

When excitement was controlled after 3 or more days, the "high dosage regime" was discontinued and haloperidol and orphenadrine hydrochloride (Disipal) were prescribed orally in diminishing doses. During this period, the patient was permitted to gradually become fully ambulant and the maintenance regimen was continued after discharge. This report covered 124 patients and, in no case, was any patient transferred from the general hospital psychiatric ward to a mental hospital because of excitement or hyperactivity.

Oldham and Bott reported that overall control was attained in 73% of patients, partial control in 22% and no control in 5%. Their patients covered a wide diagnostic spectrum and even those with "organic confusional states

---

*The parenteral form of procyclidine hydrochloride is not available in the U.S.

and dementia" responded well and did not develop severe hypotension. It is of interest that control was achieved in patients with personality disorders and aggressive symptoms and this greatly reduced ward management problems for the nursing staff. Most patients showed no soporific effects and, though confined to bed, were able to cooperate with nursing and medical procedures and to eat, drink and converse.

Oldham and Bott believed that the routine use of intramuscular injections during the initial period ensured that the patient's response could be accurately monitored without any of the doubts that might have attended the use of an oral preparation. In their experience, "an initial intramuscular injection of 20-30 mg. of haloperidol in all but the frailest of patients established control quickly and the wide safety margin of this drug enabled dosages to be given and, if necessary, to be increased without fear of adverse effect."

In 1971, Slotnick reported on the comparative symptom effectiveness profile of haloperidol and chlorpromazine in the management of the acutely agitated psychiatric patient with parenteral antipsychotics. His report combined the results of 3 controlled double-blind investigations to evaluate haloperidol. The subjects were either acute psychotic patients or chronic psychotic patients undergoing an acute exacerbation, with the majority diagnosed as paranoid schizophrenics. They were extremely agitated and most were hostile and uncooperative.

Patients received 5 mg. of haloperidol or 50 mg. of chlorpromazine. Following the first injection, drug was administered only every 6 to 8 hours as required but no more than 6 injections (30 mg. of haloperidol, 300 mg. of chlorpromazine) could be given during the 48-hour drug administration period. Blood pressure (in 3 positions), pulse and respiratory rate were determined for each patient immediately prior to, as well as 30 to 60 minutes following each injection.

Extrapyramidal symptoms constituted the majority of side effects among the haloperidol patients, about one-half occurring within 24 hours of the initiation of drug therapy. These were readily reversed with the use of antiparkinson drugs. The most significant side effects of the chlorpromazine patients were postural hypotension and excessive sedation.

About one-half the patients in each drug group had marked or moderate improvement after 48 hours of treatment with respect to the global or overall results. However, it was concluded that haloperidol appeared to be much more rapid than chlorpromazine in controlling several of the more disruptive symptoms, such as hostility, agitation, uncooperativeness and unusual thought content. Also, haloperidol would seem indicated in those patients whose cardiovascular systems are compromised. In 1 of the 3 studies it was found that parenteral haloperidol induced significantly greater improvement in patients 40 years old or older than did parenteral chlorpromazine. It was believed that this was largely because results with chlorpromazine were poorer in older patients than in younger ones.

Fann and Linton (1972) emphasized a technique for managing the severely disturbed patient without using mechanical or isolation procedures. In their concept of "chemical restraint," the patient was given a large dose of perphenazine (Trilafon) on admission to a ward or in the emergency room prior to admission if the patient's behavior warranted it. The initial dose generally was given orally in the concentrate form but the parenteral route was used when necessary. The effective oral dose range was 16 to 32 mg. initially, with 24 mg. being optimal in most cases. This was followed by a q.i.d. dosage schedule, but after 2 to 3 weeks the daily dose was given on a b.i.d. schedule. When oral medication was refused, 10 to 15 mg. was given intramuscularly. As the patient improved, the large dose of perphenazine concentrate prescribed initially (in the 2 cases cited as illustrative, one patient received 24 mg. q.i.d. and the other 32 mg. q.i.d. which was increased to 72 mg. q.i.d.) was gradually and considerably reduced to a low maintenance dosage over a period of weeks. It was reported that perphenazine, used in adequate doses, allowed control of hyperactivity without, in most cases, reducing mental clarity to the point where the patient could not respond to other therapeutic modalities. Where agitation was severe, fully adequate control was not obtained until a "parkinson-like" slowing and rigidity began, but in nearly all cases, definite inhibition of the psychomotor excitement was noted within 2 to 4 hours. Fann and Linton believed that this parkinson state, usually an undesirable side effect, actually allowed control of the more severely disturbed patients who would otherwise have required mechanical restraint or seclusion. There were a few cases where severe dystonic reactions (e.g., torticollis, truncal torsion, oculogyric crisis or pronounced "parkinson-like" states) required reducing the dose or discontinuing the medication. All cases of severe dystonic reactions responded completely to intravenous methylphenidate (Ritalin). The parkinson-like state, when too pronounced, was relieved by antiparkinson medication.

The depot-type fluphenazine preparations have been increasingly used primarily in the treatment of ambulatory psychotics in the community and for treatment-resistant patients on chronic psychiatric services. In clinical practice, depot fluphenazine in acutely psychotic patients is usually administered in combination with other antipsychotic drugs. This may be based on 2 factors: The clinician may feel insecure in giving only 1 injection every 7 to 14 days during an acute psychotic episode, or he may believe that, pharmacologically, more antipsychotic effect is needed than can be provided by a long-acting injectable phenothiazine alone.

Preliminary, uncontrolled use of fluphenazine (Prolixin) enanthate by

Chien and Cole led them to suspect that a long-acting injectable drug, administered alone, was a satisfactory medication regimen for the management of acutely psychotic inpatients. In 1973 they reported on a study to test the relative efficacy of depot fluphenazine alone, chlorpromazine alone and a combination of the 2 treatments in newly admitted acutely psychotic patients who were judged to require antipsychotic medication by the clinical treatment staff. The patients manifested intense, socially disturbing psychopathology.

One group of 16 patients received fluphenazine enanthate as the only antipsychotic medication. It was injected intramuscularly at a dosage that ranged from 0.5 cc (12.5 mg.) to 3 cc (75 mg.) at clinically determined intervals. Trihexyphenidyl HCl (Artane), 5 mg. twice daily, was given for 5 days after each injection in the hope of averting drug-induced extrapyramidal manifestations. Seven and one-half gr. of sodium amytal injected intramuscularly was administered as needed in the first 48 hours since fluphenazine enanthate was reported to take 24 to 36 hours to reach an effective blood level. A second group of 15 patients received chlorpromazine at an individually determined level with both intramuscular and oral medication available to the treating physician. A third group of 15 patients was given a combination of fluphenazine enanthate by intramuscular injections of 0.5 cc to 3 cc at clinically determined intervals and chlorpromazine daily. The dosage of chlorpromazine and its manner of administration were at the discretion of the therapist. Trihexyphenidyl was given prophylactically in the same fashion as in the first group. The average dosage of medication of the three groups were as follows: fluphenazine alone, 28.5 mg. every 11.5 days; chlorpromazine alone, 388 mg. per day; combination therapy —chlorpromazine, 249.6 mg. per day and fluphenazine, 26 mg. every 11.2 days.

All patients had their dosage regulated by the usual clinical staff with the sole specification that fluphenazine enanthate dosage should not exceed 75 mg. in a single dose. The dosage actually used therefore reflected a "clinician's choice" regimen based on the individual clinical judgements of different psychiatrists and psychiatric residents.

The incidence of extrapyramidal side effects was the highest among the groups who received fluphenazine enanthate either alone or combined with chlorpromazine. These side effects occurred despite the use of antiparkinson agents, although they were adequately controlled with additional antiparkinson medication.

It was found that a moderate dose of fluphenazine enanthate at a moderate interval was an effective treatment for acutely psychotic patients and was superior to a moderate dose of chlorpromazine during the first few weeks of hospitalization. There was very little indication that the addition of chlorpromazine increased the therapeutic efficacy of the depot fluphenazine.

In 1973, Man and Chen compared the parenteral form of chlorpromazine with haloperidol, using doses at frequent intervals until the primary unmanageable symptoms of patients were relieved. A total of 30 patients was selected for this study and the major symptoms presented were severe agitation with marked psychomotor hyperactivity, assaultiveness, mania and hostility. These patients presented a danger to other patients, to themselves, and to hospital personnel. Twenty-seven (90%) had a record of previous admissions to a mental hospital. In general, they carried a diagnosis of acute schizophrenia of various types and manic-depressive psychosis, manic type.

Each patient, initially, received either 5 mg. haloperidol or 50 mg. chlorpromazine intramuscularly and then received subsequent injections at the same dosage at 30-minute intervals until symptoms were relieved or, if symptoms were uncontrolled, until a determination was made that further injections would be of no therapeutic benefit. Patients on haloperidol received 2 to 7 injections and those on chlorpromazine 1 to 6 injections. The results showed that both drugs were rapidly effective in substantially reducing the symptoms of severe agitation, assaultiveness, hostility and mania. A 3-day follow-up showed that all patients were manageable with subsequent oral medication and most continued to improve and were transferred to the day hospital or discharged as outpatients.

No extrapyramidal symptoms were observed in any of the patients receiving either drug. However, two chlorpromazine patients had sudden, near fatal hypotensive episodes. In both instances, the blood pressure fell to zero. Man and Chen noted that severe hypotensive crisis following the use of substantial doses of chlorpromazine is well-documented and this antipsychotic may be implicated in rare cases of sudden death (Rosati, 1964; Leestma and Koenig, 1968). However, in these 2 instances the hypotensive episodes followed relatively small doses of intramuscular chlorpromazine when compared with the amount generally administered in state mental hospitals. Both patients had received chlorpromazine during prior admissions for control of their psychoses. It was hypothesized that the two patients had been sensitized previously by chlorpromazine; hence, the subsequent administration of chlorpromazine was almost fatal, requiring intensive rescue treatment to save them. Had these patients not been treated under research conditions, blood pressure readings would not have been recorded so frequently (every 30 minutes) and they might have been in shock, lying on the floor, and interpreted as being under control. Although there was no significant difference between the rapidity and effectiveness of both drugs, haloperidol appeared to be a safer drug because of the lack of severe hypotensive reaction from hypersensitivity.

Sangiovanni and his associates (1973) described the use of larger doses of intramuscular haloperidol for rapid control of psychotic excitement states. Their study included 40 acutely excited patients whose aggressive, overactive, or assaultive behavior could not be controlled by persuasion, seclusion or parenteral sodium amobarbital (250-500 mg.) intramuscularly every four hours.

Initially, 10 to 30 mg. of haloperidol intramuscularly was given, with the dosage depending on the patient's age, weight, and severity of illness. Additional injections were administered 1 to 3 times daily with the dosage and frequency based on therapeutic response and the emergence of adverse side effects. The 24-hour dosage ranged from 10 to 60 mg. of haloperidol. Oral medication was substituted when adequate symptom control was attained.

Moderate to marked clinical improvement was achieved in 90% of the patients within 72 hours. Fourteen patients (35%) were controlled by parenteral haloperidol in doses of less than 30 mg.; 14 patients (35%) were controlled by 30-60 mg.; and eight patients (20%) required more than 60 mg. Four patients (10%) responded only minimally and required other treatment.

Fifty percent of the women responded favorably with a total dose of less than 30 mg. (for the first 72-hour period), as compared to only 17% of the men. During the first 24 hours, 73% of the women improved, as compared to 44% of the men. However, there was no difference between the sexes in the control of symptoms at the end of 72 hours.

Each patient was frequently evaluated throughout the day for clinical response and adverse side effects. Blood pressure readings were taken 30 and 60 minutes after the initial injection. A drop in systolic pressure of 20 mm. Hg or more below baseline or to a level below 100 mm. Hg was considered clinically significant. Antiparkinson agents were not used prophylactically but were prescribed when extrapyramidal symptoms appeared. They occurred mainly in patients receiving injections of haloperidol at a dosage range of less than 20 mg.

Mild to moderate lethargy was the most frequent side effect. It lasted for several hours after an injection, almost always during the first day, and occurred in 35% of the patients. There were no complaints of pain at the injection site even though 2-4 cc. of solution was given.

In 1973, Hamid and Wertz reported on the problem of emotionally disturbed patients admitted to a hospital emergency room who were frequently delusional, combative, assaultive, agitated, hostile, hallucinating, incoherent and generally uncontrollable. They felt it would be preferable to find an agent that could rapidly control psychotic manifestations yet render the patient receptive to early other therapy such as psychotherapy and supportive therapy. Their study compared two chemically different phenothiazine derivatives, mesoridazine (Serentil) and chlorpromazine to determine the efficacy and safety of the compounds in controlling psychotic symptoms during a 24-hour period. Emphasis was placed on discovering the type of symptoms that would respond and the degree of sedation that would occur with each treatment during the 24-hour period.

Patients were considered for inclusion in the study if they were schizophrenics and exhibited acute psychotic symptoms sufficiently severe to warrant the parenteral administration of an antipsychotic. Ninety-one patients participated using a randomized design that provided 2 treatment groups. Each patient received an initial injection of 1 cc (25 mg/cc) of either drug by deep intramuscular injection. The patients received an additional 1 cc of their assigned treatment drug 1 hour later. Following the administration of the second 1 cc of each drug, patients were evaluated for the degree of sedation, in order to assess the sedative effects of equal amounts of the 2 drugs. Thereafter, the physician could prescribe additional injections every 4 hours when necessary, up to a 24-hour maximum of 400 mg. of chlorpromazine or 200 mg. of mesoridazine. Antiparkinson drugs were not employed prophylactically. The mean 24-hour dose of mesoridazine was 148 mg. (range: 88-200 mg.) and that of chlorpromazine was 215 mg. (range 50-400 mg.). Numerous patients in each group received the maximum permissible dosage.

Patients treated with either drug experienced relief of certain symptoms when examined after 2 and after 24 hours. However, after 24 hours, difference between treatment groups significantly favored patients treated with mesoridazine for the composites indicative of disturbances of motor activity, attitude and behavior, emotional response, and ideation and thought processes. The therapeutic effects of mesoridazine were manifested with less sedation than occurred with chlorpromazine. As a result, patients who received mesoridazine were more accessible, alert and responsive to the therapeutic, diagnostic, and custodial procedures associated with their early treatment. Mesoridazine proved to be a valuable agent for rapid control of acute psychotic symptoms.

In the community care of acute psychosis, Amdur (1974) prefers fluphenazine decanoate. His initial dose is 0.25 to 1 ml (25 mg. per ml) and usually some fluphenazine or chlorpromazine is provided to be given orally at bedtime. He has personally administered over 500 injections of fluphenazine decanoate in emergency rooms, community clinics and on home visits. In the interest of dignity, he always gives deltoid injections. However, he has found that no amount of community care will avert hospitalization of a patient whose family has a fixed expectation regarding a need for inpatient care.

Anderson and Kuehnle (1974) consider acute-onset psychosis a medical emergency that requires vigorous and immediate treatment. Because of the greater tendency to produce sedative and hypotensive effects by high-dose antipsychotics, they generally prefer the low-dose, high-potency antipsychotics. Usually, the intramuscular route is used at the start. Thus, "an initial dose of haloperidol of either 5 or 10 mg. I.M. may be given, depending on age, weight and severity of illness. This dose may be repeated hourly until satisfactory improvement occurs, the patient sleeps, or a total maximum dose of 60 mg. has been reached. Generally, optimal improvement is expected at doses between 15 and 40 mg., although on occasion higher doses are necessary. During this period, the patient is recumbent in a quiet room and accompanied by a staff member."

When other antipsychotics are used, the dosages are ajusted according to their equivalency. In the case of fluphenazine, they believe that the hydrochloride should be used rather than the enanthate, which as a long-acting drug is more difficult to titrate.

Anderson and Kuehnle reported that, while considerable improvement usually occurs, it was unrealistic to expect that all psychotic indicators will disappear within 6 hours. If no improvement was seen, hospitalization was mandatory. The goal of initial treatment was to provide a basis on which the patient could recover sufficient control to continue treatment as an outpatient. The patients selected for inpatient treatment were those in whom delirium was a possibility, whose suicidal or homicidal risk was substantial, who had no viable family or social support or whose psychosis did not clear rapidly. It was stressed that careful follow-up is required to avoid the pitfalls of reactivating the psychosis and of medication excessive in dose or duration.

Donlon and Tupin (1974) have stated that conventional low dosage schedules cause many patients to remain hospitalized for excessive periods and prolong emotional turmoil; this, in turn, interferes with psychotherapeutic and rehabilitation programs. They likened their method of rapid dosage increase as somewhat similar to "digitalization." (They later recommended that their method be referred to as "rapid neuroleptization of decompensated schizophrenic patients with antipsychotic agents.")

Following admission, the patient was given a small oral test dose of one of the "more potent, less sedating" antipsychotic drugs such as trifluoperazine, fluphenazine, haloperidol or thiothixene to uncover any idiosyncratic reactions. The dosage was increased daily until substantial clinical improvement was attained, usually within one week. The "digitalizing" daily dosage ranged between 50-100 mg. of fluphenazine or its equivalent. Since the incidence of neurologic side effects was high, an antiparkinson agent was routinely prescribed prophylactically.

Using fluphenazine (hydrochloride) as a prototype, the patient is started on 10-20 mg. on the day of admission. Then the dosage is raised by 10-20 mg. increments once or twice daily. Patients remain on a high dosage for about 6 to 8 weeks. At this time, the patients no longer require or can tolerate the "digitalizing" dosage. The dosage is then gradually reduced to "a relatively sedation-free state," while still achieving clinical improvement. This maintenance dosage is usually one-half the daily "digitalization" dosage. Most patients on maintenance medication did not require an antiparkinson drug. Through this method, the majority of psychotic patients were hospitalized less than 8 days and most schizophrenic patients could be treated in an open ward setting which was part of a community mental health center.

In discussing their "crisis psychopharmacology techniques," Thornton and Thornton (1974) stated that in acute schizophrenic or manic situations the phenothiazines with the sedative properties (such as chlorpromazine and thioridazine) are their drugs of choice. Orthostatic hypotension is a primary dose-limiting factor and the chance of its occurrence may be reduced by the addition of a barbiturate in lieu of more phenothiazines. They often begin treatment with 200 mg. of chlorpromazine or thioridazine orally and 500 mg. of sodium amytal intramuscularly. Intramuscular chlorpromazine is avoided because of the increased hypotensive hazard. In the agitated, hostile patient with paranoid delusions, they found fluphenazine and other less sedative-producing major tranquilizers to be very useful in the "post" crisis regimen where sedation may be viewed as unwanted and disabling.

Later, as a result of the interest in the low-dose antipsychotics, Thornton (1975) reported on an assessment of their use in the treatment of acute psychosis in 32 individuals. Therapeutic goals included (1) return to the level of social and interpersonal functioning that existed prior to the acute episode; (2) combined objective and subjective reports of desirable emotional comfort from the patient, nurse, family and research team; (3) the avoidance of undesirable side effects. Patients received either 5 mg. of haloperidol intramuscularly every 4 hours or this dosage of haloperidol in combination with 250 mg. of sodium amytal intramuscularly every 8 hours.

Satisfactory results were obtained for both groups. However, the patient in the combination drug group attained therapeutic goals earlier and accordingly required less total haloperidol. The incidence of dystonic reactions in the combination drug group was 40% of that in the haloperidol alone group. Hypotension was not a problem in either group. Following the onset of treatment, the combination drug patients attained sleep 10-18 hours earlier. It was concluded that a hypnotic effect was associated with an earlier return to preexisting functioning and appears to have merit.

Corbett (1975) reported about a rapid tranquilization technique using fluphenazine decanoate as "the agent of first choice for acute schizophrenic illness." When the diagnosis was established (and this was usually within 48 hours after admission), an initial dose of 0.1 cc subcutaneously was given to test for an allergic reaction. Then the principle was followed of increasing the dosage rapidly and when clinical improvement appeared, decreasing the dosage with equal speed. As a rule, 25 mg. (1 cc) of fluphenazine decanoate was given intramuscularly (IM) 2 hours after the test dose. Depending upon the patient's response and severity of his symptoms, additional doses of 12.5-25 mg. were administered either daily or every second, third or fourth day. The dose was reduced to 25 mg. weekly or every two weeks when the rate of improvement leveled off. Discharged patients were followed in a "decanoate clinic" where the range of maintenance dosage varied between 25 mg. every 2 weeks to 12.5 mg. every 8 weeks.

Patients who were management problems received the additional parenteral medication needed to prevent harm to themselves or others. Usually, haloperidol 10-25 mg. IM, droperidol 10-15 mg. IM or thiothixene 10 mg. IM, repeated on a PRN basis at the discretion of the resident or chief nurse, was used. Haloperidol 10-20 mg. as a single oral dose at night was prescribed for the patients who did not need emergency parenteral injections but were "somewhat agitated." The supplemental antipsychotic medication was withdrawn when the disruptive symptoms were brought under control. Only fluphenazine decanoate was needed in 62% of the patients.

Acutely psychotic patients who were unwilling or unable to be hospitalized received 12.5 to 25 mg. (½-1 cc) IM of the depot drug. An antiparkinson agent was prescribed and instructions were given to both the patient and his family regarding its use if certain side effects developed. Also, the family and the patient were encouraged to maintain telephone contact with the treatment team. Clinic visits at a frequency of once or twice weekly for additional injections or evaluation were scheduled until the patient's illness began to remit. The extrapyramidal side effects of acute dystonic reactions, akathisia, parkinsonism with drooling of saliva were the "major unwanted effects." They occurred in some degree in all patients who received over 4 cc in 4 weeks. However, in most cases these side effects responded to "standard remedies." Although many patients were able to discontinue antiparkinson medication 3-4 months after discharge, some began to complain about these side effects for the first time after a similar period. It was considered most important that extrapyramidal side effects be controlled since it has been shown that akathisia or akinesia appear to be associated with drug reluctance or outright refusal.

In 1976, Anderson et al. described a study in which 24 patients with acute functional psychoses were treated with intramuscular haloperidol in a 3-hour period to determine whether reversal of specific psychotic symptoms such as thought disorder would occur in this short period. The patients were assigned randomly to 2 treatment groups and both groups initially were given 5 mg. of haloperidol. A high-dose group then was treated with 10 mg. of haloperidol every 30 minutes until satisfactory remission of symptoms occurred or a maximum of 55 mg. was given. A moderate-dose group was treated with a dosage schedule of 5 mg. of haloperidol hourly for up to 2 hours or until remission occurred.

After the initial 3-hour treatment period, patients were observed for 24 hours. Those judged to require further inpatient treatment were admitted to psychiatric facilities. Those whose clinical condition warranted outpatient treatment and who had adequate family and social support were followed in the outpatient service. Dosage and choice of medication were individually adjusted thereafter by clinicians assuming ongoing follow-up care.

There were no statistically significant differences in the scores on the Brief Psychiatric Rating Scale administered hourly between the high- and moderate-dose groups who received average total doses of 33 mg. and 13 mg., respectively, in the 3-hour period. The improvement consisted not only of the calming of anxiety or other nonspecific symptoms but also in the relief of "core" psychotic symptoms (hallucinations, unusual thought content, suspiciousness, elevated mood, conceptual disorganization and grandiosity).

There were no significant differences between the high and moderate dose group in incidence of side effects. Acute dystonia, easily reversed, was the only significant side effect. Anderson et al. concluded that the study demonstrates the feasibility of bringing about rapid remission of acute psychoses; about half of the cases were substantially relieved in a few hours. Also it suggests that outpatient management may be feasible and preferable in the treatment of some acute psychotic episodes.

Levenson and his associates (1976) found that the studies reported in the literature not only fail to deal with the continued use of intramuscular administration of antipsychotic drugs to produce remission in acutely schizophrenic patients but place little emphasis on rate or speed of remission. Therefore, they conducted a double-blind controlled study comparing equipotent parenteral dosage of fluphenazine HCl, thiothixene and haloperidol for 4 days or longer to a maximum of 21 days. All agents were found extremely efficacious with this clinical approach, producing a median time to remission of 9.0 days and an average remission rate of 83%. The lack of significant differences between the drugs suggests that the efficacy of these antipsychotics is more related to the route of administration than to the innate properties of the parenteral drug form.

Although conjoint use of an antianxiety and an antipsychotic agent is generally not recmmended, Shader and his associates (1977) found that chlordiazepoxide (Librium) in doses of 200 to 500 mg. (oral or intramuscular) used daily in conjunction with antipsychotic medication (usually chlorpromazine or haloperidol), can sometimes successfully control the agitation and assaultiveness of psychotic patients. When such a combination is used, the patient must be closely observed since the pharmacologic effects of each drug may be cumulative with the maximal effect felt over the first 24 to 48 hours. To the best of their knowledge, the efficacy and side effects of this therapeutic regimen have not been systematically investigated.

Parenteral thiothixene and haloperidol administered in hourly doses of

4 mg. or 8 mg. as needed over a 4-hour period were found to be equally effective when used for the emergency treatment of acutely excited and agitated patients treated in emergency rooms of general hospitals or in the private offices of psychiatrists on an outpatient basis (Stotsky, 1977). Acutely disturbed behavior responded to treatment, usually within 1 hour, even though the other evidence of psychosis, such as hallucinations or delusions, remained conspicuous and continued to be severe. It was believed that this point needs reiteration lest it be assumed that rapid tranquilization is a substitute for a more definitive course of treatment which may take several weeks.

An acute fulminating psychosis is a crisis situation which warrants decisive intervention. Yet, as in many medical situations, there are dissenting opinions regarding the prompt institution of a rapid tranquilization method. At one medical center, there is an established rule on the psychiatric service that patients are not to receive any medication for 1 week after admission unless there are clear emergency indications that must be documented in the medical records (Klein, 1975). Thus, the automatic and immediate administration of antipsychotic drugs to disturbed patients, which often precedes and precludes even a diagnostic evaluation, is prevented.

This viewpoint further holds that the vast majority of such patients can be maintained off medication if the staff is relatively secure in its ability to handle such persons and if both nurses and doctors recognize the crucial importance of diagnosis prior to administering medications; presumably, "given the will to do so, any reasonably well staffed, closed psychiatric ward can maintain a patient under observation for 48 hours regardless of how psychotic he is." This delay allows sufficient time to gather diagnostic material and to observe the waning of any toxic episodes or hysterical outbursts. Frequently, patients with these reactions are immediately started on medication with the diagnostic rationalization that they are acute schizophrenics, although the basis for such a diagnosis does not exist; this viewpoint holds that once a patient receives emergency psychotropic medication as an "acute schizophrenic," the diagnosis remains with him the rest of his life, usually to his detriment.

Amdur (1974), another proponent of this view, believes that doing nothing (waiting and observing) can be an immensely valuable and heroic diagnostic maneuver, particularly in cases of rapid onset (days to hours), first psychotic breaks in persons with good premorbid adjustment. Heavy sedation or tranquilization of such persons may obscure important neurological or historical findings. This maneuver is "heroic" since the managing physician will be under considerable pressure from families and nurses to "do something" when the most prudent course is to wait and gain some understanding of the natural causes of the episode. Also, there may be the belief that drug treatment is undesirable because it robs the patient of the psychotic experience; it is felt that the psychotic gains knowledge of himself and others as he reaches out from his autistic world via his acute illness. In addition, a short drug-free period, for 1 week if possible, allows a patient to be initially diagnosed with all his symptoms present.

In contrast to the recommendation of initial high doses, it has been suggested that a psychotic patient should be treated with haloperidol, up to 15 mg. (or equivalent), for at least 2 to 3 months before an increase in the daily dosage, to avoid the possibility of the development of tardive dyskinesia (Baldessarini et al., 1976). However, Anderson and Kuehnle (1976) have pointed out that a patient who did not respond to the above regimen would remain psychotic for several months and would have received 1350 mg. of haloperidol with no clear benefit. The strategy of rapid administration of medication allows rapid relief in addition to minimizing the dosage required to obtain a remission.

Proponents of rapid tranquilization emphasize that every physician must accept his responsibility to relieve physical distress as rapidly as possible, before irreversible damage occurs—the faster the symptoms are relieved, the less emotional trauma the patients will suffer and the less their accustomed social and personal relationships will be disturbed. The more severe a patient's symptoms are, the more vigorous should be the therapeutic intervention. The responsibility to relieve psychiatric symptoms is equally binding on physicians. Unfortunately, for various reasons, the rapidity of psychotic decompensation is not always matched by the vigor of the intervention. As a result of delays caused by traditional practices of courts and public hospitals (i.e., leisurely preliminary interviews and procedures), immediate treatment is rare, rather than routine (Nilson, 1969).

Acute psychotic decompensation must be considered similar to an acute surgical condition for which treatment must begin at once. The pathological process must be stopped by intensive emergency treatment which should take place in a setting that emulates the medical model of temporary but total care. Only by immediately alleviating acute symptoms can there be hope to effectively rehabilitate the patient. Furthermore, it has been stated that acute psychosis is a "medical" emergency because victims of such disorders are in constant danger of acting on distorted perception or delusional ideas, with the result that injury or death may inadvertently occur. In the past, this was managed by protective custodial care until the psychotic episode subsided. It is also a "medical" psychiatric emergency in the sense that somatic therapies can bring about a rapid remission. Just as an acute condition within the abdomen deserves decisive action, so "the sun should not set" on an acute psychotic episode (Anderson and Kuehnle, 1974).

During the first decade after the introduction of antipsychotics, when large loading doses were used, there was the accusation the psychiatrists were replacing a mechanical straitjacket for a chemical one, that patients were "snowed" (i.e., rendered powerless under control and often asleep through the action of an antipsychotic drug), and that "snowing" the patient was not a satisfactory improvement on locked wards, seclusion rooms or electroconvulsive therapy (Appleton, 1965). Presently it is generally recognized that rapid tranquilization is by no means a chemical straitjacket and large doses of the high-potency, less sedating antipsychotics are effective and well tolerated by patients and, within a few hours or days, most patients are amenable to the other psychotherapeutic modalities.

Polak and Laycob (1971) found that despite the high doses initially used in their rapid tranquilization method, on the third and fourth day they are able to institute the intensive psychotherapeutic efforts. Thus, the patient may accompany his physician on a 3-hour home visit to his nuclear and extended family on the third day. Their experience has been that, far from being suppressed and chemically restrained, the patient is usually more in touch with his inner feelings and better able to synthesize psychological insights effectively than he was in his pre-admission psychotic state.

It appears that the few advocates of delay in instituting rapid tranquilization are at medical centers where the staff of the psychiatric service is well-trained and always available and where the employee-patient ratio is high. It is questionable whether they would still retain their views if they had ever witnessed an assaultive patient inflict grave injury on another patient or staff member resulting in a permanent disability, as occasionally happens in an understaffed mental hospital ward. Also, these advocates may not be aware that there are times when only one female psychiatric aide may be on duty during the night shift on some wards. Not too long ago, a paper on the use of mechanical restraints was published in a psychiatric journal with a wide circulation (Bursten, 1975). In 1976 a mental hospital received a Gold Award from the American Psychiatric Association for a staff development program, a section of which dealt with using parts of the Korean style of karate in the physical management of the disturbed patient. With the availability of rapid, safe and effective tranquilization methods for the disturbed patient, these measures may be both incongruous and anachronistic.

Some physicians are fearful of utilizing a rapid tranquilization method because of the possibility of medico-legal complications. However, it may well be that failure to institute this type of procedure in the treatment of many patients for whom it is especially indicated may result in even greater susceptibility to medico-legal involvement.

Review of these rapid tranquilization studies makes it clear that the attending physician must monitor the acutely disturbed patient much as the anesthesiologist monitors his patients during surgery. By rapidly titrating in increments that do not sedate the patient to a somnolent state, the physician can observe the underlying psychopathology as it emerges, initiate immediate psychotherapeutic exchange and, more importantly, observe the reversal of abnormal thought content and mood disorder. During this period, the physician watches for changes in vital signs or evidence of sedation or extrapyramidal signs. If the patient is not oversedated, the procedure can be directed to an end point that affords some insight for the patient as well as relief from symptoms of psychosis. The physician must be present during the procedures not only to direct its administration but to evaluate its therapeutic effects and safety.

Anderson et al. (1976) have aptly stated, "rapid tranquilization is clearly no panacea and, in fact, requires careful attention of details of diagnosis and continuing care. It is a safe means of rapid control of psychotic symptoms which allows other therapeutic measures to be employed with maximum patient participation, economy and avoidance of discomfort. Since it is clear that chemotherapy is not merely sedative but specifically antipsychotic, the patient deserves a chance for the rapid remission these antipsychotic drugs can effect."

2. ESSENTIALS OF RAPID TRANQUILIZATION

Whenever possible, a rapid tranquilization method should be instituted only after a drug history has been obtained, physical and neurological examinations have been completed and an appropriate diagnosis has been made.

Although this guideline applies to the pre-treatment workup of any psychiatric patient, it is even more important when rapid tranquilization is contemplated.

A drug history may not be obtainable for the first admission patient but the medical records would be available for the readmissions who constitute the majority of the psychotic patients seen in the admitting office. Some acutely disturbed patients refuse to be examined and some feel so threatened by physical contact they must be managed without it. In those who can be examined physically, particular attention should be given to the possibility of head injuries, deliria, endocrine and nutritional disorders, epilepsy, diabetes, hepatic and renal disease, electrolytic imbalance and psychoses associated with alcohol and poisons. Abnormal reflexes such as the grasp reflex (grasping motion of the fingers or toes in response to stimulation), sucking reflex (sucking movements of the mouth elicited by the touching of an object to lips), and palmomental reflex (when the thenar eminence is rapidly and vigorously irritated with a needle, the muscles of the chin on the same side are drawn up) are all suggestive of a neurological problem of the cerebral cortex. Tremor and asterixis (intermittent lapse of an assumed posture) may be signs of metabolic encephalopathy or impending hepatic coma. Ophthalmoplegia, nystagmus and ataxia with tremors suggest Wernicke-Korsakoff syndrome which may start with a major confusional state before ocular palsy and ataxia appear (Kiev, 1977). If feasible, the complete physical and neurological examination including pelvic, automated clinical chemistries, CBC, urinalysis and routine chest x-ray should be done on the day of admission. This type of workup will uncover, in approximately 5% of all cases, medical disease as well as psychiatric illness (Carter, 1977). In a number of cases it is recognized that a definitive diagnosis is not possible following a single interview with a patient. The team approach, in which a variety of skilled mental health workers of various disciplines are able to observe the patient's behavior on a 24-hour basis, enables the physician to arrive at a more accurate diagnosis.

Acute phencyclidine (PCP) psychosis demonstrates the importance of a drug history and differential diagnosis. Some patients may have acute PCP psychosis even without measurable urine PCP. Differentiation from a schizophrenic psychosis is vital since the pharmacological treatment is entirely different. The phenothiazines used in the treatment of schizophrenia may precipitate fatal tachycardia and hypotension in patients with PCP psychosis. It has been suggested that these patients should be observed for a period and treated only with diazepam (in doses up to 60 mg. per day) before instituting phenothiazine treatment for a presumed schizophrenic psychosis (Yesavage and Freeman, 1978).

The antipsychotic drugs are symptom-specific and thus symptoms of a psychosis, whether it be schizophrenia, an organic type of psychotic symptoms due to lysergic acid diethylamide (LSD) or amphetamines, may respond to these drugs. The major exception is the atropine-like psychoses that may occur after taking an excess of scopolamine, antihistimines or tricyclic antidepressants. Phenothiazines, as well as most other antipsychotic drugs, because of their anticholinergic properties, may worsen this picture and should not be used.

In a large number of cases, the patient is to disturbed and uncooperative, shows such intense turmoil and hostility, that only a provisional diagnosis can be made before treatment. If the patient's agitation and disruptive behavior make it impossible to do at least a cursory physical and neurological examination and if "watchful waiting" is not feasible, a 5 mg. intramuscular dose of high-potency antipsychotic such as haloperidol may be used as a remedy for this type of situation. Such injection commonly results in adequate control within 30 to 60 minutes in about 50% of the patients so that they can be examined physically and a medical history obtained without affecting vital signs adversely (Gerstenzank and Krulisky, 1977).

In general, rapid tranquilization is indicated for the acutely psychotic patient for whom rapid symptom control is highly desirable. This would include patients with such symptoms as agitation, destructiveness, hostility, assaultive or suicidal behavior, pressure of speech, incoherency, delusions, hallucinations or potentially dangerous behavior. Rapid symptom control also has been advocated for the following: mute, withdrawn psychotics who are uncommunicative and negativistic; psychotics who refuse to take or are suspected of not taking oral medications; and psychotics who have not responded to adequate trials with a number of oral antipsychotics (Ayd, 1977a). In addition, the Overview section describes various types of patients for whom rapid tranquilization was found to be effective.

The high-potency antipsychotic agents are preferable for rapid tranquilization.

Although any antipsychotic with a parenteral form (IM) available may be used for rapid tranquilization, the preferable ones are haloperidol (Haldol), thiothixene (Navane) and the piperazine phenothiazines, particularly fluphenazine (Prolixin) and perphenazine (Trilafon). These are preferred because of their milligram potency and because they seldom cause pain or tissue damage at the injection site, marked sedation or hypotension or other cardiovascular reactions. There is also some evidence that haloperidol and perhaps other high-potency antipsychotics give lower incidence of other toxic effects, including hepatic, hemopoietic, cardiovascular, skin and eye changes than do the low-potency drugs (Gerle, 1964; Shader and DiMascio, 1970).

For those patients with an acute psychosis who have a repeated history of relapse and readmissions because of failure or refusal to take oral medications, fluphenazine hydrochloride (IICl) may be the drug of choice for IM tranquilization, since, after control of their acute symptoms, they can be placed on maintenance therapy with the long-acting fluphenazine enanthate or decanoate without having to be switched from a different antipsychotic to a depot phenothiazine to reduce the risks of additional relapses.

Abuzzahab (1976) cites these relevant considerations in selecting haloperidol rather than chlorpromazine in the treatment of a psychiatric emergency: (1) Intramuscular haloperidol is available in a higher concentration per ml than other antipsychotic drugs. (2) Haloperidol produces less distress to the patient at the intramuscular site; the phenothiazines produce some pain while haloperidol does not. (3) It usually does not produce any hypotension. (4) It usually has a more rapid onset of action than the phenothiazine. (5) A shift to the oral liquid form (an advantage since it is the only tasteless, colorless and odorless liquid antipsychotic available) can be made as soon as rapport with the patient has been established.

Heavy sedation should be avoided since it may obscure medical findings that would allow a quicker diagnosis. In the past, it was common to give an agitated patient intravenous barbiturates of the short-acting variety such as sodium amobarbital. Today parenteral administration of the antipsychotic drugs is considered safer and more appropriate. These medications do not produce a rapid fall in blood pressure as do the barbiturates. It is easier to keep the patient properly hydrated while the medication is being given. Also, they minimize the frightening sense of helplessness and loss of autonomy that heavy sedation may produce.

When rapid tranquilization is started with intramuscular administration of a high-potency antipsychotic agent, the addition of a low-potency drug such as chlorpromazine or thioridazine to the regimen as is often done creates a polypharmacy situation with all its disadvantages and exposure of the patient to unnecessary hazard. The less sedative (high-potency) antipsychotics produce adequate calming of psychotic agitation when administered intramuscularly. By continuing treatment with the oral form of the same antipsychotic agent, the problem of combining different medications is avoided. Should the need to isolate the source of a side effect arise, it is far easier if one drug has been used rather than two or more. The high-potency drugs cause more undesirable extrapyramidal side effects than the low-potency drugs do, but in some violent patients, drug-induced akinesia and rigidity may not be deleterious; they may add to therapeutic efficacy if properly monitored.

Generally, the parenteral antipsychotic is best for the initiation of therapy, especially in the hospitalized psychotic patient. Previously treatment was initiated with oral preparations because the intramuscular form of chlorpromazine is highly irritating. The high-potency antipsychotics offer an advantage in that they can be injected into large muscles without significant irritation. Although the gluteus maximus and the mid-lateral thigh have been common sites due to higher blood flow, the deltoid area is the preferred site if well developed. If desirable and feasible, an explanation may be given to the patient that he will receive an injection that will help him relax and reduce his fears.

Some clinicians are beginning to use the intravenous (IV) route but this is presently in the evaluation stage. With IV administration the agitated patient may not cooperate and be still and the result could be a missed vein with the production of a hematoma or a local tissue reaction.

Select 1 or 2 methods of rapid tranquilization and become proficient in their use.

A number of excellent methods of rapid drug control of psychoses have been described in the Overview section. The empirical methods evolved by the authors consist of the use of 3 high-potency antipsychotics, haloperidol or fluphenazine hydrochloride or thiothixene (Mason and Granacher, 1976).

These have been chosen because they are highly concentrated in the parenteral form and relatively large doses may be given by intramuscular (IM) route without significant muscle trauma and they cause little local irritation on injection. Haloperidol is our drug of choice for young patients with an initial agitated psychosis, patients with uncontrollable behavior secondary to mania, agitated elderly patients, patients with known cardiovascular disease, or agitated psychoses in general. On the other hand, many clinicians prefer thiothixene as a substitute for haloperidol. Fluphenazine hydrochloride is generally selected for these patients with an acute psychosis who have a repeated history of admissions and have demonstrated poor medication compliance.

Even with rapid tranquilization, there are some acutely psychotic patients who will not respond to 1 of the 3 above-mentioned antipsychotic agents. However, haloperidol, fluphenazine and thiothixene belong to different chemical classes. Therefore, in the refractory patient, a switch to 1 of the other 2 high-potency drugs may provide rapid symptom control.

Haloperidol 10 mg. (2 cc) intramuscularly is given every hour until agitation or aggression is diminished. Most patients require 20 to 60 mg. over a 2 to 6 hour period and an occasional patient may require up to 60 to 100 mg. in the first 6 to 10 hours. Since the best yardsticks for measuring the patient's need for continued hospitalization are (1) his sleep pattern, (2) the rate at which his illness progresses, and (3) the extent of demonstrable danger to self or others, the sleep pattern and duration of sleep are closely monitored during the first week of tranquilization (Detre and Jarecki, 1971). When the florid symptoms are attenuated or sleep ensues (usually within 24 hours), injections are discontinued and the patient is switched to the liquid form of haloperidol; however, IM dosage may continue longer than 24 hours if needed.

The oral dosage is calculated in the following manner: The total IM dosage for 24 hours is used as the baseline. One and one-half times the IM dosage is given in the oral form. If 30 mg. were given by injection the first 24 hours, 45 mg. of the concentrate would be administered the following day in 2 doses, with two-thirds of the total given at bedtime. In the above example, this would consist of haloperidol 15 mg. in a.m. and 30 mg. 1 hour before bedtime, depending on the physician's judgement about the current level of agitation and sleep disruption. The concentrate is continued in the above manner for 2 to 3 days or until nighttime sleep is sustained for at least 6-7 hours for 2 consecutive nights. Then the concentrate is discontinued and the medication regimen is changed to a single nighttime dose of haloperidol in tablet form, 45 mg. h.s. During the next 10-14 days the medication is gradually reduced to the lowest effective dose, still using sleep as a monitor of improvement. Erratic or diminished sleep indicates that the psychosis is still in an acute phase and that behavioral and pharmacologic stability has not yet been attained. This requires upward adjustment of the dosage until sleep stabilizes. It is our experience that the psychosis will not improve unless sleep disturbance is corrected.

When fluphenazine hydrochloride is used, 5 mg. (2 cc) is given hourly by intramuscular injection until the patient sleeps or his symptoms abate. Experience has shown that usually 20 to 60 mg. of fluphenazine will be needed during the first 24 hours. On the second day the patient is switched to the oral elixir form. However, if behavior is still unmanageable, intramuscular injections are continued beyond 24 hours. The same formula is used as for haloperidol, namely one and one-half times the total 24-hour parenteral dose to calculate the oral dosage. If 40 mg. of fluphenazine was given during the first 24 hours by injection, then the following day 60 mg. of fluphenazine elixir is prescribed in 2 doses, 20 mg. in the morning and 40 mg. h.s. Similarly, the patient should sleep 6-7 hours per night before switching to the tablet form and adjusting the dosage downward to the lowest effective nighttime dose.

The patient is switched to fluphenazine decanoate (long-acting depot form) prior to discharge by using the rough index of 25 mg. IM every 2 weeks for up to 15 mg. of oral fluphenazine needed per day. For each 5 mg. needed above 15 mg., ½ cc (12.5 mg.) of fluphenazine decanoate is added to the biweekly regimen. For instance, if a 25 mg. dose of oral fluphenazine was required nightly for restful sleep prior to discharge, the patient would leave the hospital with an order for 50 mg. (2 cc) of the fluphenazine decanoate every 2 weeks. If 35 mg. h.s. were needed, the patient would leave the hospital on a dosage of 75 mg. (3 cc) of fluphenazine decanoate. Such large doses are rarely needed and of course should be reduced to the lowest effective maintenance level during outpatient treatment; later, the time interval between injections may be lengthened. Usually it is unwise to do this before 2-3 months post-discharge.

If thiothixene is chosen, 3 cc (6 mg.) IM is given hourly until the patient quiets. Usually 30 to 60 mg. within 24 hours will be sufficient. As with haloperidol and fluphenazine, the patient is switched to thiothixene concentrate after 24 to 48 hours of parenteral treatment. Again, the concentrate is given at one and one-half times the 24-hour parenteral dose, with one-third in the a.m. and two-thirds at bedtime. For example, if 30 mg. had been needed IM, the patient would receive 15 mg. concentrate in the morning and 30 mg. at bedtime. After a pattern of 6-7 hours of restful sleep is established, the patient can be switched to a single capsule dosage at bedtime.

Although unusual, some patients will be refractory to fluphenazine or haloperidol or thiothixene and in these cases other antipsychotics such as mesoridazine, trifluoperazine or perphenazine are given a trial. On the other hand, a complete clearing of the psychosis within 24-48 hours by 1 of the above methods points to mania, amphetamine or other drug psychoses; appropriate further evaluation for diagnosis and treatment should be undertaken.

There are two other schools of thought regarding the size of the initial dosage; one favors low initial dosages (e.g., 2 mg. haloperidol intramuscularly at hourly intervals), even though this frequently means several additional injections may be required to achieve satisfactory symptom control, especially in severely agitated, excited patients; the other favors a high initial dosage (e.g., 30 mg. haloperidol), since this often suffices and obviates the need for several repeated injections. The incidence of side effects, particularly extrapyramidal reactions, is about the same with low and high initial dosages but with high initial dosages the speed of onset is more rapid and the severity of extrapyramidal reactions is more pronounced.

Depending on response, a decision to withhold IM medication and to switch to oral dosage or to give a second injection of the same or a different amount can be made. If there is no change, the second injected dose should be at least as large as the first. If the initial dose has been adequate, an injection more often than every hour is seldom necessary. Although injections every 30 minutes may be safe and even indicated in some severely assaultive psychotics, for most patients an injection at hourly intervals is effective. Hence, most clinicians usually give injections hourly up to 6 hours or until the patient is controlled and can be switched to oral medication. The great majority of patients will be either asleep or otherwise "adequately medicated" in less than 6 hours. "Adequately medicated" means reasonably cooperative. Delusions and hallucinations usually persist and may take days or weeks to subside, but the IM medication should control assaultiveness and extreme agitation within hours. In fact, when IM antipsychotic therapy is used (i.e., total IM dose in 3 hours), improvement may consist not only of calming of anxiety or other nonspecific symptoms but often of amelioration of "core" psychotic indicators (hallucinations, unusual thought content, suspiciousness, elation, conceptual disorganization and grandiosity). An occasional patient, however, may require IM injections hourly or less frequently beyond 6 to 12 hours and up to 24 to 48 hours before this optimal therapeutic response is attained. Such patients may need 60 to 100 mg. within 24 hours of an antipsychotic such as haloperidol. Generally, if there is little or no therapeutic response after 24 to 48 hours with careful monitoring and dosage regulation, it is recommended that the rapid tranquilization procedure with parenteral antipsychotics be discontinued.

When the acute psychotic symptoms such as assaultiveness, agitation and excitement are brought under control and the patient becomes co-

operative, intramuscular medication should be changed to the oral form.

There is some variation by clinicians as to how soon to switch to the oral dosage. Ayd (1977a) believes that the intensive use of IM antipsychotics produces positive results in three stages: (1) a calming effect, (2) a change in mood, and (3) a beginning remission of psychotic symptoms. As soon as such symptomatic effects have been attained by IM therapy, oral medication should be prescribed. The dose of oral medication likely to be required in the next 24 hours should be double the IM dose in the first 24 hours that was required to achieve symptomatic control. Although it is often said that IM medication may be 5 times more potent than oral when an intensive IM program is used, such high oral doses are not necessary. If the patient becomes agitated shortly after oral therapy is instituted and this is not a manifestation of akathisia, at least one additional parenteral dose should be administered.

Carter (1977) advocates that oral medication be prescribed within 4 to 6 hours of the last injection when haloperidol is used. The total daily dose of oral haloperidol usually will be about twice the total dose of intramuscular haloperidol administered. The ratio between the intramuscular and oral doses is reduced to 1:1 when the total intramuscular dose is above 40 mg. However, he cautions that the dosage must be individualized in all cases and observed that symptoms could be controlled with the entire daily dose given at bedtime.

Some clinicians believe that the switchover to the oral form should be made early enough (within 3 to 4 hours after the last intramuscular injection) to maintain improvement in thought and mood. The early initiation of oral dosage affords maintenance of higher blood levels, continues optimal control obtained in the injectable phase and may suppress the emergence of extrapyramidal side effects. After control is achieved, other physicians calculate the amount of oral medication required during the next 24 hours by multiplying by 2⅔ the total amount of intramuscular medication needed in the first 6 hours or less (Polak and Laycob, 1971; Ketai, 1975). The switchover technique used by the authors has been effective and has not caused any problems.

In arriving at the maintenance level there is a tremendous variation from patient to patient. Some may need only 10 mg. a day, others need 20 mg., while some patients require 80 to 100 mg. per day. **Individual dosage titration is the only way to determine the adequate maintenance dose.**

The prophylactic use of antiparkinson drugs is not recommended for inpatients treated by rapid tranquilization. However, the clinical staff must be prepared to recognize and treat extrapyramidal signs and symptoms promptly.

Although it is possible that the prophylactic administration may lessen the intensity of an extrapyramidal reaction caused by intramuscular antipsychotic agents, there is no clear evidence that an antiparkinson drug will prevent an extrapyramidal reaction of sufficient severity to warrant treatment. If an extrapyramidal reaction should occur in conjunction with an incomplete therapeutic response, an antiparkinson drug should be prescribed and IM therapy continued until rapid tranquilization is achieved.

In general, extrapyramidal symptoms are dose-related. Moderate doses of the antipsychotic are more likely to cause extrapyramidal side effects than very high or low dosages. Thus, haloperidol doses such as 100 mg. may not produce extrapyramidal effects. However, when the dosage is reduced gradually to the 10 mg. dosage level, extrapyramidal symptoms may appear.

An as needed (PRN) order should be written to permit nurses to administer an antiparkinson agent.

The entire treatment team must be educated and trained in the recognition and management of acute dystonic reactions. A PRN order for an antiparkinson agent such as benztropine mesylate (Cogentin) 2 mg. or diphenhydramine (Benadryl) 50 mg. intramuscularly or intravenously will enable the nurse to institute prompt treatment for the dystonic reaction until a physician arrives. This is comparable to the coronary care nurse treating cardiac arrhythmia from a standing PRN order.

Acute dystonic reactions usually occur suddenly within 24 to 48 hours from the start of rapid tranquilization. The dystonic reactions are rarely life threatening but can be very disquieting or frightening to the patient. They can arouse anxiety in the nurses and mental health technicians unless they are trained to recognize them as extrapyramidal symptoms and have seen them respond within a matter of minutes to IV or IM administration of an antiparkinson agent

The clinical team must monitor the blood pressure and be prepared to treat orthostatic hypotension.

Orthostatic hypotension is probably the most common cause of complaints of dizziness, palpitation, tachycardia and weakness. Blood pressure should be recorded not only during admission excitement but also later when the patient is calm. When possible, record the recumbent and standing blood pressures before starting medication. Normally, systolic blood pressure is higher on standing than lying down; in orthostatic hypotension the standing systolic is lower than the lying down systolic by 20 points or more. Blood pressures should be taken 1 hour after each parenteral dose and 3 hours after each oral dose during the period of rapid tranquilization. A blood pressure flow chart should be maintained and the nursing staff must acquire competence in the technique of accurate blood pressure determination.

When hypotension follows administration of chlorpromazine, the fall in pressure almost always occurs shortly after the first dose is given. Supine and standing blood pressure readings should be taken before the second and subsequent doses are administered. Usually the hypotension is mild and transient. However, occasionally a patient will develop a severe hypotension reaction early in the course of treatment with chlorpromazine. It has been suggested that this may be true especially of persons with an acquired hypersensitivity to the drug, although in fact most persons become tolerant to its hypotensive effect. If there is concern about possible hypotension, a 10 mg. test dose of haloperidol may be given and the patient observed for 1 hour.

In general, it may be wise to withhold or reduce the dosage when the systolic drops below 90 mm Hg. until the pressure returns to its former level. At times, patients requiring temporary high dosages must be kept in bed. Hypotensive episodes may be avoided to some extent by having the patient lie down for a half-hour or so after injections. (For full details of the treatment of hypotension, see Chapter V.)

Through rapid tranquilization many psychotic patients can be treated without recourse to hospitalization or hospital stay can be shortened. The goal of rapid tranquilization may be to allow many patients to recover sufficiently so that they can continue treatment as outpatients. Although considerable improvement usually occurs during initial treatment, it is unreasonable to expect all psychotic symptoms to disappear within 4 to 6 hours. If sufficient control to continue treatment as an outpatient is attained, the patient can be given oral medication and seen once or twice weekly in the clinic.

The patient or responsible family member should be advised of possible side effects and be given a prescription for either benztropine mesylate or trihexyphenidyl in the event of an acute dystonic reaction. Both should be encouraged to maintain telephone contact with the treatment team. Patients and their families usually prefer outpatient arrangements, but no amount of community care will avert hospitalization of a patient whose family has a fixed expectation of inpatient care.

If the outpatient regimen fails, hospitalization is mandatory. Hospital care is usually necessary for patients who (1) are homicidal; are delirious or severely depressed; (3) have insufficient family or social support; or (4) have a psychosis refractory to outpatient management. The rapid control of psychosis with parenteral forms of sedating antipsychotics usually requires inpatient care with bed rest because of the tendency to produce hypotension. With rapid tranquilization it is now difficult to justify the regimen of "stair-step" increase of drug dose which takes several weeks or even months of the patient's time and staff time, and considerable monies for the hospital as well as the patient.

The control of psychotic symptoms through rapid tranquilization offers many benefits: (1) reduced duration of hospitalization, including diminished risk of institutional dependency and institutionally generated problems such as apathy, loss of contact with family, friends and job, and social stigma; (2) increased use of hospital beds through rapid turnover of patients; (3) treatment of acute psychoses in small treatment units in general hospitals, where patients may be admitted overnight or for 24 to 72 hours; (4) early engagement of the patient in psychotherapeutic and rehabilitative programs; (5) early establishment of staff-patient rapport with cooperation when the patient is treated as an outpatient; and (6) outpatient management of many patients.

With the advent of peer review, length-of-stay and utilization review committees and pressure from third-party payment sources for brief hospitalization, it is essential that physicians caring for acutely psychotic patients gain skill and experience with rapid tranquilization.

IV

Further Clinical Applications of Antipsychotic Drug Therapy

1. USE IN GERIATRIC PATIENTS

Dosages of antipsychotic agents should be reduced to below adult levels in geriatric patients. Actually, the safest rule to remember in treating elderly patients with any type of medication is "start low and go slow" (Fann and Wheless, 1976).

The present population of Americans 65 years of age or older is increasing at a far faster rate than the population at large. In 1975, Americans over 65 made up about 21 million persons while those over 60 accounted for about 27 million. The extent of significant psychiatric disease in this group has been estimated at 20-40% among aged persons living in the community. For those living in nursing homes, the prevalence of conditions requiring psychiatric intervention ranges from 62% upward (Office of Secretary, HEW,

1975). A recent government survey found that 75% of all nursing home patients are receiving at least 1 psychotropic drug (Nursing Home Care in U.S., 1974). There does not seem to be reliable data on what percentage of these are antipsychotic agents.

Previously, it was often assumed that psychiatric disorders were a natural outcome of the aging process. Since these behavioral abnormalities were felt to be inevitable, most felt they could not be successfully treated. If an elderly patient presented symptoms of a predominantly depressive or paranoid nature, these were often assumed to be prodromal to further cerebral degeneration. In the past, almost 90% of geriatric patients committed to state mental hospitals received diagnoses of "arteriosclerotic cerebrovascular disease," "senility" or "hardening of the arteries" (Fann and Wheless, 1976). Wells (1978) points out that cerebral arteriosclerosis actually affects a small proportion of patients exhibiting mental decline, even among those patients diagnosed with severe dementia.

The elderly generally have multisystem problems which alter the pharmacokinetics (absorption, distribution, metabolism, and excretion) and pharmacologic response to any given medication. Absorption from the gastrointestinal tract is often impaired. This may be due to age-related changes, such as decreased total gastric acidity, atrophy and deterioration of GI musculature producing atony, and decreased GI arterial blood supply from atherosclerosis or decreased cardiac output. With advancing age, lean body mass is replaced by fat and acts further to soak up lipid soluble antipsychotic drugs and keep them out of circulation.

Distribution of antipsychotic agents is usually impaired in geriatric patients. The elderly patient has decreased cardiac output, increased circulation time and often myocardial pathology. These factors will delay the distribution of drugs. The blood transport system is often inefficient as antipsychotics are carried by albumin and this blood fraction may be decreased in the elderly.

Drug metabolism is usually slower or impaired in elderly patients and can cause an increase or accumulation of drug blood levels. Any decrease in the number of liver cells or in the functional ability of liver metabolic systems will impair drug metabolism. Likewise, impairment of renal cells can alter certain metabolic reactions such as chemical conjugation. The older patient, even without any sign of laboratory abnormalities showing liver pathology, may have some diminished ability to metabolize drugs in the liver because of the natural consequences of aging.

Excretion of drugs is primarily via the kidneys. However, a small portion of antipsychotic drugs is lost through the bowels after excretion into the bile. Aging affects the renal excretory system by diminishing the amount of renal parenchyma and by decreasing blood flow through the kidneys. As much as 40% of renal cells may disappear by age 75. The glomerular filtration rate has been noted to decrease by 30% from age 45 to 90. It has been estimated that there is a decrease in clearance and renal absorptive ability of 6% per decade past age 30.

The elderly patient who is a candidate for antipsychotic medication will fall into two broad categories: chronic schizophrenic patients who have become elderly and elderly patients with organic brain syndromes causing severe behavior disturbances. Many other mental disorders are seen in the elderly but are often ill defined or secondary to physical illness. The chronic schizophrenic patient quite often has been stable for years. However, the aged schizophrenic may have a whole resurgence of schizophrenic symptoms when placed in a new living arrangement or nursing home. On the other hand, the patient with organic brain impairment may develop target symptoms of hyperactivity, assaultiveness, anxiety, delusions, and hallucinations.

The elderly chronic schizophrenic or involutional patient generally needs 20 to 50% less antipsychotic medication than his middle-aged counterpart. The initial starting dose should be small and upward dosage adjustments should be made gradually. Much closer monitoring of the patient's cardiovascular status, blood pressure, bowel function, urinary output, and mental status is required. Nursing orders should reflect the need to more carefully monitor these potential problem areas. Particular care must be taken to prevent orthostatic syncope when the patient arises in the morning or gets up at night to go to the bathroom. If the patient is managed at home, family members must be educated in the observation for potential problems.

The choice of antipsychotic drug in the elderly patient should reflect the patient's ability to swallow, level of agitation, sleep disturbance, concomitant medications, and physical disease. For example, a drug should be chosen that is available in a liquid and parenteral form as well as tablet or capsule. Elderly patients will often have difficulty swallowing or, due to paranoia, will refuse tablet forms. Parenteral dosing may occasionally be needed for particularly severe problems. For the patient with cardiovascular disease, the high potency antipsychotics such as haloperidol, fluphenazine, thiothixene or triflouperazine seem preferable (Branchey et al., 1978). The patient requiring sedation may do well on mesoridazine or thioridazine. Chlorpromazine should be a second-line drug due to risk of hypotension, and thioridazine can be limited in these situations by lack of parenteral form. Table 10 gives oral dosage guidelines for antipsychotic agents in elderly schizophrenic patients.

In the geriatric patient with an organic brain syndrome (OBS), antipsychotic drug dosage will generally be even less than for the elderly schizophrenic. The compromised cerebral function of the elderly patient with an organic brain syndrome generally will not tolerate the usual or expected dosages of antipsychotic agents. Moreover, management can often

TABLE 10
Recommended Oral Antipsychotic Dosages* for Elderly Schizophrenics

Drug	Acute Daily Starting Dose	Daily Maintenance Dosage Range	Sedation	Hypotension	EPS**
Mesoridazine (Serentil)	25-75 mg.	50-200 mg.	moderate	moderate	mild
Thioridazine (Mellaril)	50-150 mg.	100-400 mg.	moderate	moderate	low
Haloperidol (Haldol)	1-6 mg.	2-15 mg.	low	low	high
Thiothixene (Navane)	2-10 mg.	5-30 mg.	low	low	moderate
Trifluoperazine (Stelazine)	2-8 mg.	4-20 mg.	low	low	high
Fluphenazine HCl (Prolixin HCl)	1-5 mg.	2.5-15 mg.	low	low	high
Chlorpromazine (Thorazine)	50-150 mg.	100-500 mg.	high	high	mild

*In rare cases, higher dosages may be necessary
**Extrapyramidal Syndrome

be obtained with dosages that would be considered homeopathic for a person with schizophrenia.

One of the more frequent management problems seen is the hyperaroused and agitated geriatric patient. These individuals often decompensate following admission for routine medical or surgical problems. These nonspecific behaviors can often be treated using parenteral antipsychotic agents. Since much lower dosages are generally needed, these medicines must be titrated. Readily available U-100 insulin syringes seem to make this easier.

To avoid overdosing an already compromised individual, start with tiny doses. As an example mesoridazine has shown efficacy in elderly patients. Start with 5 mg. by muscular injection. This is 5/25 ml or 20 units (5/25 × 100 units) in a U-100 insulin syringe. Give this dose every hour until the patient quiets. One may then switch to concentrate forms when the patient responds. Generally, especially if the patient is quite old, 3 to 4 doses is sufficient. If the physician wishes to use haloperidol, the same principles apply. For instance, start with ½ mg. IM every hour. This is 10 units in a U-100 insulin syringe (.5/5 × 100 units). Patients will usually respond to 2 or 3 mg. and can then be switched to the concentrate form.

As it is difficult to measure less than 1 ml of medication, nurses unfamiliar with psychotropic agents find insulin syringes to be easily mastered. This allows the psychiatrist or physician to titrate the dose upward until control is achieved and avoids overdosing the elderly individual (Granacher, 1979). If the patient does not respond to these small doses, the principles in Section 5, Use in Psychiatric Emergencies, should be tried.

The same principles of geriatric pharmacology apply to the older patient with organic brain syndrome, except more so. Thus, start with very low dosages and increment the dosage upward very gradually until target symptoms recede. The physician must watch for the physical side effects noted above and pay particular attention to the patient's mental status.

Based on palatability of liquid forms and lesser side effects, thioridazine or mesoridazine is recommended if sedation is needed or neurologic side effects are troublesome, and haloperidol, thiothixene, fluphenazine HCl or trifluoperazine if hypotension or cardiac disease is a problem. Chlorpromazine is a second-line drug if the patient is not responsive to the others; however, hypotension will be usually more troublesome with this agent (Table 11).

Due to the aging process, antipsychotic drugs are prone to certain side effect profiles or altered pharmacologic response in the elderly. Hamilton (1966) has pointed out that the aging nervous system affects drug activity.

TABLE 11
Recommended Oral Antipsychotic Dosages for Elderly Persons with Organic Brain Syndrome

Drug	Daily Starting Dose	Daily Maintenance Dose	Anticholinergic Potency	Hypotension
Mesoridazine (Serentil)	20-50 mg.	10-150 mg.	moderate	moderate
Thioridazine (Mellaril)	25-100 mg.	50-200 mg.	very high	moderate
Haloperidol (Haldol)	½-3 mg.	½-5 mg.	low	low
Thiothixene (Navane)	2-6 mg.	2-10 mg.	low	low
Trifluoperazine (Stelazine)	2-6 mg.	2-10 mg.	low	low
Fluphenazine HCl (Prolixin)	1-2.5 mg.	1-5 mg.	low	low
Chlorpromazine (Thorazine)	25-100 mg.	50-200 mg.	high	high

The neuronal loss with aging seems to be the primary mechanism responsible for the altered reactivity and sensitivity to antipsychotic agents. Moreover, parkinsonian effects are more frequent in the elderly and may be related to the aging basal ganglia. Old age lowers the tolerance to antipsychotic side effects. These compounds have also been noted to decrease certain aspects of cerebral metabolism, which may compromise the often marginal abilities of the geriatric brain.

The most serious gastrointestinal side effect in the aged individual is paralytic ileus or megacolon. Antipsychotic drugs are capable of this and it is probably related to their anticholinergic nature. Likewise, the addition of anticholinergic antiparkinson agents will often have an additive effect. The aliphatic and piperidine phenothiazines are the most likely to cause this problem, with the piperazine phenothiazines, butyrophenones and thiothixene the least likely.

The most troublesome cardiovascular effect of antipsychotic agents in geriatric patients is orthostatic hypotension. Again the aliphatic and piperidine phenothiazines are the worst offenders, with the higher potency antipsychotics, such as haloperidol, less prone. Elderly patients often have systolic hypertension and show a great lability of blood pressure. They may be especially sensitive to the hypotensive effect of antipsychotic drugs. Likewise, the antihypertensive effect of drugs such as guanethidine (Ismelin) or clonidine (Catapres) may be blocked by antipsychotic agents (see Drug Interactions section in Chapter V). All elderly patients and their families should be warned about rising too quickly from chairs and should be advised to dangle their feet over the bedside before rising. This may prevent a sudden orthostatic drop in blood pressure. Elastic support hose may be worthwhile and prevent blood pooling in the distal extremities.

Parkinson side effects are more likely with the high potency phenothiazines, butyrophenones and thiothixene. These neurologic effects seem more common in older than younger patients and 50% of all patients between 60 and 80 develop at least some extrapyramidal effects with antipsychotic drugs (Hamilton, 1966).

Whether or not tardive dyskinesia is more common in elderly patients with the same duration of antipsychotic drug exposure as younger patients is not fully answered. Treatment of parkinsonism in the elderly is with the anticholinergic antiparkinson agents or amantadine. However, dosages should be lower than for younger adults and caution used to prevent anticholinergic toxicity. If the aged patient seems particularly sensitive to anticholinergic effects, amantadine may be used, as it is largely devoid of anticholinergic activity. Dosage should probably not exceed 200 mg. daily in patients over 70 and **good renal function is necessary**.

Other rarer side effects may occur. Seventy percent of all cases of agranulocytosis occur in patients between ages of 48 and 70. Fatalities increase with age (DiMascio and Shader, 1970). Open-angle glaucoma tends to be a disease of later years and caution with the more anticholinergic antipsychotics such as the aliphatic and piperidine series of phenothiazines is advised. (See Chapter V.)

The elderly male may be particularly sensitive to urinary obstruction because of an unrecognized prostatic disorder. Again, the highly anticholinergic agents, including the antiparkinson agents, are likely to be the worst culprits. Therefore, a good urinary flow history should be taken, if possible, before starting antipsychotics in elderly patients. The management of urinary outflow problems with bethanechol (Urecholine) is described in Chapter V.

If careful consideration is given to the particular needs of the elderly patients, many can have an improved quality of life and greater social acceptance through judicious use of antipsychotic agents.

2. USE IN CHILDREN

Antipsychotic agents for pediatric use are recommended primarily in the management of psychotic children. They seem useful in the behavioral control of hyperactivity, assaultiveness, destructiveness, self-injury and stereotypies in mentally retarded children. They are less effective in treating hyperkinetic children than stimulants and tricyclic antidepressants. There is no sound evidence that they are useful in the management of neurotic children (Winsberg and Yepes, 1978).

The philosophical approach to the drug treatment of behavior problems in children is presently ambivalent and polarized. The extreme view sees psychopharmacology in children as a form of chemical social coercion, since children generally don't make their own decisions for treatment (London, 1969). Eisenberg (1972) holds that psychotropic drugs in children "promise neither the passport to a brave new world nor the gateway to the inferno." The authors hold that view and feel that a sound multimodal treatment program, including psychotropic agents if indicated, offers many children hope for a more successful life.

The pharmacology of antipsychotic agents in children is poorly developed. There are almost no data available. Most explanations are based on the assumptions that these drugs are qualitatively the same in children as in adults. Moreover, the usual pharmacologic explanations rely on assumed quantitative differences. These may or may not be warranted and further research and clinical studies are required before concrete statements about pediatric pharmacology of antipsychotic agents can be made.

Some recent progress in dosage studies of antipsychotics in children has been made. These suggest that previous poor responses of children to these agents could be secondary to underdosing. For instance, Rivera-Calimlim et al. (1979) have found that children need larger doses of chlorpromazine than adults in order to attain comparable plasma concentrations. Their studies suggest that children may autoinduce their liver metabolism system to degrade chlorpromazine more rapidly than adults. This study is the first of desperately needed research in this important pediatric area.

In the developing child, educators have questioned the ability of behavior modifying agents to disrupt cognition and learning. A study by Gittelman-Klein et al. (1976) finds that thioridazine neither enhances nor disrupts scores on various measures of learning performance in hyperactive children. It was inferior to methylphenidate (Ritalin) in this regard. On the other hand, Helper et al. (1963) found that chlorpromazine diminished paired associate learning and scores on a motor test among a group of hospitalized children. Haloperidol has been found effective in low doses (0.025 mg./Kg.) at facilitating performance in hyperactive children, but at higher doses (0.05 mg./Kg.) a slight deterioration of performance was noted (Werry and Aman, 1975). A complete review of the literature on classroom learning effects of antipsychotic agents was done by Winsburg and Yepes (1978). They find that laboratory-type tests show a possible depression of performance in children exposed to clinical doses of antipsychotic agents. **However, in clinically prescribed doses these antipsychotics do not seem to interfere with classroom learning**.

The symptoms of psychosis in the child are varied and not the same as signs and symptoms of schizophrenia in an adolescent or adult. Target symptoms vary with the age of onset of illness and present as disorders of speech and language, relationships, emotions and physiologic functions. The physician should have an accurate diagnosis before prescribing antipsychotic agents in children. Likewise, drugs alone never suffice and other concomitant therapies should be included (e.g., remedial education, individual psychotherapy, parental counseling and possibly hospitalization). Table 12 gives dosage guidelines for those antipsychotic agents that are FDA approved for use in children.

As can be seen, only chlorpromazine, triflupromazine, thioridazine, or prochlorperazine is approved for use in the preschool child. Trifluoperazine and chlorprothixene can be used for ages 6 to 12 but IM chlorprothixene is not recommended. Fluphenazine, thiothixene and other antipsychotic agents have been successfully used in the management of childhood psychosis, but the approval by the FDA has not been completed.

The side effect profile of these agents in the child is essentially the same as for adults (see Chapter V). Children may be more susceptible to dystonic reactions than adults, particularly with prochlorperazine and trifluoperazine. As in adults, thioridazine would be the least likely to cause neurologic

TABLE 12
Recommended Dosages of Antipsychotic Drugs* for Children Under 12 Years of Age

Drug	Comments
Chlorpromazine (Thorazine)	Oral: ¼ mg./lb body wt. q 4-6 hr. prn Rectal: ½ mg./lb body wt. q 6-8 hr. prn IM: ¼ mg./lb body wt. q 6-8 hr. prn Note: Maximum IM Dosage up to 5 years or 50 lbs. 40 mg. daily; 5-12 years (50-100 lbs) not over 75 mg. daily except in severe cases.
Triflupromazine (Vesprin)	Oral: 1 mg./lb (2 mg./Kg) up to maximum daily dose of 150 mg. in divided doses. IM: ¹⁄₁₀-⅛ mg./lb (0.2-0.25 mg./Kg) up to a maximum daily dose of 10 mg. Note: Do not use in children under 2½ years of age.
Thioridazine (Mellaril)	Oral: 1-6 mg./lb total daily dose depending upon size (0.5-3 mg./Kg daily). Starting dose generally 10 mg. b.i.d. to t.i.d. Note: Not intended for children under two years of age.
Prochlorperazine (Compazine)	Oral or Rectal: 2½ mg. b.i.d. or t.i.d. starting dose, ages 2-5, do not exceed 20 mg. daily. Ages 6-12 do not exceed 25 mg. daily. IM: 0.06 mg./lb (e.g. 50 lbs = 3 mg.) each dose. Note: Do not use under 20 lbs or 2 years.
Chlorprothixene (Taractan)	Oral: 10-25 mg. t.i.d. or q.i.d. IM: *Not* to be used in children under 12 Note: Oral use not indicated under age 6
Haloperidol (Haldol)	Dosage guidelines not given

*Approved by FDA as of 1978.

dysfunction, with the remaining compounds somewhat in between. Children with a history of epilepsy require cautious management. Drowsiness is a common and often unwanted side effect in children. Chlorpromazine and thioridazine are worse than the others for this effect. Excessive weight gain from increased appetite can be a problem. Drug interactions are the same as for adults. One of the more important for children is the combination of the antihelminth piperazine citrate (Antepar) with the phenothiazines. Convulsions have been reported with this combination. The major complication of these medications is the child who overdoses with antipsychotic agents. **Vomiting should not be induced when a child has overdosed, as a dystonic reaction might be precipitated with resulting aspiration**. Controlled gastric lavage is preferred, as all antipsychotics, with the exception of thioridazine, are antiemetic.

Antipsychotic agents have usefulness in the total management of the psychotic or behaviorally deviant retarded child. They should be incorporated into a complete psycho-social management program. They are only symptom specific. They tend to make the psychotic child less active, anxious and agitated but, compared to their action with adults, do not seem truly antipsychotic. In the retarded child they are useful in controlling some deviant behaviors. These agents are probably not as efficacious in children as in adults, and in this age group may tend to be overused.

3. USE IN ANXIETY REACTIONS

By leafing through any of the myriad advertisements for treating anxiety, the physician will note a large number devoted to the use of antipsychotic agents. These displays are always quite colorful and often frankly misleading. While they cajole the practitioner to use them for "chronic neurotic anxiety," the fine print usually states that for most antipsychotics, a review by the National Academy of Sciences has found this drug "possibly effective for the control of excessive anxiety, tension and agitation." This disclaimer usually points out that "final classification of the less-than-effective indications requires further investigation" (PDR, 1978).

Many antipsychotic drugs have been evaluated in controlled antianxiety studies and none seems equal to the benzodiazepines in efficacy (Rickels, 1978). Some have been found to be totally ineffective. Even in low dosages akathisia or motor restlessness can be a disturbing side effect and can actually increase the patient's perception of anxiety. **The usefulness of antipsychotic agents in treating anxious neurotic symptoms has still not been clearly established after almost 25 years of experience with these agents.**

For most anxious conditions, psychotherapy, benzodiazepines or a combination of these approaches should be tried first. In a few situations, antipsychotic agents may be tried in low doses (Shader and Greenblatt, 1975). Specifically, these are patients showing distractibility with anxiety, anxious patients with thought-blocking or racing thoughts, and anxious obsessional patients with magical thinking or faulty reality testing. Obviously, these are all thought disorders in one form or another and probably not true anxiety in the first place.

The use of antipsychotics in anxious neurotic patients probably presents a risk of tardive dyskinesia. This side effect does not require that the patient by psychotic and therefore antipsychotic agents should be generally avoided in nonpsychotic conditions such as anxiety (Cole, 1977; van Praag, 1978).

However, if a neurotic patient does not respond to therapeutic doses of other medication, an antipsychotic may be tried despite the possible side effects. Its use should be limited to a brief period and rationale documented in the patient record.

4. USE IN DEPRESSION

The drug literature that passes the physician's desk continually points out the usefulness of certain antipsychotic agents in the treatment of "neurotic depression." Many studies comparing tricyclic antidepressants and antipsychotic agents in groups of relatively unselected cases of serious depressions have found little differences in the efficacy of either drug group. From some of these early studies, thioridazine to this day has an exaggerated reputation concerning its usefulness in depressive syndromes (Overall et al., 1964). The natural history of depressive episodes must be kept in mind or treatment responses to certain drugs may seem more beneficial than is the case. Prior to the development of electroconvulsive therapy or antidepressant drugs, Alexander (1953) found from extensive studies that 40% of hospitalized depressed patients recovered spontaneously within the first year and 60% recovered within 2 years. Obviously, spontaneous recovery will have an effect upon drug outcome studies. The difficulty with most early drug studies in depression was that all depressions were lumped together and not clearly separated into diagnostic subtypes.

Most psychotropic drug authorities today agree on some basic principles in using antipsychotic agents in depression. **Antipsychotic agents have the greatest benefit in those depressions that are psychotic or involutional in type with delusional morbid ruminations. Tricyclic antidepressants seem more beneficial in those depressions that are motorically retarded and displaying quiet, ruminating depressive thoughts without delusional content** (Baldessarini, 1977; van Praag, 1978). Manic-depressive depressions usually fall into this latter group. Moreover, the neurotic depressions seem as likely to respond to adequate doses of the antianxiety benzodiazepine agents such as diazepam (Valium) or chlordiazepoxide (Librium) as to tricyclic antidepressants or antipsychotics.

To use antipsychotic agents in a psychotic depression, the management principles are similar to those followed with a schizophrenic psychosis (see Chapter II). If rapid control of arousal signs such as agitation, motor hyperactivity, or insomnia is needed, early use of injectable antipsychotic medication may be helpful. The target symptoms displaying relief in psychotic depression are the same as for any psychosis, namely arousal signs will come in control first, with affective and cognitive changes following in that order. Cognitive and perceptual changes may require 6 weeks or longer to improve in particularly severe cases.

Much has been written in the last few years about post-psychotic depression following the use of antipsychotic agents in schizophrenia. Patients with clear-cut mood changes may be benefited by the addition of antidepressant agents but this remains controversial. On the other hand, physicians must be aware that many "post-psychotic depressions" are actually akinetic motor disorders secondary to the antipsychotic drug (Van Putten and May, 1978). These disorders are recognized by motor retardation, emotional withdrawal, lack of initiative, hypersomnia, and overwhelming fatigue. All of these signs and symptoms have been reported with antipsychotic drug-induced akinesia (Rifkin et al., 1975).

These findings are exactly those often seen in true Parkinson's disease. Depressive symptoms with suicidal ideation may be seen in combination with neurologic symptoms but disappear following appropriate treatment. Having the patient write a sentence can be a useful aid in diagnosis. The handwriting may show the constriction noted in parkinsonism. A test dose of benztropine (Cogentin) 2 mg. IV will usually be diagnostic. If it is a true parkinson disorder, relief will be obtained within 15 minutes and this patient should then receive continuing antiparkinson medication. Further improvement may be obtained by reducing the antipsychotic dosage or switching the patient to a drug with few neurologic side effects, such as mesoridazine (Serentil) or thioridazine (Mellaril).

The addition of a tricyclic antidepressant to patients seemingly depressed from antipsychotics can fool the physician into thinking he is treating a mood disorder. All tricyclic antidepressants are highly anticholinergic and will improve signs of parkinsonism in a manner similar to the antiparkinson agents. If, after starting a tricyclic antidepressant, the patient shows improved facial expression and an apparent activation within a day or two, drug-induced akinesia is a more likely diagnosis than depression.

Another common treatment in depression is to use a fixed combination of amitriptyline and perphenazine (Triavil, Etrafon). This has developed a reputation of being useful in "anxious depression." However, Hollister et al. (1967) were unable to show that this combination is superior to amitriptyline alone in depressions. This is particularly important as an examination of their data shows only an average amitriptyline dose of 111 mg./day, which many authorities would consider inadequate for depressed patients. On the other hand, the average dose of perphenazine was 19 mg./day, a significant dose for nonpsychotic patients. Amitriptyline has also been compared with thiothixene in the treatment of endogenous depression and the response favored amitriptyline (Simpson et al., 1972). For the nonpsychotic depressions, tricyclic antidepressants or ECT seem the present treatments of choice.

5. USE IN PSYCHIATRIC EMERGENCIES

There are, of course, many forms of psychiatric emergencies. A large majority of these are best served by psychosocial or legal intervention rather than pharmacologic means. However, two emergencies in particular require incisive treatment with psychotropic agents: acute agitation in ambulatory patients and agitated delirium in surgical and medical patients.

The severely agitated patient often presents a management dilemma for general hospital emergency rooms, admission areas of state mental hospitals and community mental health centers. Droperidol (Inapsine) has been found to be an effective, quick and safe agent for many of these patients (Granacher and Ruth, 1979). Unlike the barbiturates, droperidol causes no respiratory depression and is much less likely to cause severe hypotension. Moreover, it is not additive in effects with alcohol or drugs of the sedative-hypnotic group.

Droperidol is somewhat of an unique agent. It is structurally similar to haloperidol (Figure 4) but it is much more potent and higher in sedative activity (Janssen and Van Bever, 1976). In the United States, no oral form exists and this product is only used intramuscularly or intravenously. It has enjoyed use almost entirely in anesthesia as a preoperative medication and is neuroleptanalgesia. For neuroleptanalgesia it is often combined with the potent narcotic fentanyl (Innovar). **This combination should never be used for psychiatric therapy**.

One advantage of droperidol seems to be its relative lack of toxicity and most pharmacologic reviews stress this point. When tested in a controlled fashion it is superior to placebo in its ability to quell excitement and agitation and seems somewhat specific for arousal signs (Van Leeuwen et al., 1977). It has shown usefulness in combating the occasional psychosis secondary to ketamine HCl (Ketaject) anesthesia (Neff et al., 1972) and in gaining rapid control following methamphetamine intoxication (Gary and Saidi, 1978).

Another advantage of droperidol is its extremely rapid absorption from intramuscular administration. The uptake from the injection site is so rapid that it is difficult to distinguish the intramuscular response from the intravenous response. The distribution phase is likewise very rapid (134 ± 13 minutes) and explains the need for frequent injections (Cressman et al., 1973).

Droperidol is highly potent (more than 100 times as potent as chlorpromazine) and is commercially available in a parenteral solution of 2.5 mg./ml

HALOPERIDOL (Haldol)

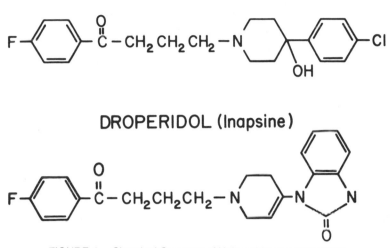

DROPERIDOL (Inapsine)

FIGURE 4.   Chemical Structure of Haloperidol and Droperidol

(droperidol, Inapsine, McNeil). The usual starting dose for an agitated patient is 5-10 mg. (2 to 4 cc) IM depending upon body size and level of
agitation. A useful guide is 1 ml (2.5 mg.) for every 50 lbs. body weight.
For very severe agitation, slow intravenous infusion can be used. If the
patient remains agitated after 15-20 minutes, another 5-10 mg. may be
given. **If the first dose was intravenous, the second dose should be by
intramuscular injection**. van Praag (1978) suggests that the maximum dose
in 24 hours should not exceed 45 mg.

The acute side effects of droperidol are similar to those of other antipsychotic agents. Namely, these are neurologic effects and hypotension.
Neurologic effects are rare when this agent is used briefly. Hypotension will
be more of a problem if the intravenous route is chosen. The management
of these problems is outlined in Chapter V.

Droperidol is recommended for short-term control of agitation (Granacher
and Ruth, 1979). Other measures are necessary for guaranteeing the safety
of patient and staff. Seclusion or restraint may be indicated. A definitive
diagnosis must be sought. If the patient is psychotic, an appropriate antipsychotic should be chosen (Chapter II). Until further knowledge is gained,
droperidol cannot be recommended for long-term management of agitation.

The use of antipsychotic agents in acute delirium in medical or surgical
settings has received even less scientific examination that droperidol. However, some recent uses of haloperidol deserve mention. Ayd (1976c) advises

that intravenous haloperidol might be a desirable method of safe and rapid symptom control in acute delirium tremens, very severe mania or severe and malignant catatonic excitement. He further suggests its use in controlling acute agitation following myocardial infarction or postoperative psychosis.

Two studies on intravenous haloperidol were presented at the 1978 annual meeting of the American Psychiatric Association. Cassem and Sos (1978) evaluated haloperidol given intravenously to patients after cardiac surgery or myocardial infarction. Many of the post surgical patients were intubated, had indwelling arterial, left atrial, pulmonary arterial and central venous pressure lines. Moreover, they were monitored by E.K.G. leads, pacing wires in the right atrium and left ventricle, Foley catheters and intra-aortic balloon pumps. Obviously, agitation per se is a threat to the stability of these patients. Likewise, cardiovascular status might be compromised by increased myocardial oxygen demands and Valsalva effects of agitation.

Ten of these patients received IV haloperidol. Intravenous dosages ranged from 2 to 135 mg. in 24 hours. Immediately upon injection no observable changes were noted. When calmness occurred, it came at 10 to 40 minutes following injection. No significant changes were noted in systolic blood pressure, cardiac rhythm or left atrial pressure. However, all patients received morphine sulfate and hydantoin (Dilantin). Five of the 10 patients showed unequivocal tranquilization following IV haloperidol while the remainder derived partial benefit.

Cassem and Sos summarized their recommendations and conclusions as follows:

(1) Intravenous haloperidol seems to have a benign effect on blood pressure and heart rate.
(2) There exists a wide variation in dose/response as high as 1000fold among patients.
(3) Clinical effects are usually not seen before 10 minutes or after 40 minutes.
(4) Rate of administration should not exceed 5 mg./30 seconds.
(5) Extrapyramidal effects were *not* seen.
(6) Postoperative delirium should be rapidly and vigorously treated with most of the dose given in the first few hours and sharply tapered down thereafter. If most of the drug is given early, accumulation of the drug is less likely. Haloperidol should be given intravenously every one-half hour until quiet. The patient will then be controlled with booster doses every 12 hours. When no agitation is evident, switch to a small bedtime dose. This should be continued at least 2 nights after the patient is clear. Giving doses every 6 hours may cause excessive somnolence. Because of wide individual variation in response, no formula is available to direct the physician and vigilant titration is required.

A second study was independently conducted at the University of Washington Hospitals. Dudley and Rowlett (1978) treated patients with serious or life-threatening illness who were impeding their appropriate medical or surgical treatment because of significant psychiatric pathology. Most of their 20 patients suffered from schizophrenia, organic brain syndrome, or mania. Medical surgical diagnoses in these individuals ranged from upper GI bleeding to burns or trauma. The dose to achieve calming varied from 2.5 to 25 mg. of haloperidol intravenously over a 20-minute period. They reported that every case responded to a level where medical treatment could be given. These patients differed qualitatively from those of Cassem and Sos in that most were psychotic or had organic brain pathology. The former cases were primarily post-myocardial infarction or postoperative delirium.

The response and side-effect profile of European investigators using haloperidol has paralleled the American experience. Maximum sedative-calming effects are seen the first hour. If extrapyramidal effects occur, they are most likely at 12-16 hours with falling blood levels (Forsman, 1976; Dencker, 1976).

Thus, intravenous haloperidol may be safe for use in seriously delirious medical-surgical patients and in psychotic or organic brain syndrome patients who are impeding needed medical-surgical treatment. It should be noted that the use of droperidol in agitation or of intravenous haloperidol in the delirium and agitation complicating medical-surgical treatment has not received official approval by the FDA. Therefore, it is advisable that clinicians accurately document a need for these treatments before using and reserve these applications for patients in the specific clinical categories mentioned.

6. USE IN OTHER DISORDERS

In view of the present day concern regarding tardive dyskinesia, the risk-benefit factor must be carefully weighed when antipsychotic drugs are used for disorders other than relief from disabling systems of schizophrenia and other psychoses. Therefore, antipsychotics should be prescribed *only* when a patient has symptoms known to be responsive to such medication.

Alcoholism

In evaluating the effectiveness of various agents used in the treatment of alcohol withdrawal states, a review of the literature reveals a substantial controversy. There are numerous reports about the use of antipsychotic agents for these disorders. Although early reports were extremely favorable, most of the recent studies have not generated enthusiasm for a wide range.

Chlorpromazine, 100 mg. intramuscularly every 2 to 4 hours, has been advocated in the management of alcoholic delirium tremens (Chapel, 1973). In reply, Kalda (1973) stated that chlorpromazine was contraindicated for delirium tremens because of increased mortality and the danger of further compromising hepatic functioning thus leading to cholestatic jaundice. He claimed that other undesirable effects of chlorpromazine might complicate the medical management of already seriously ill and dehydrated patients. Many have concomitant congestive heart failure, bronchitis or emphysema while others may show tachycardia, quinidine-like electrocardiographic changes, hypotension and lowering of the convulsive threshold.

In a cooperative V.A. study both chlorpromazine and chlordiazepoxide produced symptom improvement in a great majority of patients suffering from acute withdrawal symptoms. However, chlorpromazine was associated with a much higher incidence of both delirium and seizure (Kaim et al., 1969, 1971). In spite of other unfavorable reports, Cade (1974) has stated that, in Australia, chlorpromazine has been found to be an extremely safe and effective drug in the management of the restless alcoholic, especially the patient with delirium tremens. His psychiatric hospital treats many hundreds of alcoholics each year and over a period of many years its use has never been cause for alarm. The mortality rate for patients with delirium tremens treated at his hospital is "nil" but he attributes this primarily to the prompt use of massive doses of thiamine plus adequate oral rehydration as well as effective sedation.

Thioridazine has been reported to be safe and efficacious in the treatment of anxious-depressive symptomatology among hospitalized chronic alcoholics and as effective as chlordiazepoxide (Librium) in controlling symptoms attributable to alcoholic withdrawal. Thioridazine also has been recommended as a therapeutic agent for the depressed alcoholic patient who is a high suicidal risk (Penna-Ramos, 1977). The dosage range may vary from 25 to 200 mg. Usually the depression does not represent a primary effective disorder but appears to be the consequence of the depressant action of alcohol plus the life stress associated with alcoholism. The depressive effect tends to lift with the passing of withdrawal (Schukit, 1975). Mesoridazine, perphenazine and other phenothiazines also have been used for alcohol withdrawal states but none has proved to be superior to the others.

Palestine and Alatorre (1976) reported on the results of a double-blind 4-hour study of parenteral haloperidol and chlordiazepoxide in 49 alcoholic adults who were experiencing acute withdrawal symptoms. Patients were given an initial injection of ahloperidol 5 mg. or chlordiazepoxide 50 mg. If symptoms were not controlled, subsequent injections of haloperidol 5 mg. or chlordiazepoxide 50 mg. were repeated hourly until symptoms were controlled or until the end of the 4-hour study period. During the 4-hour period, the mean total dose of haloperidol administered was 16 mg. with a dose range from 5 to 20 mg. The mean total dose of chlordiazepoxide administered was 182 mg. with a dose range from 50 to 200 mg. Patients who did not respond within 4 hours were considered treatment failures and alternative medication was given.

Seventy percent of the haloperidol group was successfully controlled in contrast to 44% of the patients treated with chlordiazepoxide. The psychiatric symptoms of the haloperidol group were most rapidly controlled (thus fewer injections needed) and the patients were not oversedated and were able to communicate with the nurses and physicians. These effects were in marked contrast to the relatively slower onset of effect, deep sedation and residual tremors observed with chlordiazepoxide. In addition, haloperidol showed significant antiemetic effects not seen with chlordiazepoxide. Palestine and his associates concluded that haloperidol could have a vital role in the establishment and maintenance of an acute care detoxification center where early discharge to continuing care of a rehabilitation facility is desirable. They recommended haloperidol as a useful and safe pharmacotherapeutic agent for the primary care physician who is called upon to treat patients in various states of alcoholic withdrawal. However, it is now known that the uptake of intramuscular chlordiazepoxide is poor and erratic. Thus this study favors haloperidol.

Presently, for most clinicians, the phenothiazines and the butyrophenones are no longer considered appropriate for treatment of withdrawal of alcohol. It is believed that the hypotensive side effects of these drugs may further compromise a cardiovascular system already damaged by alcohol. In addition, there is the fear of their epileptogenic and hepatotoxic side effects. It is a basic principle to treat drug withdrawal with pharmacologically equivalent or cross-tolerant drugs and therefore the benzodiazepines, pharmacologic equivalents of alcohol, are the preferred drugs. In addition, the benzodiazepines, such as chlordiazepoxide (Librium) and diazepam (Valium), are the primary drugs of choice because of their relatively low level of undesirable side effects. A survey of selected, experienced physicians' preferences in the chemotherapy of delirium tremens found the benzodiazepines the favorite drugs of choice (86%) with paraldehyde in second place and the phenothiazines in third (Farazza and Martin, 1974).

Chorea

A current concept regarding the mechanism of abnormal movements holds that chorea and parkinsonism are opposing disorders. Since trifluoperazine (Stelazine) produces a high incidence of a Parkinson-like syndrome as a side effect, it seemed likely that trifluoperazine might be useful in this disorder. This antipsychotic is effective in the symptomatic relief of chorea of different etiologies, including genetic-degenerative (Huntington's), vascular inflammatory (Sydenham's), and vascular occlusive. The effective dose range usually varies from 4 to 16 mg. The drug is generally well tolerated and dose-related side effects of nausea and parkinsonism respond to decreased dose levels (Stokes, 1975).

Oral fluphenazine (Prolixin), at a mean daily dosage of 6.4 mg. after an escalation schedule of 1 mg. weekly until the chorea is diminished and parkinsonism appears, has been reported to decrease choreoid activity in 62% of patients with the diagnosis of Huntington's chorea (Whittier and Korenyi, 1968). Haloperidol also has been reported to be of symptomatic benefit in some cases of chorea.

Nausea and Vomiting

Phenothiazine antipsychotics with the exception of thioridazine are almost universally accepted as effective antiemetics for nausea and vomiting from causes other than motion sickness. Prominent side effects include sedation and potentiation of opiate-depression action. Other acute or chronic side effects rarely occur with short-term pre- or postoperative use, but sedation, dystonia and dyskinesia may be undesirable during this period.

Prochlorperazine (Compazine) is probably the phenothiazine most widely used specifically as an antiemetic. It produces minimal hypotension and tolerable sedation but there are significant extrapyramidal effects. To control nausea and vomiting, the usual adult oral dosage recommended is 5 or 10 mg. 3 or 4 times a day or rectal dosage 25 mg. twice daily. Intramuscular dosage recommended usually is "5 to 10 mg. (1-2 ml) injected *deeply* into the upper outer quadrant of the buttock. If necessary, repeat every 3 or 4 hours. The total intramuscular dosage should not exceed 40 mg. per day. *Subcutaneous administration is not advisable because of local irritation.*" For severe nausea and vomiting associated with adult surgery, intramuscular dosage consists of "5 to 10 mg. (1-2 ml) 1 to 2 hours before induction of anesthesia (repeat once in 30 minutes, if necessary), or to control acute symptoms during and after surgery (repeat once if necessary)" (*Physicians' Desk Reference*, 1978).

Perphenazine (Trilafon) is another reliable postoperative antiemetic and produces some sedation but no hypotension. "For rapid control of severe nausea and vomiting in adults, 5 mg. (1 ml) IM should be given; in rare instances it may be necessary to increase the dosage to 10 mg. In general, higher doses should be given only in hospitalized patients" (*Physicians' Desk Reference*, 1978).

Chlorpromazine is also effective for the control of nausea and vomiting. Like other antiemetics, it may mask signs of overdosage to toxic drugs and may obscure conditions such as intestinal obstruction and brain tumor. Oral dosage for nausea and vomiting is 10 to 25 mg. every (q) 4-8 hours, PRN, increased if necessary. Intramuscular dosage recommended is 25 mg. (1 ml). If no hypotension occurs, 25 to 50 mg. (q) 4-6 hours, PRN may be given until vomiting stops. Then a switch can be made to oral dosage. Rectal dosage is 1 suppository (100 mg.) every 6-8 hours, PRN. In some patients, half this dose will do (*Physicians' Desk Reference*, 1978).

Haloperidol has been found to be an effective and safe prophylactic against nausea and vomiting. It is equipotent with other antiemetics and has fewer unpleasant side effects (Shields et al., 1971). Since it is a potent antiemetic, anesthesiologists and surgeons use it to abolish or minimize postoperative vomiting and obstetricians prescribe it for morning sickness, hyperemesis gravidarum and for neuroleptanalgesia at delivery (Ayd, 1972).

When the antipsychotic drugs are used for nausea and vomiting, therapy should begin with the lowest recommended dosage which can then be adjusted in accordance with the response of the individual.

Gilles de la Tourette's Syndrome

This disorder is characterized by: (1) sudden involuntary movements, including vulgar gestures (copropraxia), (2) explosive utterances—both inarticulate noises (barks, yelps, grunts, coughs) and articulated obscenities (coprolalia), and (3) imitative phenomena—verbal (echolalia) and behavioral (echopraxia). Diagnosis is based on the first 2 symptoms. Almost all patients develop motor and verbal tics and about half develop coprolalia (Woodrow, 1974).

The syndrome usually begins with involuntary tic-like muscular movements in patients between the ages of 2 and 14 years (mean age of 7). The tics are coordinated, rhythmical, purposeless, rapid (less than 1 minute in duration) and may vary from 1 to thousands of tics per hour. They are usually multiple, involving more than one muscle group. However, a simple, single facial tic usually occurs first, although other parts of the body or vocalization may be involved. The illness has a fluctuating and insidious course and although there are rare remissions for varying periods, the symptoms usually wax and wane (Shapiro et al., 1972, 1973).

The treatment of choice is haloperidol, which results in marked improvement in about 90% of the patients. The dosage of haloperidol can be rapidly titrated in increments of 2 to 10 mg. daily or weekly against an end point of symptom relief or the occurrence of incapacitating side effects. With this regimen the dosage varies between 6 and 180 mg. daily during acute treatment with a mean stabilization dosage of about 9 mg. The acute period lasts from 1 to 3 months before the dosage, effectiveness of the drug, and side effects become stabilized. The dosage can be lowered against an end point of symptom relief and ability to tolerate side effects. Dosage usually can be decreased to very small amounts over a period as long as 1 to 4 years with increased symptom relief (Shapiro et al., 1973).

A maintenance dosage of from 2 to 4 mg. may be reached within several years and the symptoms decrease until they reach a plateau. The symptoms almost always return within 2 to 7 days if the patient stops the medication. Side effects most often encountered are dyskinesias, akathisia, akinesia and parkinsonism. Almost all patients on doses above 2 mg. of haloperidol per day require antiparkinson medication for control of the extrapyramidal symptoms from the antipsychotic drug.

A dosage regimen presently recommended for most young children consists of starting with a very low dose (¼ mg. daily) and increasing the dosage slowly (¼ mg. every 4 days) to an end point of maximum improvement and minimal side effects. To prevent dystonia, Cogentin is given at the beginning of treatment. The average dose of patients on haloperidol through this regimen is 5 mg. a day (Shapiro et al., 1978). However Shapiro and Shapiro (1977) have identified a group who can be successfully treated only if the dosage of haloperidol is titrated more slowly, perhaps in increments of ¼ mg./day every 3 weeks.

Bruun et al. (1976) found that as the length of treatment increases, the amount of improvement also increases. They discovered that patients with an average dose of 6.3 mg. of haloperidol a day for less than 2 years (7-23 months) showed an average improvement in symptoms of 74.3%; those with an average dose of 16.9 mg. a day for 2-4 years (24-47 months) reported an average improvement of 80.6%; a group of patients (with average daily dose of 8.1 mg. a day) treated for more than 4 years reported an average improvement of 93.4%. The dosage of haloperidol showed no consistent relationship with length of treatment or degree of improvement, although many patients, especially older ones, were able to decrease dosage with increasing length of treatment.

Akinesia seems to occur in all children on dosage over 4 to 8 mg. of haloperidol. It is experienced as depression, loss of vivacity or spontaneity, feeling sad or "down," or as nonspecific dysphoria. Treatment often becomes very complicated because of this side effect, since it may not respond to antiparkinson, antidepressant or stimulant drugs, although they should be tried if reassurance does not work.

Phenothiazines have been used in Tourette's Syndrome and found to be much less effective than haloperidol, which appears to be the most effective medication available. Its effectiveness is severely hampered by side effects that often force patients to compromise between the maximum relief of symptoms and minimum discomfort from side effects or to discontinue the drug completely and live with their symptoms even though disabling. It appears that a clinician experienced in the use of high dosages of antipsychotic drugs and who is able to recognize and manage their side effects is necessary for successful treatment. Psychotherapy or behavior modification alone fails to result in any substantial improvement (Bruun et al., 1976; Shapiro et al., 1978).

Pain

The phenothiazines, chlorpromazine in particular, potentiate the effects of analgesics and may be singularly effective in chronic illness with severe pain. The pain is perceived but the emotional reaction is of less distress and discomfort, particularly in young children. Chlorpromazine 25 mg. combined with acetylsalicylic acid 300 mg. may replace demerol or morphine in conditions such as burns or hemophilia. It has been found helpful in the relief of the neurasthenic musculoskeletal pain syndrome (fibrositis syndrome).

In the treatment of cancer and severe pain, chlorpromazine may be prescribed as follows: orally—10 mg. t.i.d. or q.i.d. or 25 mg. b.i.d. or t.i.d.; intramuscularly—25 mg. (1 ml) b.i.d. or t.i.d. Concomitant narcotics and sedatives should be reduced to ¼ or ½ (PDR, 1978).

In certain patients, haloperidol is a very effective pain relief drug and no other analgesic is needed. In other patients, haloperidol may be used to potentiate small doses of narcotics and thus obviate excessive usage. With haloperidol, addiction or tolerance is not a problem. When heavy doses of a narcotic are required, the potential for addiction is always present. In cases where the patient has a terminal illness, addiction is not a great clinical concern but in other non-lethal pain syndromes it may be a major worry. Haloperidol is not obtunding or constipating and it does not produce respiratory depression. The patient is not "drugged" and is able to enjoy conversation and other social interactions without any marked narcotic effect. A dosage regimen that has proven effective starts at 5 mg. at bedtime with a rapid increase to 25 mg. at bedtime.

With a pain syndrome patient who is prone to abuse medication or to take more than is prescribed, haloperidol is a safe drug. The patient will not take more haloperidol than is ordered because no "high" is produced, as in the case with narcotics. The only serious side effects are extrapyramidal, which respond to antiparkinson medication (Cavenar and Maltbie, 1976).

Spinal Cord Injury

Side effects of psychotropic medication present a special threat to patients with spinal cord injuries because the paralysis involves the autonomic nervous system. If necessary, the anticholinergic effects of the antipsychotic agents can "unbalance" the already compromised function of the neurogenic bladder. The alpha-adrenergic properties of these medications can be dangerous because quadriplegics have tenuous control of their blood pressure due to the disruption of thoracclumbar sympathetic outflow. The result could be serious hypotension (Stewart, 1977).

Thus, when antipsychotic medication is required in a patient with condom drainage, it is important to select agents with fewer anticholinergic effects, e.g., haloperidol or piperazine phenothiazines. However, if an antiparkinson drug with anticholinergic properties is used, this advantage is lost.

If injection is required, haloperidol is recommended because it appears to be less irritating than injectable chlorpromazine. The irritated site could lead to a bed sore. Haloperidol should not be used in acute cervical injury since it creates substantial risk for an oculogyric crisis, particularly when injected in young men.

Stuttering

Haloperidol has been found useful in the treatment of young adult stutterers. The drug had a significant effect on the percentage of time the patients were dysfluent but not on the number of dysfluencies per minute (Rosenberger et al., 1976). The hesitation and phonemic stoppage of the severe stutterer may be most dramatically affected by haloperidol. The characteristic facial contortion found under the condition of severe stuttering almost completely disappears. Dosage of haloperidol recommended is 1 mg. 3 times a day. Teenagers have shown an inability to tolerate the side effects and discontinuation of medication results.

Vertigo

Oral haloperidol may be effective for the control of vertigo (Duberstein, 1977). The phenothiazines as a class are not generally very effective in the treatment of emesis due to vestibular disturbance, despite its action upon the "vomiting center."

Mental Retardation

Although the antipsychotic drugs, especially chlorpromazine and thioridazine, are extensively prescribed for the mentally retarded, the efficacy of pharmacotherapy has not received the adequate objective testing that is required to permit firm conclusions of the behavioral and cognitive effects of these medications. However, it seems likely that the antipsychotic drugs may be effective in reducing such behaviors as hostile-aggressive-outbursts, self-mutilation and stereotyped movements. The efficacy of thioridazine is most firmly established, followed by chlorpromazine and more questionably by trifluoperazine and haloperidol.

Some pediatric psychopharmacologists recommend that only 2 phenothiazines, chlorpromazine and thioridazine, be recognized as effective for the treatment of mentally retarded children on the basis of the available scientific literature. Their recommendation stresses the use of these medications mainly for the treatment of severe behavior problems such as persistent hyperactivity, combativeness, self-mutilation and nonprovoked explosive excitability. There is very little evidence to suggest that doses higher than 500 mg. of chlorpromazine or 400 mg. thioridazine are required and efficacy has not been established for periods longer than 6 months. They believe that these drugs may cause a possible reduction in learning performance and periodic discontinuation once or twice a year to assess the effects of the medication on the behavior problem is suggested (Sprague, 1975).

During the past decade, there has been a shift of mentally retarded individuals from institutions into the community. This change has been accompanied by a reduction in the use of antipsychotic drugs and less polypharmacy prescribed for the mentally retarded. There are still large numbers receiving these drugs unnecessarily and, all too often, the medication is given for staff convenience. For example, if restlessness is observed, commonly that person will soon be receiving an antipsychotic agent.

The prevalence of psychosis among the mentally retarded is believed to be about the same as among the population in general. The target symptoms of their psychoses do not respond as well to antipsychotics as those of the schizophrenic patient. It has been found that the dosage of antipsychotic drugs prescribed for many mentally retarded can be markedly reduced or even discontinued. However, in the mental retardate with psychotic symptoms or severe behavior problems, especially of the type mentioned above, a trial on a substantial dose of an antipsychotic agent often results in striking improvement.

It has been noted that the vast majority of the population in many mental retardation facilities are adults rather than children. Most of the residents have had thioridazine and, to a lesser extent, chlorpromazine in small (pediatric) or moderate doses prescribed for them for long periods of time. This may account for the lack of therapeutic optimism with antipsychotic drugs in management of behavior problems in mental retardation. However, psychopathology or behavior problems such as hostilities, aggressions, self-mutilation, assaultiveness, hyperactivity, agitation, destructiveness, uncooperativeness and other such target symptoms are just as likely to respond to antipsychotic drugs in adults regardless of the presence or absence of mental retardation.

These residents deserve trials on the newer antipsychotics (i.e., mesoridazine/Serentil; loxapine/Loxitane) or the low-dose drugs (i.e., haloperidol/Haldol; thiothixene/Navane; fluphenazine/Prolixin; perphenazine/Trilafon), with the dosage carefully titrated upward to attain optimal therapeutic results. An effective response then will give these individuals the opportunity to participate in and benefit from non-drug programs such as behavior modification, special education and other learning and habilitative modalities.

Acute Intermittent Porphyria

Chlorpromazine is effective for the control of acute intermittent porphyria. Oral dosage consists of 25 to 50 mg. t.i.d. or q.i.d. Medication can usually be discontinued after several weeks but maintenance therapy may be necessary for some patients. Intramuscular injection of 25 mg. (1 ml) t.i.d. or q.i.d. may be used until patient can take oral therapy (*PDR*, 1978).

Intractable Hiccups

Chlorpromazine has been found to afford relief for intractable hiccups. The recommended oral dosage is 25 to 50 mg. t.i.d. or q.i.d. If symptoms persist for 2 or 3 days 25 to 50 mg. (1-2 ml) intramuscularly can be given. Should symptoms still persist, the use of *slow* IV infusion (with the patient flat in bed) of 25 to 50 mg. (1-2 ml) in 500 to 1000 ml of saline is recommended. The blood pressure should be closely followed (*PDR*, 1978).

Tetanus

Chlorpromazine may be used as an adjunct in the treatment of tetanus. Intramuscular dosage consists of 25 to 50 mg. (1-2 ml) given 3 or 4 times daily, usually in conjunction with barbiturates. The total doses and the frequency of administration must be determined by the patient's response, starting with low doses and increasing gradually. Intravenous dosage recommended consists of 25 to 50 mg. (1-2 ml). The IV medication should be diluted to at least 1 mg. per ml and administered at a rate of 1 mg. per minute (*PDR*, 1978).

7. COMBINED WITH OTHER THERAPEUTIC MODALITIES

It is generally recognized that antipsychotic drugs constitute the primary treatment for acute and chronic schizophrenia. However, the most effective regimen for the treatment of schizophrenia is an integrated effort combining an organic, psychological and environmental therapeutic approach which is carefully individualized. Many chronic patients have been removed from social activity for years and there is atrophy of basic personal and interpersonal skills. Their pre-illness baseline may have been characterized by social isolation and inadequate role performance in school, at work, or at home. Improvement on drugs may simply indicate that patients are more manageable and tractable in the hospital but may not indicate that they have become more socially responsible and self-sufficient human beings. Drugs can never serve as a substitute for psychological attempts to solve the array of problems which contributed to the original hospitalization of individual patients and which continued to make them fearful about leaving the hospital. It should be recognized that while antipsychotic drugs may enhance coping behavior, they cannot resolve financial and employment difficulties, poor socialization skills, family conflicts and personal fears and anxieties (Ludwig, 1973).

It has been shown that individual psychotherapy alone (even with experienced psychotherapists) does little or nothing for chronic schizophrenic patients in 2 years' time (Grinspoon and Shader, 1975). Psychotherapy for a much longer period is rarely feasible because of the expense and time involved. For acute schizophrenic patients, individual psychotherapy given once or twice weekly, either with or without drugs, seems to offer little advantage over the usual "drugs alone" state hospital treatment. The value of insight or uncovering therapy is, at best, dubious. For all practical purposes, psychotherapy cannot be considered an acceptable treatment for schizophrenic patients in general (Lehmann, 1975).

However, group psychotherapy in conjunction with drug therapy is of some benefit. This type of therapy must center around reality or a group activity. Group activity aimed at psychological understanding and the promotion of insights is usually ineffective. Beneficial results can be obtained from outpatient psychotherapy when the focus is on social and occupational rehabilitation, on problem-solving and on cooperation with pharmacotherapy (May, 1976). Claghorn and his associates (1974) found that group therapy, when added to antipsychotic medication in the treatment of outpatient schizophrenics, did not alter patients' symptomatology. According to projective test results, it did deepen the subject's awareness and insight into his own behavior. Many clinicians have recommended that aftercare programs shift to much greater use of group therapy of a supportive, reality-oriented type, accompanied by appropriate use of pharmacotherapy. Instead of seeing an endless succession of patients one after another for brief periods of time, therapists should spend a much larger block of time with one group of patients. In this way, patients gain a sense of belonging and have an opportunity for increased socialization.

The question has been raised whether milieu therapy really adds to the treatment of schizophrenics, once optimal drug therapy is used and gross neglect corrected. Particularly for the chronic schizophrenic patient, the addition of milieu therapy fails to produce significant improvement (Van Putten, 1973). The case for adoption of "therapeutic community" measures found in an enriched milieu rests on general humanitarian ground rather than on the therapeutic benefit to be derived in chronic schizophrenic patients (Letemendia et al., 1967).

Milieu therapy with its emphasis on active treatment may be of some value in preventing institutionalism. The therapeutic atmosphere of many milieu wards is characterized by very high stimulus input. The emphasis is on liveliness and spontaneity and the patient is forced to interact with a large staff and various groups. The possibility that social withdrawal may serve as a protective mechanism against excessive stimulation is not considered. An enriched milieu environment may be toxic for over-aroused schizophrenic patients with disturbed attention. In lively group meetings, they often become worse as reflected by increasing agitation, bewilderment or withdrawal. However, inpatient milieu treatment has been shown to be effective when there is a concentration on real life problems and on planning for discharge (May, 1976).

Depending upon the individual needs of the patient, the rehabilitation programs should be geared to recognize the need for social rehabilitation and preparation for community adjustment. Retraining and reeducation should include diet, exercise, personal hygiene, good grooming and etiquette, caring, selecting and purchasing clothing, the use of cosmetics and general health suggestions. Through group discussions, films, role-playing, bus schedules, restaurant menus, teaching telephones and other pertinent material, the patient can become acquainted with specific situations he may encounter in the community. The objective of resocialization programs should be to raise the level of social competence.

Social competence is unlikely to improve unless the chronic patient is offered some kind of long-term social retraining. The patient must learn to bathe regularly, dress with some decorum, eat inoffensively and respond appropriately to simple requests. Sheltered workshops, social clubs, bibliotherapy, music and dance therapies, when properly prescribed and structured, can help the patient maintain his ability to interact with others, remain interested in the outside world and retain his ties with the larger community. Day hospital care, halfway houses, night hospitals and many other types of community placement programs may help ease the transition to life outside the hospital (Detre and Jarecki, 1971).

Aftercare programs can help the patient remain in the community after discharge from the hospital. It has been shown that day care or home care programs, when feasible and practical, may serve the patient as well as or even better than inpatient programs, provided adequate drug treatment is continued. Successful programs focus mainly on problem-solving, social adjustment, living arrangements, obtaining employment and facilitating cooperation with maintenance drug therapy. Both inpatient and outpatient social rehabilitation classes can help prepare patients for community living.

Hogarty and associates (1975) have demonstrated that sociotherapy can augment drug therapy to some extent for the patient in the community. The sociotherapy which they called Major Role Therapy (MRT) was a combination of intensive individual social casework and vocational rehabilitation counseling. MRT was administered by master's degree social workers with an average of nearly 7 years of experience. It was viewed as a problem-solving method designed to respond to the interpersonal, personal, social and rehabilitative needs of both patients and their families. The primary goal was the resolution of personal or environmental problems that directly influenced the patient's major role performance, either as a homemaker or as an actual or potential wage earner. Otherwise, therapeutic objectives ranged from improving the quality of interpersonal relationships and avoiding social isolation to such rudiments as self-care, financial assistance, housing and taking medication. However, MRT had a positive influence on adjustment only after 18 and 24 months following hospital discharge and then only in combination with drug therapy. MRT had some effect beyond antipsychotic drugs in preventing relapse, particularly for female schizophrenic patients.

Stein and Test (1976) have demonstrated that a "unique" treatment model, "Training in Community Living," virtually eliminated hospitalization or readmissions. A staff of psychiatrists, psychologists, social workers, occupational therapists, nurses and aides were retrained to work with patients, families, community agents and individuals to mobilize all possible support systems for the patients' benefit. Every effort was made to avoid hospitalization except for patients who were suicidal or homicidal or who required such high doses of medication that a structured environment was necessary.

The patients lived in independent settings scattered through the community. In addition to pharmacotherapy (usually a depot phenothiazine), treatment consisted of participation in a full schedule of daily activities. The therapeutic staff motivated and supported the patients by being present or available at all hours. Staff members were visitors in the patients' homes and neighborhoods. They taught patients daily living techniques such as laundry upkeep, shopping, cooking, using restaurants, grooming, budgeting, and using transportation facilities. Patients were given intensive assistance in finding jobs or sheltered workshop placements and the staff continued daily contact with the patients and with their supervisors or employers to help with on-the-job problems. Leisure time was enhanced through the development of the patients' social skills; the staff arranged relevant community recreation and social activities. Patients in the program were superior to control patients on all measures of adjustment. Only 18% required hospitalization during the first year. This was in contrast to 89% of the patients who did not receive the benefit of this program.

There is scant evidence that the effect of electroconvulsive therapy (ECT) in schizophrenic patients is enhanced by antipsychotic drugs. Occasional serious complications and even deaths have been reported with the combined therapy. There may be the additional risk of tardive dyskinesia. Therefore, it seems prudent to avoid combining antipsychotics with ECT unless the patient does not respond to either treatment alone. When antipsychotic therapy is used to manage severely agitated or excited patients during the early phase of a course of ECT, the drug should be withdrawn when no longer needed (Abrams, 1975). If the combined therapy is deemed necessary, it is recommended that the morning dose of antipsychotic be omitted before ECT treatment. If the drug dosage is high, it is also wise to omit the evening dose prior to the ECT treatment day. Some severely ill patients will require continued drug therapy during a course of ECT to maintain symptom control on inter-treatment days. Although conjoint treatment may be necessary, it does not provide any evidence for a synergistic effect of ECT and antipsychotic drugs.

It has been stated that the psychological, economic, vocational and social environments of the patient are as important as drugs in the long-term treatment of schizophrenia (Davis, 1975). They should be used jointly with drug therapy but it is clear that in no sense are they substitutes for adequate drug treatment. To a lesser or greater extent, modalities such as social and rehabilitation therapy, group psychotherapy, milieu therapy, family therapy, behavior modification, day care, partial hospitalization and other programs can augment the therapeutic response to antipsychotic drugs. However, if optimal results are to be obtained, comprehensive and intensive efforts must be directed toward changing basic maladaptive attitudes and behaviors of the chronic schizophrenic patient to alter elements of the patient-staff culture in mental hospitals conducive to the perpetuation of chronicity and to an extensive retraining and rehabilitation program designed to enhance the coping, interpersonal and economic skill of patients. Some person must have a relationship with the schizophrenic patient to help him in the practical affairs of everyday living. This individual, whether called a "case manager" or by some other title, must have the responsibility and accountability on an ongoing basis to arrange for follow-up, drug intake, regular medical review and to coordinate the necessary supportive and rehabilitative services for the patient in the community. Traditionally and otherwise, the professional social worker is best suited for this role. However, with the present inflationary budget crunch, volunteers will have to be recruited and trained so that they can become successful "support" personnel under the guidance and supervision of the mental health professional.

8. THE DEPOT FLUPHENAZINES

The long-acting injectable phenothiazines, fluphenazine enanthate and fluphenazine decanoate are commonly referred to as the depot fluphenazines. The introduction of these drugs constitutes one of the milestones in the development of psychopharmacology. This major advance in the antipsychotic drug treatment of schizophrenia has the potential of ensuring continuous medication and stimulating the development of adequate community care service that can result in significant reduction of relapses and readmissions.

Fluphenazine and perphenazine are the only 2 commonly used phenothiazines that possess an alkyl-piperazine side chain that allows them to be esterified with a long chain of fatty acid (Sanseigne, 1970). The effective duration of orally taken fluphenazine hydrochloride is about 24 hours. When it is dissolved in sesame oil and injected parenterally, the duration of effect is doubled (Laffan et al., 1965). If the fluphenazine hydrochloride is esterified with a long chain fatty acid, such as heptanoic acid (see fluphenazine enanthate—Figure 5) and dissolved in a sesame oil vehicle, the duration of effect following a single intramuscular injection is 1 or 2 weeks or longer (Burke et al., 1962). The prolonged effect of the ester reflects the low rate of absorption of the esterified phenothiazine from the sesame oil vehicle, as aqueous solutions of the enanthate do not have prolonged activity.

The successful experience with fluphenazine enanthate stimulated the search for other long-acting drugs. A logical variation stemmed from the use of decanoic acid as the esterifying agent. Apparently, because of the greater number of carbon atoms of the decanoic acid ester, the resulting molecule is even more complex and even slower to hydrolize. Van Praag and Dols (1973), in a double-blind study, found that the therapeutic effect of the decanoate ester lasts longer and is less provocative of untoward motor effects than the enanthate ester. Both of these depot antipsychotics can be given subcutaneously as well as intramuscularly without producing pain, burning or other local reactions.

Many years of clinical experience with fluphenazine enanthate and decanoate have shown that almost any drug can be co-prescribed with them with little or no risk of harmful potentiation or of other forms of adverse interaction. Even the potentiation of barbiturates, sedatives and alcohol declines rapidly, so that after a few weeks most people treated with a depot

FLUPHENAZINE HCL

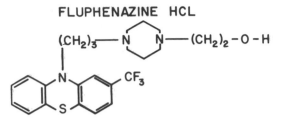

FLUPHENAZINE ENANTHATE

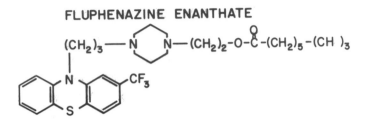

FLUPHENAZINE DECANOATE

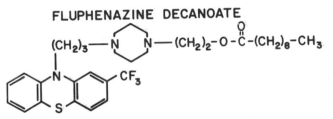

FIGURE 5. Chemical Structure of Fluphenazine HCl, Fluphenazine Enanthate and Fluphenazine Decanoate

antipsychotic can take reasonable doses of any of these agents with only a slight risk of harm (Ayd, 1975b). Thus, depot fluphenazines can be combined safely with a majority of the drugs most commonly prescribed by physicians.

The intramuscular administration of long-acting antipsychotics may be more effective than oral medication since drugs administered orally may be less therapeutic because of poor absorption from the gastrointestinal tract, incompatibility with food or other ingested substances, rapid gastrointestinal motility or inactivation in the intestinal wall. In addition, injected anti-psychotics may reach the central nervous system, their presumed area of therapeutic activity, before passing through the liver where they may be deactivated by microsomal enzymes (Cole, 1970). A double-blind clinical trial of oral chlorpromazine and injectable fluphenazine decanoate has shown a statistically significant difference in favor of the injectable preparation in a group of patients selected for their inability to absorb chlorpromazine effectively. Furthermore, it has been demonstrated that up to 40% of chronic drug-refractory schizophrenics treated with oral chlorpromazine have low serum levels of chlorpromazine and many of these patients improved when given parenterally administered phenothiazines (Adamson et al., 1973).

When patients are switched from fluphenazine enanthate to the same dose levels of the decanoate, the interval between injections can usually be lengthened from 2 weeks to 3 weeks (Lambert and Marcou, 1970). The decanoate causes fewer side effects than the enanthate. It also seems that the therapeutic activity of the decanoate is of better quality, especially as regards passivity in certain schizophrenic patients. There are, however, no significant differences in the therapeutic efficacy for the 2 depot drugs. Both are highly similar in therapeutic effectiveness, dosage levels, prevention of relapse during maintenance therapy and incidence of extrapyramidal symptoms. The decanoate patients require a lower dose to produce symptom remission and maintenance, but, again, the differences are not significant. Antiparkinson agents are much less successful in reducing or preventing parkinsonism and akathisia caused by depot fluphenazines than acute dystonia (Donlon et al., 1976). The decanoate preparation is perhaps somewhat better tolerated and is the depot fluphenazine more often prescribed. However, some patients who fail to respond to the decanoate form may improve when given fluphenazine enanthate.

Ayd (1978a) has emphasized that as part of the art of depot fluphenazine therapy, the therapist, before initiation of injections, should brief the patient and, whenever possible, the family on the possible side effects, especially extrapyramidal reactions, and take steps to minimize the risk of the latter and to have them treated promptly should they occur. This briefing of patients and relatives on the possible side effects of a depot fluphenazine and what can and should be done in the event they occur has many advantages. Should an acute extrapyramidal reaction occur in an outpatient, the forewarned patient and relatives do not panic and can institute appropriate remedial action promptly. In addition, if the severity of an acute extrapyramidal reaction can be minimized and particularly if it can be relieved quickly, patients and families do not become disenchanted and stop treatment but remain willing to continue. On the other hand, the occurrence of an unexpected acute dystonic reaction or of moderate to severe akinesia or akathisia after the first injection is one of the principal reasons for the rejection of depot fluphenazine treatment by patients and families.

There is no standard method of initiating fluphenazine decanoate therapy. The *Physicians' Desk Reference* (1978) suggests the following regimen:

For *most patients*, a dose of 12.5 mg. to 25 mg. (0.5 to 1 ml) may be given to initiate therapy. . . . Subsequent injections and the dosage interval are determined in accordance with the patient's response. . . . When administered as maintenance therapy, a single injection may be effective in controlling schizophrenic symptoms up to 4 weeks or longer. It may be advisable that patients who have had no history of taking phenothiazines should be treated initially with a shorter-acting form of fluphenazine before administering the decanoate to determine the patient's response to fluphenazine and to establish appropriate dosage. Since the dosage comparability of the shorter-acting forms of fluphenazine to the longer-acting decanoate is not known, special caution should be exercised when switching from the shorter-acting forms to the decanoate.

With poor risk patients (those with known hypersensitivity to phenothiazines or with disorders that predispose to undue reactions) therapy may be initiated cautiously with oral or parenteral fluphenazine hydrochloride. When the pharmacologic effects and an appropriate dosage are apparent, an equivalent dose of fluphenazine decanoate injection may be administered. Subsequent dosage adjustments are made in accordance with the response of the patient.

The optimal amount of drug and the frequency of administration must be determined for each patient, since dosage requirements have been found to vary with clinical circumstances as well as with the individual response to the drug. Dosage should not exceed 100 mg. If doses greater than 50 mg. are deemed necessary, the next dose and the succeeding doses should be increased cautiously in increments of 12.5 mg.

Fluphenazine decanoate is usually prescribed on a very empirical basis. Therapy may be initiated according to the patient's body weight, giving 1/100 ml per pound of body weight. Thus a 100-pound person would receive 1 ml (25 mg.), 150-pound person would get 1½ ml (37.5 mg.), etc. This guideline is used to calculate the initial dose for the average psychotic patient, one who may be severely psychotic but is relatively calm and reasonably cooperative. However, if the patient is agitated or hyperactive, the dose might be doubled, going to 2/100 ml per pound. The dose is adjusted according to severity of symptoms, agitation and behavior. In the violent patient, the dose is raised more drastically. This type of agitated patient may be given a minimum of 2 ml and the dosage might rise as high as 2½ or 3 ml, regardless of body weight.

Goldberg (1976) has found that 90% of his patients receive between 1 and 2 ml with about 1½ ml as a starting dose. However, the acutely psychotic patient would receive 2 to 3 ml of fluphenazine decanoate on admission, usually in the admitting room. He is reevaluated on the ward and if a supplemental drug is needed, the patient is given 5 mg. of fluphenazine hydrochloride orally to be repeated every 4 to 6 hours for the first day if necessary. If the patient is still out of control, the dose might be doubled on the second day, but this is rare. By the third day, the oral medication is no longer necessary, since the injected depot drug has usually begun its antipsychotic effect.

The vast majority of patients show significant improvement by the end of the first week. With the less agitated, less psychotic patient who begins to respond, calms down and can be discharged in a week, a schedule of an injection every 3 weeks on the same dose is prescribed. No problems have been encountered with this regimen. The more agitated patient is given 2 or 3 ml a week after the initial injection and seen again in a week but not given another dose until at least 10 days have elapsed. The patient is then placed on a 2-week interval regimen. Usually, if the patient fails to respond to adequate doses injected weekly for 3 or 4 weeks, consideration is given to a switch to another drug.

When the patient becomes compensated and only requires a maintenance regimen, the time interval between injections is lengthened. If the patient is getting injections every 3 weeks, a change is made to a 4-week interval for 3 visits. If this regimen is successful, a 5-week interval regimen is instituted. Slow, gradual reduction of dosage is started (¼ ml each time an injection is given) after the patient remains symptom-free on a 4 to 6 week interval schedule. The objective is to give the drug as infrequently and at as low dosage as is possible to maintain compensation. Some patients can be maintained on 25 mg. every 6 to 10 weeks.

With a more conservative approach, the starting dose and the intervals between injection are carefully selected for each individual and such factors as age, physical condition, the nature and severity of the illness and the drug history of the patient and his family are taken into consideration. The lowest possible dose may be best to inaugurate treatment. Ayd (1975b, 1976a) believes that it is prudent to initiate depot fluphenazine therapy with a test dose of 1/10 ml (2.5 mg.). If this dose is tolerated, the dose can be increased at short intervals. The dose may have to be repeated 24 hours later but more often 2/10 ml is given after 18 to 72 hours. In 4 to 5 days, 3/10 ml will be given; after a wait of 5 days, another 3/10 ml injection is given. With this regimen, in 14 days the patient has received about 1 full ml. The immediate objective with this method is not to achieve a true antipsychotic effect but sufficient symptom control so that the patient suffering from a chronic illness can function outside of a hospital and be treated as an outpatient.

A variation of this technique for initiation of therapy is as follows: Give .1 ml of the drug on days 1, 3, 5, and 8; .2 ml on day 12; .5 ml on day 19; and 1 ml on day 26. Thereafter, for several months, 1 ml or more is given every 14 days, always balancing clinical effects against side effects (Bakke, 1973).

Ayd (1976a) is convinced that a substantial number of the adverse reactions noted at the beginning of depot fluphenazine therapy are a direct consequence of initiating therapy with too high a dose, especially for patients whose tissues retain much of previously administered antipsychotic agent(s). These reactions can be avoided by a drug holiday and by starting low dose injections to a chronic patient for whom there is no rush to achieve immediate therapeutic response.

Although acutely psychotic schizophrenics can be treated successfully from the outset with depot fluphenazines (see Chapter III), most clinicians still prefer to start therapy with a short-acting antipsychotic (either oral or injectable). After clinical stabilization for a week or two, a switch is made to long-acting fluphenazine, usually the decanoate form (the conversion from oral antipsychotic to the depot fluphenazine is discussed under Section 2 in Chapter III). After control has been maintained for 3 months with no significant change in clinical status, the dosage per injection can be reduced or the interval between injections can be lengthened. Thus, the patient may need 25 mg. every 2 weeks for the first 6 months of treatment, 25 mg. every 3 weeks for the next 3 months and so on until the interval is increased to 4 weeks or longer.

By gradually adjusting dose and interval, the risk of distressing side effects which might cause the patient to discontinue medication is minimized. The family members see the patient far more in terms of time than the physician and, if they see the patient is very stiff or very restless, they will be reluctant to persuade him to continue with injections. The physician should listen very carefully to family members and have them particularly note what happens in the 48 to 72 hours after an injection when the more troublesome side effects may occur.

Grozier (1973) recommends fluphenazine enanthate or fluphenazine decanoate therapy in chronic schizophrenics as follows:

(1) Pretreatment with oral fluphenazine is usually not necessary.
(2) Initial dose: 0.5 ml (12.5 mg.); range: 0.25 ml (6.25 mg.) to 2 ml (50.0 mg.)
(3) Second injections: 0.5 ml (12.5 mg.) to 3 ml (75 mg.) after 1 week, depending on the clinical situation.
(4) Subsequent injections: 1 ml (25 mg.); range: 0.5 ml (12.5 mg.) to 4 ml (100 mg.) at intervals of 1 to 5 weeks, depending on individual patient response and sensitivity.

To minimize the risk of inadvertent overdose and severe side effects, especially extrapyramidal reactions, at the outset of depot fluphenazine therapy for chronic patients being switched from oral antipsychotics, it may be wise to first place the patient on a drug holiday for at least a week. A substantial number of adverse reactions noted in the beginning of depot fluphenazine treatment are a direct consequence of initiating therapy with too high a dose which superimposes the fluphenazine on the accumulated oral antipsychotic in the patient's tissues.

Some therapists, especially in Europe, use high doses of the depot fluphenazines in the treatment of the chronic schizophrenic patient. Doses ranging from 100 to 500 mg. have been used and the clinicians experienced with this high-dose therapy believe that it is remarkably safe and does not cause a significantly higher incidence of extrapyramidal reactions than low-dose therapy. Short-term high-dose depot fluphenazine therapy has been and is being used effectively for the treatment of acute schizophrenic, manic and other severely disturbed psychotic patients with moderate or marked agitation. Bakke in Scandinavia (1973) reported treatment of 30 acute patients with 200 to 500 mg. (usually 200 to 250 mg.) of fluphenazine enanthate. In France, Ropert and his associates (1973) treated acute manic patients whose ages ranged from 27 to 62 years with 75 to 300 mg. of fluphenazine enanthate or with 100 to 300 mg. of fluphenazine decanoate. The use of the above high dosages is cited only to suggest the relative safety of the depot fluphenazines.

In this country, Owens (1978) has reported on the use of dosages up to 150 mg. of fluphenazine enanthate in chronic schizophrenics who had not responded to lesser dosages with favorable results. During the past 2½ years, doses up to 250 mg. of fluphenazine enanthate weekly have been used. Occasionally, doses as high as 500 mg. a week have been given for short periods of time ranging from 1 to 6 weeks with no alarming side effects and with remarkable amelioration of symptoms. Some of these patients require high maintenance doses in the range between 75 mg. and 125 mg. a week and rapidly show regressive symptoms on lower doses or on the same number of milligrams in the decanoate form. However, for most outpatients, the intervals between injections is gradually increased, so that 6 months after hospital discharge a patient is typically receiving only 6.25 to 75 mg. of the depot fluphenazine every month. In general, Owens has found that the decanoate form seems to be more advantageous in low to moderate maintenance doses when the injection interval is increased beyond 3 weeks. There are some patients on dosages as low as 6.25 mg. of fluphenazine enanthate who rapidly regress on the decanoate form. At the end of 1 year, the typical patient is receiving 50 mg. of fluphenazine decanoate at intervals of 4 to 8 weeks. This type of schedule assures medication individualized to control symptoms; a low lifetime dosage if long-term maintenance is required, compared to oral fluphenazine or the other low-dose antipsychotics such as trifluoperazine and haloperidol; and the total 1-month or 2-month dose in 1 injection provides a drug holiday 6 to 12 times a year so that dyskinesia is noted early if it occurs.

It is recommended, however, that, generally, high-dose therapy be reserved for those chronic schizophrenics most likely to benefit from it. These are physically fit patients under 40 with acute onset rather than a slow evolution of their psychosis, who have been ill less than 10 years, who have had some response to antipsychotic therapy and who are still reacting with affect to their delusions and hallucinations rather than accepting them complacently. When maximum improvement is reached in these patients (which may not be for 4 to 6 months), the depot fluphenazine should be reduced gradually to the lowest effective individual maintenance dose.

Oral fluphenazine hydrochloride in combination temporarily with a depot fluphenazine may be necessary to control the acute psychotic symptoms initially. However, a faulty prescribing practice consists of maintaining the patient on both forms of the drug for weeks and months. Often the dosage of either medication is inadequate. At other times, the oral antipsychotic agent is other than fluphenazine hydrochloride, thus creating a polypharmacy situation.

Some schizophrenic outpatients receiving maintenance depot fluphenazine therapy fail to return for further injections. The majority of these relapse, and for many, hospitalization is necessary. At the time of readmission, these patients can be given either fluphenazine enanthate or decanoate immediately and usually respond to the depot fluphenazine in the same way they had previously. Some clinicians now reinstate depot fluphenazine therapy promptly in relapsing outpatients and have learned that quick administration of proper doses of a depot antipsychotic can produce sufficient symptom amelioration to obviate the need for rehospitalization.

A depot fluphenazine regimen for outpatients in non-emergent situations that has proved successful consists of initiating treatment with .125 ml. A second injection of .125 ml or .25 ml is given 5 to 7 days later. Patients are seen at least weekly. If side effects are manageable and symptoms so indicate, dosage is increased by .25 ml per week. After 6 to 8 weeks, if the clinical picture is stable, the patient may be switched to a bimonthly schedule, receiving the same dosage or 1½ times the weekly dosage. Most patients are scheduled for injection every 1 or 2 weeks unless their work situation interferes with such frequent clinic visits. Frequent appointments encourage habit formation and facilitate close monitoring for detection and management of side effects (i.e., depression) and change in mental status (Amdur, 1978).

A common error consists of maintaining the patient on a fixed dosage and time interval indefinitely. It is emphasized that the dose and the interval between injections must remain flexible to establish optimal maintenance dosage and demonstrate the need for continued medication. During periods of stress and evidence of psychotic decompensation, the dose and frequency of administration may have to be increased.

Geriatric patients are possibly the most unreliable takers of tablets. They often have a distrust and dislike of drugs, specifically in the form of tablets; they may be forgetful; they may have difficulty in swallowing and periods of confusion. Paranoid symptoms in the elderly may contribute to drug deviation or refusal. When initiating depot phenothiazine therapy for chronic patients over the age of 50, it is wise to start with a .1 cc dose. The older the patient, the less tolerant of oral and depot antipsychotics he is likely to be. The risk of antipsychotics causing extrapyramidal reactions is highest in the geriatric population. Therefore it is especially important that elderly patients not be given high doses of a depot fluphenazine at the beginning of therapy. The majority of these patients are best treated with low doses at short intervals, for example, .1 to .2 cc every week or 10 days rather than higher doses at 2- or 3-week intervals (Ayd, 1975b).

Some clinicians will start the elderly patient with a larger dose (usually ¼ ml) and gradually increase the dosage if necessary. Usually 1 ml is the maximum. However, if the initial ¼ ml injection ameliorates some symptoms but the patient is still symptomatic, a second dose of ½ ml may be given in 2 weeks. This 2-week interval regimen is maintained unless the patient is in a nursing home and is disruptive. In such instances, the dosage would have to be raised to control the target symptoms and avoid a transfer to a mental hospital.

Raskind and his colleagues (1976) have demonstrated that low dose depot fluphenazine for outpatient geriatric psychotics can be practical, safe and effective. To cope with the variety of acute psychoses in the elderly, they start treatment at the patient's home with a 5 mg. (0.2 ml) dose and monitor the patient's status daily for the first week. They have found that this low dose frequently markedly relieves psychotic symptoms and that, although periodic repeat doses are usually necessary, several patients have been treated successfully with 1 injection and have not had recurrence of severe psychosis at a 6-month followup.

In view of their relatively slow onset of action (24 to 96 hours) the depot fluphenazines are not generally recommended as the initial treatment of acute conditions. Usually they should be employed with inpatients who are first stabilized on oral doses or with outpatients who are unreliable about taking daily medications. A prime candidate is the patient who lives alone and has no family or friends to ensure that he is taking the medication properly. Without proper drug therapy, these chronic schizophrenic patients would be confined to mental hospitals for part or all of their lives. Other types of patients who benefit from the long-acting fluphenazines are the patients who are resistant to oral medication because of poor absorption or rapid enzyme induction, patients requiring long-term medication, those refusing all oral medication, and patients inadequately treated because of the high cost of drugs or the unavailability of treatment facilities. In addition, the patient who sequesters drugs with the consequent possibility of suicide is prevented from doing so.

Grazier (1973) has pointed out that the advantages of the long-acting fluphenazines include: (a) adequate continuous therapy without the need for frequent administration of oral or injectable doses; (b) full control and full knowledge of treatment by the physician (knowing immediately when the patient has discontinued treatment); (c) lower doses of drug are required, resulting in safer and less expensive treatment. Thus, drug holidays, which may sometimes be confusing to the patient and family, are not required. (d) Controlled studies with fluphenazine enanthate and fluphenazine decanoate have shown that the number and duration of hospital readmissions have been significantly reduced when treatment with these drugs was compared with standard oral therapy.

In the United Kingdom and more recently in the United States, some community mental health clinics have been converted to decanoate clinics, wherein discharged schizophrenics in remission routinely receive injections of either fluphenazine enanthate or fluphenazine decanoate. When patients are unable to attend the clinic, the local public health nurse gives them the injections at home.

The period immediately following discharge from the hospital may be a critical time for the schizophrenic. The necessity of readapting himself to the community, family and friends may impose a stress and strain unlike anything experienced in the protective environment of the hospital. Yet this is a time when many patients abandon the very drug therapy that brought them to the point of discharge. Goldberg et al. (1976) estimate that approximately 50% of all discharged psychotic patients fail to take even the first dose of their outpatient medication. The often difficult responsibility imposed on family members to supervise outpatient medication is also avoided by the use of these long-acting drugs. During these periods, fluphenazine decanoate enables the physician to monitor the patient's medication to a degree not possible with oral therapy. In spite of a high incidence of akinesia, it still may be preferable to use fluphenazine decanoate rather than an oral antipsychotic because extrapyramidal side effects are observable, especially when the clinician is sensitive to their emergence, whereas covert noncompliance with pill-taking is not. The long-acting injectable, therefore, offers an advantage in patient management particularly applicable to community mental health programs.

For inpatient settings, the use of daily doses of oral medication is inconvenient and annoying, constantly reminding the patient of his need for medication and is an uneconomical use of staff time. The nursing staff welcome relief from this situation through the use of depot fluphenazines, which enables them to spend more time with patients. The disadvantage of the depot fluphenazines is that some patients object to being injected.

The depot fluphenazines have proven to be as safe as any potent oral antipsychotic, if not more so. Even after years of use, absorption of successive injections is most satisfactory, without any occurrence of inflamation or local induration. Differences in results or frequency of an adverse effect more likely reflect differences in the skill of the clinician than any other factor. In addition, these agents have the ability to control the symptoms of chronic schizophrenic patients at doses significantly lower than oral doses of the same or other antipsychotic drugs.

It is stressed the depot fluphenazines, just like the other antipsychotics, are not a substitute for careful and frequent patient observation. Despite their safety, all patients treated with them should be carefully followed for reactivation of illness or occurrence of side effects. However, the potential risk of these side effects should not prevent the use of these drugs in adequate doses for the time required to achieve the maximum therapeutic effect. This treatment may be required for many years or a lifetime.

As Grozier (1973) has aptly stated: "**These drugs are not curative and only control a patient's symptomatology and, therefore, it is more important that the physician not rely completely on the long-acting depot antipsychotics for treatment, but continue to use his diagnostic judgement and clinical acumen in adjusting the dosage in response to the individual patient's physical characteristics, diagnosis, environment and lifestyle, along with initiating whatever other forms of therapy a patient may require.**" With an organized system of drug maintenance and essential aftercare including social and vocational supports, patient and family education, vigorous follow-up and a therapist-patient relationship, the depot fluphenazines may appreciably slow down the revolving door syndrome of mental hospitals.

9. ANTIPSYCHOTIC DRUG THERAPY AND THE NURSING STAFF*

The nursing staff should be informed and trained for their specific duties in regard to patients on antipsychotic drug therapy.

The nursing personnel play a very important role in the administration of antipsychotic agents for several reasons: (1) Patient response to medication requires 24-hour per day observation by nursing personnel and (2) astute and accurate observation of side effects in the patient provides vital information for the physician. Some patients may be unable to verbally state that they are having problems because they cannot communicate or may be

---

*Adapted with permission from *Introductory Clinical Pharmacology*, by Shearer, J. C., J. B. Lippincott, 1975.

delusional or are unaware of physical changes. For example, their illness may prevent them from relating to the physician or nurse that they have a rash that itches or are constipated or feel restless. It is the nurse then who must closely observe these patients for any physical or mental changes. Observation of patient activities may also lead one to suspect the occurrence of side effects; for instance, the appearance of a tremor of the hands, a change in gait or posture or smacking or licking of lips may indicate extrapyramidal involvement.

Patient response to medication should be noted throughout the day and night. Daily activities—eating, occupational therapy, interactions with others—should be closely observed. All activity and patient responses are important, as drug therapy may be changed or adjusted according to changes (or lack of changes) seen. It is also important to stay with the patient when medications are taken. If there is any doubt as to whether the patient is swallowing the drug or possibly vomiting (self-induced) immediately after the drug is taken, the physician should be told, as other routes of administration may be necessary.

Contact dermatitis due to the handling of liquid forms of chlorpromazine and other phenothiazines has been reported. Rubber gloves should be worn while preparing the solution and gloves, dropper and bottle should be washed after each handling. Persons with known sensitivity to phenothiazine drugs should avoid direct contact with the liquid preparations of these drugs.

The nursing staff can help reinforce the explanation made by the physician to the patient that this drug will help him and that taking the medication at regular intervals is essential if he wants to get well and stay well. They can reassure the patient that sometimes he will experience annoying side effects while on medication, that these are only temporary and that, if necessary, the doctor can take steps to relieve the condition. Members of his family should be given an explanation and reassurance beforehand when they come to visit the patient who is displaying prominent symptoms of a side effect.

It is important for the nursing staff to encourage the patients to move around and engage in ward activities even though participation may be limited at first. As the patient improves, he should be helped to improve personal appearance and to socialize. The handling of these patients often involves working closely with them, creating constructive activities to keep them occupied and emphasizing the social amenities.

Because drug therapy is just as important to the outpatient or the discharged patient as it is to the hospitalized patient, the nurse must stress the need for continuing medication to both the patient and his relatives. The family must be made to understand that, regardless of how "well" the patient may seem, skipped or forgotten doses may lead to unpleasant symptomatic outbreaks and that discontinuance of the drug may result in a relapse and readmission to the hospital.

In the hospital situation it is important to be aware of the potential hazards associated with the use of antipsychotics. The first step in recognizing side effects is knowing what they are. Listing the side effects of these agents on cards which can be posted in the medicine room will remind personnel. The second step is to take routine precautions for each type of drug.

Precautions

(1) Avoid exposure to sunlight (due to photosensitivity reactions).

(2) Vital signs monitored, especially during the early phase of therapy (hypotension, cardiac irregularities).

(3) Bed patients—assist in and out of bed or chair slowly (postural hypotension).

(4) Maintain blood pressure chart. Obtain the recumbent, sitting and standing blood pressures if possible.

(5) Parenteral form of these drugs—give deep IM and keep the patient flat one-half hour after administration (postural hypotension).

(6) Take blood pressure before each intramuscular injection of an antipsychotic and 30 to 60 minutes later—after 3 minutes in the standing position if possible. Notify physician if the systolic blood pressure falls below the 90-100 mm Hg range or there is a fall of more than 20 mm HG in the systolic blood pressure.

(7) Parenteral form of these drugs, especially with the high-potency antipsychotics or with a rapid tranquilization procedure—be alert for the sudden appearance of an acute dystonic reaction (such as laryngospasm and difficulty in breathing).

(8) Inspect skin for redness, rash, color changes, pigmentation daily.

(9) Those with history of seizures—watch for convulsions, keep airway handy (but not necessarily in the patient's room).

(10) Supervise routine activities if excessive drowsiness is apparent.

(11) Suicide risk if patient appears depressed; suicide precautions may be necessary.

(12) Observe sleep pattern of patients closely, especially during the night, for sleep is a vital clue if an effective therapeutic dose has been reached.

(13) When a drug order reads h.s., the antipsychotic agent should be given 1-2 hours before bedtime.

(14) When dispensing tablets of antipsychotic drugs, make certain they are swallowed, not "cheeked" and later disposed.

(15) Be especially alert regarding drug-defaulting by patients who do not respond to adequate doses or who improved on medication and have begun to relapse.

(16) Since more than one-half of the side effects caused by psychotropic drugs occur during the first week of treatment, carefully observe patients during this period for the most frequent side effects: drowsiness, slurred speech, dry mouth, constipation, rigidity,

restlessness, hypotension and dystonic reactions.

(17) Be alert for the reappearance of extrapyramidal symptoms when antiparkinson medication is discontinued.

(18) When giving fluphenazine enanthate or fluphenazine decanoate intramuscularly or subcutaneously, use a dry syringe and a needle of at least 21 gauge. The use of a wet needle or syringe may cause the solution to become cloudy.

10. ADMINISTRATIVE MEDICATION GUIDELINES*

It is recommended that the following administrative medication guidelines be adopted by psychiatric facilities where antipsychotic drugs are administered.

(1) Medication shall be administered only at the order of a physician. (Emergency phone orders may be used provided the physician countersigns the order within 24 hours.)

(2) The rationale for the medication (i.e., target symptoms) shall be included in the patient's treatment plan.

(3) The drug regimen of a newly admitted patient or an acutely psychotic patient will be reviewed at least weekly by the attending physician.

(4) Administration of antipsychotic medication and related drugs for the chronic patient shall be reviewed not less than every 30 days to determine the appropriateness of continued care.

(5) Medication shall not be used as a punishment or for the convenience of the staff.

(6) Original periods of administration should not exceed 30 days per prescription before it is represcribed on the basis of the patient's response.

(7) The physician shall specify the number of days for a PRN order if it is to exceed 48 hours.

(8) Medication should be administered by qualified and trained facility personnel.

(9) The administration of medication shall be recorded in the patient's medical record.

(10) Medication cards or other approved systems shall be used in the preparation and administration of medication.

(11) Medication errors and adverse drug reactions shall be immediately reported to a physician and shall be recorded in the patient's clinical record. The facility director and chief of staff should be informed.

(12) Nursing units shall be equipped with adequate medication areas

---

*Adapted from guidelines for the use of psychotropic drugs issued by the Michigan Department of Mental Health, 1976.

    providing appropriate and sufficient spaces for dosage preparation
and setup.

(13) Medications shall be given to patients upon leave or discharge
only on written authorization of a physician.

(14) Medications given to patients upon leave or discharge shall comply with state rules and federal regulations pertaining to labeling
and packaging.

(15) Medication should not exceed United States Food and Drug
Administration standards (as in *Physicians' Desk Reference, American Medical Association Drug Evaluations*, second edition, and/or
Hospital Formulary Service) unless the medical rationale is documented in the patient's clinical record in accordance with written
review procedures established by the hospital staff.

11. ECONOMIC FACTORS

**Millions of dollars can be saved annually if certain general guidelines
are followed whenever possible.**

Mental health care costs, just like other health care costs, are escalating
at a constantly accelerating rate, far outpacing inflation, and are now a matter
of urgent national concern. Funding sources, whether local, state or federal
government bodies, as well as the general public and its consumer advocates,
are becoming increasingly active in attempting to monitor and, in some
cases, control the cost of health care (Sider et al., 1976). The cost of hospital
care is rising 3 times as fast as the cost of living. The mental health profession,
like the rest of the medical profession, has not been, and to a significant
extent, still is not interested in the cost-effectiveness of the health care it
delivers.

Antipsychotic drug therapy is unique in that effective and safe psychopharmacotherapy is also the most economical. When the antipsychotic drugs
are used skillfully and with sophistication, incorporating the latest scientific
findings, not only does maximal patient benefit ensue but there also is
substantial savings in hospital costs, staff time and drug expenditures. This
section will concentrate mainly on the economic facets of antipsychotic drug
therapy, since the clinical aspects have been discussed in the previous chapters. Most of these general guidelines may seem repetitious, yet not only
from the therapeutic standpoint but also from the view of cost-effectiveness,
they warrant repeated emphasis.

**Use a rapid tranquilization or a rapid titration method in appropriate
patients to reduce length of hospital stay.**

Hospital care is the most expensive item in the treatment of the mentally
ill. In some psychiatric units of general hospitals or private mental hospitals,
the daily cost is reaching $200. Even in many state mental hospitals (some

now called community mental health centers) the per diem may amount to over $75. While formerly with the slow "stair-step" increase of oral anti-psychotic medication or with fixed dose schedules the patient remained in the hospital for many weeks or months, rapid tranquilization or aggressive antipsychotic drug intervention now can shorten the hospital stay to 1 week or 10 days. It has even made possible 24-hour or 3-day periods of hospi-talization for many patients. The shorter length of stay reduces significantly by far the most costly factor in psychiatric treatment.

Use rapid tranquilization techniques in suitable patients for ambulatory treatment as outpatients and thus avoid the cost of hospitalization.

Rapid tranquilization methods, usually through the initial use of the short-acting parenteral form of the high-potency antipsychotics, can eliminate hospitalization for a large percentage of patients even though they present acute psychotic symptoms.

Avoid polypharmacy whenever possible. Use combinations of psycho-tropic drugs only when there is conclusive evidence that the combination is more effective than an appropriate single drug. Use one antipsychotic at a time.

The practice of administering 2 or more psychotropic drugs is widespread and without scientific support or solid clinical corroborating evidence. In some state mental hospitals, patients are prescribed on the average 2.8 psychotropic drugs (DiMascio, 1975). Instances of 4 to 6 psychotropic drugs prescribed simultaneously are not uncommon. Obviously, reduction in the number of drugs prescribed unnecessarily will result in substantial savings.

When conjoint antipsychotic drugs are used, the dosage of each anti-psychotic is usually low. If only 1 antipsychotic drug is prescribed, drug costs can frequently be cut in half or more with no loss of clinical benefit to the patient.

After the patient's illness has been stabilized, reduce dosage to the lowest maintenance level for retaining therapeutic gain.

All too often patients are maintained on a fixed high or moderate dosage of their antipsychotic for months or years, even though their florid symp-tomatology has been controlled. In the residual state, overdosage is probably more of a problem than underdosage. The schizophrenic process is not static. Patients who needed moderate to high doses of antipsychotic drugs a few years ago may be currently functioning at a level which requires less medication.

When the patient's clinical condition is stabilized, administer the anti-psychotic drug on a once-a-day (q.i.d.) or, at most, a twice-a-day (b.i.d.) schedule.

The administration of total daily dosage on a q.i.d. or b.i.d. schedule allows for the use of a proportionately less expensive size tablets with a

TABLE 13
Price Range—Chlorpromazine Tablet Comparison

Tablet Size	Cost/tablet
10 mg.	3.1¢
25 mg.	3.6¢
50 mg.	4.2¢
100 mg.	5.1¢
200 mg.	6.2¢

considerable potential in savings. It is less costly because the cost of the drug is not directly proportional to the amount of medication in a tablet.

Table 13 gives a price range of chlorpromazine tablets and it can be noted that it costs less than twice as much to give 10 times the active medication (10 mg. vs 100 mg.) and exactly twice as much for 20 times medication (10 mg. vs 200 mg.).

In Table 14, the cost of a 400 mg. daily dose of thioridazine is used as the example. The data show that the cost of the same amount of this medication may vary from 36¢ to $1.50 per day, depending upon the tablet sizes that are prescribed. Furthermore, if a patient was treated with the first regimen (four 25 mg. tablets four times a day), he would have to swallow 16 tablets compared to 2 tablets if he were on the last regimen listed (one 200 mg. tablet twice a day, or both tablets at bedtime). The greater number of tablets a patient is required to take, the more likely he is to deviate from the prescription instructions—thus ingesting less medication that is prescribed

TABLE 14
Cost of Medication—A Tablet-Size Comparison
(400 mg. daily dose of thioridazine) with varying dosage units*)

Prescription Schedule	Daily Cost
(Tablet size)	
4 (25 mg.) q.i.d.	$1.50
2 (50 mg.) q.i.d.	.82
1 (100 mg.) q.i.d.	.48
1 (100 mg.) + 2 (150 mg.)	.43
1 (100 mg.) + 1 (100 mg.	
& 200 mg.)	.42
1 (200 mg.) b.i.d.	.36

*The cost figures in Tables 13 and 14 are from the 1977 Drug Topic Red Book published by Medical Economics Co., Oradell, N.Y. They are average wholesale prices when purchased in 1000-tablet quantities by retail pharmacies.

and potentially, therefore, causing a return of symptoms, relapse, and re-hospitalization (DiMascio, 1975).

At one of the state hospitals in Massachusetts several years ago a study showed that by merely switching the directions and strength sizes of out-patient prescriptions, the hospital would save over $7,300 a year in drug costs (Marder and DiMascio, 1973). Furthermore, there was an average savings of about $4 per prescription if the patient purchased the drug in a retail pharmacy.

Mason (1976) showed by cost analysis of 100 outpatients on antipsychotic drugs followed by several mental health centers that there would be an annual savings of $3,094 if they were placed on a once-a-day medication schedule. An analysis of 365 patients on the rolls of a comprehensive care center indicated that an annual savings of $11,470 would ensue with a similar change in the medication scheduled (as in Tables 13 and 14, the calculations were based on the wholesale price guide for pharmacists). Marder et al. (1971) surveyed the staff time consumed in preparing and dispensing psychotropic medication in a public state hospital. They found that daily administration of drugs on a 3 times a day or 4 times a day basis took about 53 minutes of staff time per week for each patient, but twice a day/weekend free schedules required only 14 minutes. Considered economically, staff time for giving medication to 375 patients was about $26,000 annually. This sum could be reduced 43% for a savings of $11,000 a year with a twice-a-day schedule. A bedtime only medication regimen could cut down staff time still further. This saving in time would free staff members for vocational, psychological and counseling activities and therapy which should further benefit the patients.

By giving the antipsychotic 1-2 hours before bedtime (or the bulk of the daily dosage in a b.i.d. schedule), there are fewer side effects including extrapyramidal reactions and the sleep-inducing action of the drug becomes a desirable effect. Thus the costs involved in purchasing and dispensing antiparkinson and sedative-hypnotic drugs can be reduced.

Prescribe an antiparkinson drug only after extrapyramidal symptoms appear to a degree where such medication is necessary; do not prescribe an antiparkinson drug prophylactically.

There are only 1 or 2 published articles in the scientific literature demonstrating that the antiparkinson drugs prevent the occurrence of antipsychotic-induced extrapyramidal reactions. Instead, there are numerous reports on the results of studies verifying that antiparkinson drugs do not prevent the emergence of extrapyramidal reactions in patients treated with antipsychotics. Accordingly, the use of antiparkinson drugs prophylactically in most instances is considered an unnecessarily costly practice in psychiatric facilities.

Discontinue antiparkinson drugs after 3 months and then reinstate only in those patients whose extrapyramidal symptoms return.

The application of this general guideline and the 1 above referable to antiparkinson drug use can result in substantial savings. When the staff physicians altered their prescribing of antiparkinson agents, the use of such medication in 1 state was reduced from 3,500,000 in 1968 to less than 1,500,000 in 1973; this amounts to a reduction of 2,000,000 tablets and a saving of over $20,000 in 1 year (DiMascio, 1975).

Trihexyphenidyl hydrochloride (Artane), biperidine hydrochloride (Akineton) and benztropin mesylate (Cogentin) are called "universal agents" in that they are equally effective in the management of reversible extrapyramidal symptoms caused by antipsychotic drugs. Using the maximal level of the daily dosage as stated in the *Physicians' Desk Reference* (1978), the cost per day of these drugs is shown in Table 15.

As can be noted in Table 15, trihexyphenidyl hydrochloride (Artane) is far less expensive than most of the other antiparkinson agents and the lower cost ratio would apply when smaller oral doses are prescribed. Table 16 demonstrates the substantial savings differential between trihexyphenidyl and benztropine.

TABLE 15
Comparative Cost of Antiparkinson Drugs

Antiparkinson Drug	Maximal daily dosage	Cost*
Trihexyphenidyl hydrochloride (Artane)	15 mg (three—5 mg tablets)	2¢
Biperiden hydrochloride (Akineton)	6 mg (three—2 mg tablets)	16¢
Benztropine mesylate (Cogentin)	8 mg (four—2 mg tablets)	19¢
Procyclidine hydrochloride (Kemadrin)	20 mg (four—5 mg tablets)	10¢
Diphenhydramine hydrochloride (Benadryl)	200 mg (four—50 mg capsules)	3¢
Orphenadrine hydrochloride (Disipal)	150 mg (three—50 mg tablets)	21¢†
Amantadine hydrochloride (Symmetral)	300 mg (three—100 mg tablets)	52¢

*Based on F. Y. 1977-78 contract prices in one state (when purchased in 1000 tablet quantities).
†From American Druggist Blue Book, 1978 (100 tablet quantity).

TABLE 16

Cost Comparison Between Benztropine (Cogentin) and Trihexyphenidyl
(Artane) Prescribed for 1,000 Patients for 365 Days

Drug	Daily Dose	Cost/Year
Benztropine	4 mg.	$29,200
Trihexyphenidyl	10 mg.	$ 4,876

A savings of $24,324.00 per year is realized when trihexyphenidyl is prescribed when clinically indicated.

From: *Psychotherapeutic Drug Manual*, prepared by New York State, Department of Mental Hygiene, November, 1977.

If an antiparkinson drug is necessary, reduce sodage to the lowest effective level for control of extrapyramidal symptoms.

Review of thousands of medication orders for antiparkinson drugs reveals that it is common practice to prescribe moderate to high doses of these drugs initially and leave this dosage unchanged for months or years, regardless whether it is given to an inpatient or outpatient. Occasionally the daily dosage is increased but a reduction is uncommon. Most clinical studies reported in the literature involving the combination of an antiparkinson agent with an antipsychotic utilized a fixed daily dose of the antiparkinson drug.

It appears that usually the recommendations in the manufacturer's insert or the *PDR* is unheeded. Regarding the prescription of trihexyphenidyl hydrochloride (Artane) in drug-induced parkinsonism, the *PDR* (1978) states as follows: "The size and frequency of the dose of Artane needed to control extrapyramidal reactions to commonly employed tranquilizers, notably the phenothiazines, the thioxanthines and butyrophenones, must be determined empirically. The total daily dosage usually ranges between 5 and 15 mg. although, in some cases, these reactions have been satisfactorily controlled on as little as 1 mg. daily. It may be advisable to commence therapy with a single 1 mg. dose. If the extrapyramidal manifestations are not controlled in a few hours, the subsequent doses may be progressively increased until satisfactory control is achieved." With respect to benztropine mesylate (Cogentin), the *PDR* states, "**Dosage must be individualized according to the need of the patient**. Some patients require more than recommended; others do not need as much." Especially with long-term use of an antiparkinson agent, titration to the smallest dose needed to control the extrapyramidal side effects results in improved patient care as well as reduced drug costs.

Try intermittent drug holidays, especially with the chronic hospitalized patient.

It has been shown that if only half the patients (about 900) in a study hospital were switched to a twice daily (b.i.d.) and weekend free schedule, there would be a saving of over $65,000 a year in nursing time costs, without reducing the clinical benefit derived by patients on antipsychotic medication. Dispensing the drugs 5 days a week instead of 7 days a week would obviously reduce drug expenditures by 28% in a high percentage of patients (Marder et al., 1971).

Use the Forrest Urine Tests routinely when the phenothiazines are prescribed (especially the low-potency phenothiazines) to make certain the drug is truly ingested.

The Forrest Urine Tests are the only practical objective method of determining whether the patient is truly ingesting phenothiazine medication. Even when the concentrate is used, patients have been known to go immediately to the ward bathroom and regurgitate the medication. This guideline is especially important in the care of the outpatients on phenothiazines. Failure to use these tests routinely during clinic visits to check on drug compliance results, for many patients, in relapse, in another period of costly hospitalization and wasted medication.

After the first week or two or as soon as the patient has been stabilized, discontinue as-needed (PRN) orders, unless there is a special indication.

The cost in staff time of a PRN order may amount to $.47 per order (Mason and DeWolfe, 1974). Thus the many thousands of unnecessary PRN orders throughout a year constitute a substantial waste of costly staff time.

Do not waste oral forms of antipsychotics when patients have demonstrated repeated poor drug compliance. Switch to and stabilize these patients on the long-acting depot injectables.

Maintaining patients on low doses of prolixin decanoate or enanthate at 1 month to 3-month intervals is less costly than the smallest oral doses of any antipsychotic drug given daily. With higher doses, there is less difference in cost. If one considers that about half of all oral medications dispensed are somehow discarded, the cost benefits of the depot phenothiazines are incalculable (Owens, 1978).

Consider the comparative cost of the antipsychotic prescribed, all other factors being equal.

Table 17 shows the comparative costs of the various antipsychotics. It is more important to choose the drug that is clinically right for the patient rather than the one that is least expensive. However, a number of studies in the past have found that chlorpromazine and thioridazine are, by far, the most commonly prescribed drugs for the treatment of schizophrenia (Laska et al., 1973; Sheppard et al., 1969; Altman et al., 1972; Mason et al., 1977a). Thioridazine is a widely used antipsychotic for all the other psychiatric disorders in many mental hospitals. Yet it should be noted that the monthly

TABLE 17
Comparative Dosages and Costs of Antipsychotic Drugs

Generic name	Tradename	Defined dosage* (mg.)	Dose equivalent† (mg.)	Average cost‡
Chlorpromazine	Thorazine	100	100	$15.31
Thioridazine	Mellaril	97 ± 7	100	37.29
Mesoridazine	Serentil	56 ± 6	51	30.68
Chlorprothixene	Taractan	44 ± 8	100	18.03
Triflupromazine hydrochloride	Vesprin	28 ± 2	28	38.71
Carphenazine maleate	Proketazine	25 ± 1	19	23.34
Prochlorperazine	Compazine	14 ± 2	15	30.09
Piperacetazine	Quide	11	14	22.27
Butaperazine maleate	Repoise maleate	9 ± 1	13	19.63
Perphenazine	Trilafon	9 ± 6	10	27.11
Molindone hydrochloride	Moban	6 ± 9	10	12.06
Thiothixene	Navane	4.4 ± 1	3	22.39
Trifluoperazine hydrochloride	Stelazine	2.8 ± 4	5	16.91
Haloperidol	Haldol	1.6 ± 5	2	28.04
Loxapine Succinate	Loxitane		15	17.45
Fluphenazine hydrochloride	Prolixin (5 mg.)	1.2 ± 1	2	15.84
Fluphenazine hydrochloride	Permitil (10 mg.)	1.2 ± 1	2	6.92
Fluphenazine enanthate	Prolixin enanthate	.67	—	20.91
Fluphenazine decanoate	Prolixin Decanoate	.61	—	18.24

*Empirically defined dose in milligram equivalent to 100 mg. chlorpromazine.
†Average dose in milligrams equivalent to 100 mg. chlorpromazine, as defined by experts.
‡Average cost for one month at acute dose schedule.
From: Davis, J. M.: Comparative Doses and Costs. *Arch. Gen. Psychiat.* 33: 858-861, 1976. Copyright 1976 American Medical Association.

cost of thioridazine is more than twice that of chlorpromazine. The average monthly cost of thioridazine medication is the highest of all antipsychotics listed in Table 17, with the exception of trifluopromazine, which is infrequently prescribed. During the past few years there has been a growing trend to use the high-potency antipsychotics, which are also less expensive than thioridazine.

When the patient is on a substantial daily dose of an antipsychotic, use tablets instead of the concentrate.

This guideline does not apply to the patient who has swallowing difficulties. The experienced nurse knows that one cannot be certain that the patient took the medication unless water is swallowed after taking the tablet and then the mouth is inspected. Relatives of patients should be taught the same technique if there is reason to suspect that a nonhospitalized patient is not reliable in taking medication. Crushing pills before offering them to the patient is another way of preventing the outpatient from jeopardizing his treatment (Lehmann, 1975).

The concentrate, especially when adequate doses are prescribed, may cost 2-3 times as much as the equivalent tablet dose when purchased at retail prices. Tablets, if available, are often soluble in fruit juices and are a cheaper alternative to liquid medication. However, there is no monetary advantage between the 2 forms when small doses are used. Nursing time costs for dispensing antipsychotic medication can be appreciably reduced with the use of tablets or capsules instead of the concentrate. A 40 mg. dose of haloperidol in the concentrate form, for example, requires the careful measuring out of eight 5 mg droppers (the capacity of the dropper packaged with the 120 ml bottle) into a medicine cup in contrast to placing four 10 mg. pills in the cup.

Prescribe the largest possible tablet or capsule size necessary to obtain the desired dose.

There is considerable financial advantage gained by following this guideline. DiMascio (1975) states this rule as follows: **Prescribe the highest dose unit the patient can tolerate.** For example, if a physician prescribed equal total daily doses of the average antipsychotic drug, 2 tablets twice a day vs 1 (larger size) tablet at bedtime, it would cost the patient roughly 50% more to take his medication in a divided dose. If 1 tablet 4 times a day is prescribed rather than 1 tablet at bedtime, it would cost the patient roughly 2.5 times as much.

Do not prescribe delayed release oral forms (Spansules).

These are expensive formulations and offer no advantage over the standard tablet preparations. They cost 2 to 3 times more than an equivalent amount of the drug in a tablet form.

Consider the use of generic preparations instead of the proprietary antipsychotic if there is clear evidence of bioequivalency, clinical efficacy and if they are appreciably cheaper.

When the patient on chlorpromazine expired, generic forms of this compound became available. Two investigations (Simpson et al., 1974; Ota et al., 1974) have demonstrated that either generic form of chlorpromazine, Chlor-PZ and Promachel, is clinically comparable to the proprietary chlorpromazine (Thorazine) and can be prescribed as an adequate substitute for the latter. It is stressed that those who wish to prescribe generic chlorpromazine should do so only for Chlor-PZ or Promachel until other generic forms have been proven to be bioequivalent to and as efficacious as Thorazine (Ayd, 1975c).

Do not use antipsychotic drugs purely as sedatives.

Not only are antipsychotic poor sedatives that may produce a variety of side effects, but there are many sedative-hypnotics which are more effective, do not produce serious side effects and are less expensive.

Use lithium for preventive action in manic-depressive psychosis.

An outpatient clinic where patients on lithium carbonate can receive specialized attention for the treatment and prevention of recurrent affective disorders will eliminate many episodes of costly hospitalization (Cusano et al., 1977). Outpatient lithium therapy can be of economic value to the patient, his family and the community. A lithium clinic may be able to handle 400 patients a year at a cost of $350 per client per year for a total cost of $140,000; these same patients may require an average of 20 days of hospitalization at $100 a day for a total cost of $800,000 (Treffert, 1978).

Develop educational or training program in the art of psychopharmacology for physicians of psychiatric facilities, community mental health centers and make them available to the physician in private practice.

Additional emphasis should be placed on the subject of psychopharmacology in the medical school curriculum and in psychiatric residency training programs. At any one time, it is estimated that there are probably at least 1,000,000 schizophrenics in active treatment or sufficiently symptomatic as to merit such treatment. Thus, any educational program which results in increased skill and effectiveness in the use of antipsychotic drug therapy by physicians may be reflected in huge savings.

Institute periodic audits, monitoring or peer reviews of the prescription practices in psychiatric facilities, outpatient clinics, community health centers and alternative programs and living situations in the community.

Wherever these measures have been instituted there has been substantial cost reduction as well as improvement in patient care. Monitoring the prescribing patterns of physicians and psychiatrists treating the psychiatric patient is a necessary and challenging professional responsibility. It makes the physician more familiar with the state of the art of psychopharmacology, constitutes a form of continuing education and yields vastly reduced drug costs (Diamond et al., 1976; Mason et al., 1977b). A peer review system established in 1970 led to a 70% reduction in costs through use of alternatives to individual psychotherapy such as group psychotherapy, brief medication visits and the formation of support-resocialization groups (Ozarin, 1977). Partial hospitalization is underutilized even though its clinical effectiveness for a variety of psychiatric patients and fiscal advantage have been demonstrated (Fink et al., 1978). An intensive outpatient treatment program incorporating drug-intake supervision with partial hospitalization or day care (or family care where practical) has the potential of savings as high as $100 per day compared to full-time hospitalization.

The specific savings mentioned in this chapter were derived mainly from studies conducted several years ago. With the inflationary spiral since then, current savings would be much greater. If the psychiatric profession will adopt or institute these cost-saving measures, procedures and programs where feasible and assume some fiscal accountability, it can help put the brakes on the skyrocketing price of an adequate mental health care delivery system.

V

Side Effects of
Antipsychotic Drugs
And Their Management

There are no drugs in medicine which do not have at least some side effects. The antipsychotic drugs are no exception. However, very few of their side effects are dangerous and these should be respected but not feared. Knowledge and understanding of the management of side effects secondary to these agents will separate the truly artful clinician from the routine prescriber.

Usage of the term "adverse effects" is purposefully being avoided. What is an adverse effect for one physician may become an adjunct in drug therapy to another. For instance, the anticholinergic effect of chlorpromazine causing urinary retention in one individual may be useful in preventing unwanted extrapyramidal effects in another. Or, orthostatic hypotension from chlorpromazine may cause difficulty in schizophrenic patients, while it may be a wanted effect for the neurosurgeon managing post-traumatic hypertension. Most of the clinically relevant side effects seen with antipsychotic agents will be reviewed and management guidelines offered. This knowledge may then be applied to the previous principles of antipsychotic drug therapy to enable the physician to become truly expert in the use of these agents.

1. NEUROLOGIC SYNDROMES

Neurologic side effects have long been recognized as one of the most common outcomes with the use of antipsychotic agents. Many physicians are familiar with acute dystonias, akathisia, and parkinsonism. More recently, tardive dyskinesia is being recognized and a few reports of antipsychotic drug-induced catatonia or akinetic mutism have appeared (Table 18). All of these syndromes can be classified as drug-induced movement disorders.

Acute Dystonias

Of all the side effects attributed to antipsychotic agents, the acute dystonias are the most likely to strike dread and fear into the hearts of nursing

TABLE 18

Neurologic Syndromes Associated with the Use of Antipsychotic Agents

A. Reversible	
Acute dystonias	Prolonged tonic contractions.
	Torsions, twistings and drawing of muscle groups, e.g. torticollis, retrocollis, opisthotonos, trismus, oculogyric crisis and laryngospasm.
Akathisia	Motor restlessness.
	Subjective internal feeling of incessant need to move.
	Seen as pacing, rocking, foot stomping and shuffling feet while sitting
Parkinsoniam	Similar in appearance to true Parkinson's disease.
	Shuffling gait, difficulty with starting and stopping movement, bradykinesia, muscular rigidity, masked facies, tremor, postural instability, and drooling.
Catatonia or Akinetic Mutism	Usually have associated extrapyramidal signs and cogwheel rigidity.
	May show waxy flexibility, emotional withdrawal, posturing, mutism and negativism.
B. Possibly Irreversible	
Tardive Dyskinesia	Constellation of involuntary hyperkinetic movements.
	Usually involves face, tongue, and oral area.
	Can be a variety of tics, chorea, athetosis, and dystonias.

staffs and physicians who are unprepared for or do not recognize their occurrence. In fact, the appearance of acute dystonic reactions during the use of antipsychotic agents is the factor most likely to cause nursing staffs to be afraid of using a particular agent. This underscores the necessity of education for the recognition and management of these disorders.

Acute dystonic reactions are sudden in onset and can be bizarre in presentation. These are involuntary turning or twisting movements (torsion spasms) produced by massive and sustained muscle contractions. They usually involve the back, neck muscles, and oral area. Thus, one may see extension of the back (opisthotonos) or the head arching severely backwards (retrocollis). The eyes may be pulled vertically upward in a painful manner (oculogyric crisis). Often the staring appears to be directed at the ceiling and some may erroneously conclude that the patient "is avoiding eye contact." The mouth may contort into a puckering form such that the tongue protrudes. This dystonia of the oral area can be severe enough to prevent swallowing and on rare occasion may interfere with proper breathing. The affected patient often sweats profusely due to the increased muscle tone. In fact, this may be a useful sign when combined with a sudden change for the worse in a previously active patient. The onset of a dystonic reaction usually occurs within 24-48 hours of starting antipsychotics and is seen more often in young people than old and more frequently in males than females. Prediction of likelihood of occurrence in the individual patient is difficult and somewhat idiosyncratic. However, a previous history of acute dystonic reactions may be predictive and high-potency antipsychotics are more prone than aliphatic or piperidine phenothiazines.

Treatment of acute dystonic reactions should be prompt and vigorous. As previously outlined in Chapter II, benztropine 2 mg. (Cogentin) IV or diphenhydramine 25 mg. (Benadryl) IV will reverse most acute dystonias within 5-10 minutes. However, other equally effective antiparkinson agents are available. Table 19 lists these agents and their dosage forms. It should be noted that the only other injectable form available for acute use is biperiden (Akineton) and will be effective in a 1 ml dose (5 mg.) IM or IV. The patient should then be placed on one of these agents for 2-3 weeks with an automatic stop order so the physician will have a reminder to see if the continued use of the antiparkinson agent is warranted. Other treatments for acute dystonia have been employed. These include caffiene sodium benzoate, diazepam and methylphenidate (Ritalin), but they are not widely used at the present time.

Akathisia

Akathisia is a subjective desire to move and is a syndrome of motor restlessness. The physician using antipsychotic agents must carefully evaluate this complaint and not merely diagnose anxiety. This could mislead the physician and cause an unneeded increase in dosage. The patient with akathisia often feels "nervous" or "jittery" in the inner abdominal area and is compelled to pace the floor or, if seated, to shift his legs or tap his feet. When standing he may march in place. Maltbie and Cavenar (1977) feel that a useful adjunct in the diagnosis of akathisia is the ability to show cogwheel rigidity. This is a jerky resistance felt by the examiner when passively moving the patient's arms through a range of motion. If cogwheeling is not present with this maneuver, it can often be elicited by recruitment. This involves instructing the patient to perform rapid alternating movements simultaneously in the extremity opposite the one being passively tested.

Akathisia may occur early in treatment, after years of therapy or upon a change in drug regimens. It is often refractory to treatment and may not respond to antiparkinson agents. The frequency of akathisia is not well documented but has been reported to vary from 12.5% to 45% in patients receiving antipsychotic drugs (Van Putten, 1975). Ayd (1961) has reported a frequency of 21.2% at some time during antipsychotic treatment in 3,775 patients.

A vigorous attempt should always be made to treat akathisia, since its unpleasant nature often causes patients to discontinue their medications. Patients may feel that the physician is trying to "poison them," or feel that "their nerves are getting worse." Treatment involves first trying the addition of universal antiparkinson agents such as benztropine (Cogentin), trihexyphenadyl (Artane), biperiden (Akineton), or procyclidine (Kemadrin). A switch to an antipsychotic agent such as thioridazine, mesoridazine, or chlorpromazine may be helpful. In some, a mere reduction in the dosage of the offending agent may suffice. Other patients will remain refractory to all of these approaches but may show a response to diazepam (Valium) 5 mg. t.i.d., oxazepam (Serax) 15 mg. t.i.d. or another benzodiazepine with or without an antiparkinson agent. **As stressed in the previous section on antiparkinson medications, many feel the prophylactic use of these agents is to be avoided. In fact, Swett et al. (1977) reported frequency of extrapyramidal symptoms attributed to chlorpromazine in 86 patients who received prophylactic benztropine was 9.3%, while those patients receiving chlorpromazine alone had a frequency of 10.6%. This suggests no prophylactic value for benztropine in the reduction of extrapyramidal symptoms.**

Parkinsonism

Drug-induced parkinsonism is probably the most common neurologic syndrome that will confront the physician using antipsychotic medications. This is to be distinguished from idiopathic parkinsonism or post-encephalitic parkinsonism. Drug-induced parkinsonism is often clinically indistinguishable in appearance from these entities and its diagnosis rests upon a temporal relationship with the concurrent use of antipsychotic agents. Its appearance is described in Table 18.

The manifestations of drug-induced parkinsonism are many and any combination of signs may be seen. One of the more distressing features may be postural instability, especially in the older patient. In fact, a few patients may actually walk backwards due to this condition and this sign may be mislabeled as a manifestation of their psychosis or even interpreted psychodynamically. Other features of drug-induced parkinsonism such as rigidity, bradykinesia, and drooling may interfere with dressing, eating, and other purposeful movement. Tremor is seen at rest and generally disappears upon volitional movement. It is more likely to appear in the upper extremities or head and may be unilateral in either hand. Vague aches and pains may accompany the tremor and fine motor activity is often impaired.

The management of drug-induced parkinsonism centers around the use of universal anticholinergic agents. However, often these agents will synergistically add to other drugs with anticholinergic properties. Recently amantadine (Symmetrel), an agent without significant anticholinergic properties, has been shown useful in drug-induced parkinsonism. It seems equal to benztropine or trihexyphenidyl in effectiveness at relieving parkinsonian side effects, but is much lower in anticholinergic effects. It is most effective in relieving akinesia and parkinsonian rigidity. It is least effective with akathisia. The usual daily dose is 100 mg. b.i.d., with rare patients requiring up to 400 mg. daily. In fact, its half-life is long enough (24 hours) that once-a-day administration can be tried. The clinical effectiveness of amantadine is partially lost after 6-8 weeks of continuous treatment.

Side effects of amantadine are infrequent. It can produce psychosis in toxic amounts (greater than 1 gram) and reversible loss of vision has been reported in 1 patient (Ayd, 1977d). In cases of overdose, amantadine is poorly removed by hemodialysis. Long-term use has reportedly caused livido reticularis, a net-like purplish discoloration of the lower extremities. This seems cosmetically undesirable but not harmful. Confusion from amantadine has reportedly been reversed by physostigmine.

At the present time, amantadine is quite expensive when compared with standard antiparkinson agents. Furthermore, few clinical studies have examined its long-term effects. Amantadine is not metabolized and more than 90% is excreted unchanged in the urine. Therefore, caution should be exercised when using this drug in the elderly. Until more is known about amantadine, it should probably be a second choice to the other antiparkinson agents in treating drug-induced parkinsonism (Ayd, 1977d).

TABLE 19
Antiparkinson Drugs

TRADE NAME	GENERIC NAME	DOSAGE FORM	DAILY DOSAGE RANGE
Artane	trihexyphenidyl HCl	Tablets—2 mg., 5 mg. Elixir—2 mg. per 5 ml. Sequels**—5 mg.	4-15 mg. p. o.
Akineton	biperiden HCl	Tablets—2 mg. Parenteral—5 mg. per ml.	2-6 mg. p. o. 1-2 mg. i. m. or i. v.*
Cogentin	benztropine mesylate	Tablets—2 mg., 5 mg. Parenteral—1 mg. per ml.	2-8 mg. p. o. 1-2 mg. i. m.
Kemadrin	procyclidine HCl	Tablets—2 mg., 5 mg.	6-20 mg. p. o.
Benadryl	diphenhydramine HCl	Capsules—25 mg., 50 mg. Elixir—12.5 mg. per 5 ml. Parenteral—10 mg. per ml., 50 mg. per ml.	25-200 mg. p. o. 10-50 mg. i. m. or i. v.
Disipal	orphenadrine HCl	Tablets—50 mg.	50-150 mg. p. o.
Symmetrel***	amantadine HCl	Capsules Syrup—50 mg. per 5 ml.	100-400 mg. p. o.

*May be repeated every half-hour until resolution of symptoms is effected, but not more than four consecutive doses should be administered in a 24-hour period.
**Sustained release capsules.
***Good renal function necessary for use.

Akinesia

Akinesia, another reversible neurologic syndrome, usually takes the form of decreased movements and psychosocial withdrawal. The patient is often thought to be depressed. On neurologic examination, the physician will usually find muscular rigidity, cogwheeling and often tremor. These signs are useful in differentiating drug-induced akinesia from true isolation or depression.

The most severe forms of akinesia can resemble catatonia. The features of these reactions include negativism, mutism, withdrawal, and occasionally bizarre posturing and waxy flexibility (Gelenberg and Mandel, 1977). In general, these syndromes seem more likely on high-potency, low anticholinergic activity antipsychotic agents such as fluphenazine and haloperidol.

The most severe form of these catatonic disorders is frank akinetic mutism.

This syndrome must be differentiated from true catatonia or other neurologic entities. The history of antipsychotic therapy and the presence of associated extrapyramidal signs such as bradykinesia, muscular rigidity, cogwheeling, tremor and drooling rule out true catatonia. Failure to make the differentiation may result in raising the antipsychotic dosage with a resultant increase in the catatonia.

Treatment of akinetic catatonia is sometimes difficult. A decrease or discontinuation of the offending agent may not cause an immediate change. Some patients will not respond to benztropine or other anticholinergic agents. However, amantadine has shown a rapid alleviation of signs in those patients in whom it has been tried (Gelenberg and Mandel, 1977).

There seems to be an inverse relationship between the anticholinergic potency of an antipsychotic agent and its ability to produce reversible neurologic syndromes. Table 20 demonstrates the anticholinergic activity of these agents and contrasts them with agents, such as trihexyphenidyl or benztropine, used to treat neurologic side effects from antipsychotic medications. In other words, antipsychotic drugs that are highly anticholinergic are less likely to produce acute dystonias, akithisia, parkinsonism, or catatonic-akinetic reactions. From Table 20 it can be seen that atropine is very anticholinergic. Thioridazine is a more potent anticholinergic agent than haloperidol on an equivalent basis and is much less likely to produce acute neurologic dysfunction than drugs below it in the table. By going from top to bottom in Table 20 it can be predicted that thioridazine would be the least likely to produce neurologic dysfunction while haloperidol would be

TABLE 20
Anticholinergic Potency of Antipsychotic and Antiparkinson Agents

AGENT	POTENCY	EPS
Atropine	+ + + + +	
Trihexyphenidyl (Artane)	+ + + +	
Benztropine (Cogentin)	+ + + +	
Thioridazine (Mellaril)	+ + +	+
Chlorpromazine (Thorazine)	+ +	+ +
Triflupromazine (Vesprin)	+ +	+ +
Acetophenazine (Tindal)	+	+ + +
Perphenazine (Trilafon)	+	+ + +
Fluphenazine (Prolixin)	+	+ + +
Trifluoperazine (Stelazine)	+	+ + +
Haloperidol (Haldol)	+	+ + + +

Modified from Snyder et al. (1974).

the most likely. Thus, the other antipsychotic agents in this table become more likely to induce neurologic side effects as one moves down the table from thioridazine to haloperidol. However, it must be recognized that agents such as haloperidol or fluphenazine should not be rejected merely because of their greater likelihood to cause neurologic side effects. The lack of anticholinergic activity may be very desirable in some patients where sedation is to be avoided and those with medical problems that might be exacerbated by anticholinergic side effects.

Most of the neurologic side effects are treated successfully with antiparkinson agents such as trihexyphenidyl, biperiden, benztropine or even amantadine. However, another problem is emerging with the use of anticholinergic antiparkinson agents such as trihexyphenidyl or biperiden. They are frequently being abused by patients and seem to cause a type of psychological dependence. Many youngsters are using trihexyphenidyl to induce "highs" or "trips."

Psychiatrists will often find that they can reduce the dosage of antipsychotic drug in a given patient or even discontinue its use later to find that patient refusing to stop his antiparkinson agents. Jellinek (1977) has noted that these agents have mood-elevating properties and speculates that this is the reason for their dependence in some patients. However, there is presently no data to show that these compounds will elevate mood. **In any event, antiparkinson agents should not be used indiscriminately, especially in young patients with a history of alcohol or drug abuse (Ayd, 1978c).**

The term of tardive dyskinesia (TD) often has been simply and rather loosely applied to all patients who develop involuntary tic-like and choretiform movements, mainly perioral, after having taken antipsychotic medication (tardive means "late blooming" since originally the disorder seemed to be a geriatric syndrome). TD has also been called "irreversible," "permanent," "terminal extrapyramidal insufficiency," "complex dyskinesia" and "persistent." None of these appellations coincides with irrefutable facts or can even be considered valid with any substantial degree of conclusiveness.

The reports in the literature regarding the prevalence and the various etiological factors possibly linked to the production of TD are unclear, highly contradictory and controversial. For example, the incidence of TD in chronic hospitalized psychiatric patients on antipsychotic drug therapy has been reported to range from .5-2% to as high as 56-60% (Crane, 1973; Quitkin et al., 1977; Tarsy and Baldessarini, 1976). The incidence among outpatients shows a disparity just as great. In a group of 575 schizophrenic patients, only 3 cases of TD developed during 15 years of outpatient antipsychotic drug therapy (Hansell and Willis, 1977). Another group of clinicians found a 43.4% frequency of TD in a random sampling of 250 outpatients receiving a variety of antipsychotic drugs. Later, this frequency was qualified with the statement that only 4% of the patients surveyed had severe dyskinesia while the remaining cases were of minimal or mild severity (Asnis et al., 1977; Asnis, 1978).

From the above, it can be concluded that the incidence of TD is not well established. It is rarely seen in acute psychiatric units, even in patients with recurring schizophrenia. An FDA Drug Bulletin (1973) states that "incidence rates of about 20% have been reported in older institutionalized, chronically ill patients" and that "perhaps 3% to 6% of patients in a mixed psychiatric population receiving neuroleptics exhibit some aspects of the syndrome at one time or another."

Age is generally acknowledged to be a crucial factor with most TD patients observed in the over 50 age group who have been taking antipsychotic drugs for a long period of time. Yet it has been demonstrated that TD can occur in young patients treated for relatively short periods of time with moderate doses of antipsychotics (Tarsy et al., 1977). It has been reported that the high-potency low-dose drugs are more prone to produce TD, despite the finding that the great majority of cases of TD in mental hospitals are commonly found among the geriatric patients who have been given the older low-potency high-dose antipsychotics (chlorpromazine and thioridazine) for years. Large dose therapy has been stated to increase the risk of TD; yet thousands of schizophrenics have been treated for 10 to 20 years with massive doses of various antipsychotics (and combinations of them) and show no signs of TD.

Antiparkinson agents have been suggested as having a possible role in causing TD (Kobayashi, 1977). While this possibility has been suggested as another reason why physicians should avoid the prophylactic use and minimize the long-term use of antiparkinson agents, other investigators have found no causal relationship between TD and these drugs. Other factors previously reported to have an influence on TD—previous history of brain damage, electroshock therapy, insulin treatment or tricyclic antidepressant intake—have not been substantiated. Similarly, factors such as the type of schizophrenia, initial syndrome, present psychotic state, dosage of antipsychotics received in the past or currently prescribed have not been significantly correlated to the production of TD.

Although drug holidays are advisable for a number of valid reasons, there are contradictory reports as to whether they prevent the development of TD. Jeste et al. (1977) reported that they were "surprised" to find in their study that patients have irreversible or what they termed "persistent" TD had significantly more drug-free intervals in treatment than those with reversible dyskinesia. On the other hand, it has been strongly advocated that outpatient schizophrenics be taken off antipsychotic medication for 4 to 6 week periods from time to time; it is thought that these drug holidays will uncover most cases of "covert dyskinesia" who possibly represent a subgroup of early tardive dyskinesia potentially reversible with drug cessation (Carpenter, 1978; Ayd, 1978b). The rationale for these drug-free periods is the belief that early tardive dyskinesia cases are not detected because of the masking effect of the dopamine-blocking action of the antipsychotic drugs. The risk of relapse may be minimal during a drug holiday of such length.

It has been observed that TD of mild or minimal severity may be readily reversed by discontinuing antipsychotic medication or lowering the dosage. However, even severe, long-standing TD may improve considerably if the maintenance dose is reduced and if one waits long enough. Instances of marked improvement in the long-standing TD raises questions about the permanence of the symptomatology (Solomon, 1977a).

In view of these disparate factors, it is not surprising that some clinicians have concluded that identification of a single etiologic factor, including the use of phenothiazines, in case analyses of TD is impossible and the etiology of TD remains a puzzle (Turek, 1975). The paradoxical phenomenon of symptoms that may become manifest after the withdrawal of medication and may subside after the inreinstitution of treatment even raises the question of the wisdom of describing TD as a side effect of antipsychotics (Curran, 1973).

Clinically, TD is a constellation of involuntary hyperkinetic movements and may represent an irreversible neurologic syndrome in some patients. These movements may take the appearance of dyskinesias which are acquired involuntary movements superimposing upon or replacing normal motor activity. They may be further subdivided. Chorea (increased speed, amplitude and frequency of body movements) is the term for quick, "dancing" movements of a body part. Athetosis may be seen with writhing, "worm-like" contortions of tongue, fingers, wrists, arms, or ankles. Prolonged contractions of muscle groups can occur to produce a dystonia (prolonged tonic contraction). Dystonias can appear as severe arching of the back (oposthonos), arching the head backwards (retrocollis), rotational twisting of the neck (torticollis) or numerous bizarre contorted postures. Very quick flinging or flailing movements of the arms may appear. These are called ballistic movements (e.g., hemiballismus = flinging of one arm). An individual muscle in an arm or leg may twitch and contract in a rapid fashion (myoclonus) Many other nonspecific bizarre movements or postures may be seen (Table 21).

Abnormal movements of the mouth and face are the most common signs of TD. They are more likely to be seen in older rather than younger patients, while younger patients tend to show movements in the trunk musculature or extremeties. These orofacial dyskinesias usually appear with quick, repetitive tongue protusions ("fly catching") which are not unlike those of a frog after insects. Other oral-facial movements can be pouting, sucking, chewing, or twisting of the lips. Some patients may continually press their tongue against their buccal area and appear as if they have hard candy in their mouth (bon-bon sign). A rabbit syndrome may appear where the upper lip repeatedly elevates.

Extremity movements are more restless in nature than the orofacial disorders and often choreiform or athetotic in the hands or feet. These movements tend to amplify in the hands as the patient walks. If the patient is sitting, dorsiflexion and tapping of the feet may be present. This may sometimes be confused with the restless legs of akathisia. Younger patients (20s and 30s) may have very exaggerated and bizarre postures with marked truncal and extremity movements (Tarsy et al., 1977). These can be severe enough to impair employment and cause social disfigurement. Abnormalities of posture such as severe lordosis, shoulder shrugging or swaying and rocking while standing may be seen. Abnormal pelvic movements may resemble copulatory thrusting. Less common features of TD can be grunting vocalizations, myoclonic jerks of individual muscle groups, asynchronous breathing, and upward deviations of the eyes due to dystonias of the yoke muscles.

TABLE 21
Frequent Signs of Tardive Dyskinesia

FACE
  Blepharospasm (spasm of the eyelids, eyelid fluttering)
  Tremor of upper lip (rabbit syndrome)
  Pouting, puckering, smacking of lips
  Chewing movements
  Sucking movements
  Buccal pressing of tongue (bon-bon sign)
  Tongue protrusion (fly catching syndrome)

NECK
  Retrocollis (head arches backwards)
  Spasmodic torticollis (head and neck twist to right or left)

TRUNK
  Axial hyperkinesia (rocking, pelvic thrusting, copulation movements)
  Torsion or athetotic movements (twisting or writhing)

EXTREMITIES
  Ballistic movements (flinging or flailing)
  Chorea of hands or toes (quick, dancing movements)
  Athetosis (worm like, writhing movements)
  Rotation and/or flexion of ankles

OTHER
  Grunting vocalizations, asynchronous breathing (diaphragmatic dyskinesia),
  Myoclonus (rapid contractile jerking of individual muscle groups)

All of the previously described dyskinetic features may be seen alone or in combination with dystonias (prolonged tonic contractions). Dystonias are more frequent in the axial musculature of the neck and spine and can be present as torticollis, retrocollis or truncal torsion. Severe dystonias in TD, as with acute dystonias, are more commonly seen in persons less than 50 years of age (Tarsy and Baldessarini, 1976).

Tardive dyskinesia in children is generally far more florid than in adults. The movements are primarily confined to the extremities and chorea, athetosis, hemiballismus and myoclonus predominate (Polizos et al., 1973). Paulson et al. (1975) have described the emergence of tardive dyskinesia in 21 institutionalized mentally retarded children who have been exposed to long-term phenothiazines. Twenty of these patients were followed for 4 years. When reevaluated at that time, 6 children showed no change in severity of their dyskinesia, 4 had worsened movements, 5 had diminished movements, and 5 were lost to follow-up. However, the abnormal movements tended to remain visible at some level while maintained on the antipsychotic regimen. Browning and Ferry (1976) have likewise reported TD in a 10-year-old autistic child exposed to 20 mg. daily of prochlorperazine (Compazine). **Generally speaking, it seems advisable to avoid the use of antipsychotic medications in children unless management is impossible without them**.

The onset of TD is usually insidious. However, often the first sign of this syndrome will be vermicular (wormlike) movements of the tongue observed with the tongue lying in the floor of the mouth. Many factors can change the appearance of TD from time to time in the same patient. Abrupt withdrawal of antipsychotic medication can produce abnormal involuntary movements where none were previously present or can increase the amplitude of movements already present. Even a reduction in dosage might produce a breakthrough of TD. In other patients, the movements may insidiously appear over time while the antipsychotic drug dosage remains stable. Regardless of the time and manner of onset, the rate and severity of the abnormal movements may vary during the waking hours. Many physicians are unaware of this fact and may erroneously claim the patient is "hysteric" or "in control" of his symptoms. Asking a patient to focus on a mental task usually worsens the movements. Likewise, performing repetitive motor acts such as finger-tapping or walking will increase the severity of TD. Having the patient suppress movement in one body part usually increases remaining movements. Reduction of movements is seen with drowsiness or sedating drugs such as barbiturates or benzodiazepines. Movements cease altogether during sleep.

The differential diagnosis of tardive dyskinesia includes many potential causes of abnormal involuntary movements (Table 22). The diagnosis of TD should be considered in any patient who has more than a few months' exposure to any one of the phenothiazines, butyrophenones, thioxanthenes, dibenzoxazepines, or dihydroindolones. **Suspicion of TD should be especially keen if the onset of the abnormal movements coincides with either a reduction in dosage or a discontinuation of the antipsychotic medication.** The diagnosis of TD may be further confused by other drug-induced neurologic symptoms such as akathisia, parkinsonism, or acute dystonias. However, tremor is not a part of TD and is usually associated with other parkinson signs such as rigidity and bradykinesia.

Extrapyramidal dysfunction has many causes and most of these can be distinguished from TD on the basis of medical history, family history, drug history, laboratory study or physical and neurological examination. A confusing aspect of abnormal movements in psychotic patients is their variable nature. Spontaneous movements have been reported as a part of psychosis since Bleuler and Kraeplin and these obviously antedated the antipsychotic drug era. However, spontaneous movements seem qualitatively different from those in TD and are usually manneristic, stereotyped, repetitive and purposeless (Marsden et al., 1975). The most likely adult movement disorder to be confused with TD is Huntington's disease. This spontaneous extrapyramidal disease usually has less oral-facial involvement while the movements are often incorporated by the patient into other voluntary movements. Important clues to diagnosis are family history of abnormal movements, early associated dementia, and premature death. Usually an autosomal dominant inheritance pattern can be demonstrated. Three other spontaneous movement disorders can have certain features which resemble TD. Torsion dystonia generally begins between ages 5 and 15. There is less associated chorea and athetosis while severe axial torsions and dystonias predominate. Usually a familial pattern is apparent and a long progressive history is characteristic. Gilles de la Tourette's syndrome also occurs early in youngsters between 7 and 15 years of age. It is more common in boys than girls and can be separated from TD in children by the occurrence of facial grimacing, obscene vocalizations and facial tics. Like TD, however, it is treated with haloperidol, which may diminish or suppress the movements; these may reappear or worsen upon withdrawal of the drug. The last spontaneous movement disorder is Halervorden-Spatz syndrome. This has a peak age of onset of 10 years. There may be a family history of the illness and rigidity and paresis are the cardinal signs. Death usually occurs within 10 years and brain tissue findings show pigmentary deposits in the globus pallidus (McDowell and Lee, 1976).

Many infectious processes have caused extrapyramidal dysfunction; however, the most likely causes are rheumatic fever and post-encephalitic syndromes. Sydenham's chorea is the most common neurologic outcome of rheumatic fever. Most patients are less than 20 years of age and women outnumber men 2 to 1. Antipsychotic drugs will suppress the chorea and chlorpromazine has been the one most widely used for this purpose. Extrapyramidal disorders following encephalitis are reported but apparently are rare. These are more likely to occur in younger adults (McDowell and Lee, 1976).

Of the metabolic and toxic causes of abnormal involuntary movements, the one most likely to be confused with TD is hepatolenticular degeneration. (Wilson's disease). This inherited disorder of copper metabolism is primarily seen in adults. Abnormal movements are associated with lesions in the basal ganglia and signs of liver cirrhosis are generally present. A greenish deposit can often be seen in the corneal limbus of the eye but generally requires slit lamp examination for adequate demonstration. Patients with Wilson's disease should have diminished serum ceruloplasmin and total serum copper. On the other hand, albumin bound serum copper increases. Kernicterus (elevated serum bilirubin) at birth may leave adults with athetoid posturing and grimacing. These victims are mentally retarded and may have eighth nerve deafness. This syndrome is irreversible and diagnosis is made by history. Manganese toxicity can present with extrapyramidal signs. Usually an associated dementia is present. Elevated manganese levels will be found in urine, serum and hair shafts (Banta and Markesbury, 1977). Metabolic disorders can produce abnormal movements. Chorea may be seen in hyperthyroidism and differs from the usual find tremor in this disorder (Klawans and Shenker, 1972). Occasionally hypoparthyroidism will produce calcification of the basal ganglia with a resulting chorea (Tarsy and Baldessarini, 1976).

Other drug-induced abnormal involuntary movements are not that uncommon. The drug which causes an oral-facial dyskinesia most commonly is L-dopa. These movements caused by L-dopa are the most similar to TD of all reported drug-induced movement disorders. However, differentiation is fairly simple as this agent is almost exclusively used in the treatment of idiopathic or post-encephalitic parkinsonism. Alphamethyldopa, used in antihypertension therapy, has been reported to induce choreo-athetoid movements which reverse upon its discontinuation. Amphetamines, whether used licitly or not, can produce chewing movements but generally the movements are repetitious and stereotyped and do not resemble TD. Anticholinergic drugs (e.g., diphenhydramine) can induce abnormal movements in some patients and will generally worsen the movements of TD (Granacher, 1977). Tricyclic antidepressants, which are highly anticholinergic, have produced myoclonus at high or toxic dosages. Toxic amounts of phenytoin (Dilantin) have produced choreiform syndromes (Shuttleworth et al., 1974).

Antipsychotic agents have been used to control vomiting in pregnancy.

This could potentially cause diagnostic confusion with TD as chorea gravidarum (chorea of pregnancy) is a rare condition of pregnancy. It is reported to occur 1 in every 2000 to 3000 pregnancies. In the psychotic woman who is maintained on antipsychotic agents and then becomes pregnant, careful observation would be required in order to differentiate chorea gravidarum from TD. Generally, this chorea of pregnancy disappears following delivery.

Presently, one of the most confusing issues in the diagnosis of TD may be its differentiation from senile oral-facial dyskinesia. The aging process causes severe losses of enzymes important in the synthesis of basal ganglia dopamine. This in turn may predispose aged individuals to develop spontaneous oral-facial dyskinesia (McGeer et al., 1977). Therefore, in the elderly individual, one may have a chicken-egg dilemma. Did antipsychotic medication induce oral dyskinesia, hasten its appearance in a predisposed individual, or is the dyskinesia a consequence of an aging extrapyramidal system? These questions are presently unanswered.

TABLE 22
Differential Diagnosis of Tardive Dyskinesia

1. Spontaneous movements of psychosis

2. Spontaneous extrapyramidal disease
    a. Huntington's chorea
    b. Torsion dystonia (dystonia musculorum deformans)
    c. Gilles de la Tourette's Disease
    d. Hallervorden-Spatz Syndrome

3. Infectious or postinfectious extrapyramidal dysfunction
    a. Sydenham's chorea
    b. Post encephalitic syndromes

4. Metabolic or toxic causes of extrapyramidal dysfunction
    a. Hepatolenticular degeneration (Wilson's disease)
    b. Kernicterus
    c. Manganese poisoning
    d. Hyperthyroidism
    e. Hypoparathyroidism with basal ganglia calcification

5. Drug-induced extrapyramidal dysfunction
    a. Dihydroxyphenlalanine (L-dopa)
    b. Alpha-methyldopa
    c. Amphetamines
    d. Drugs with anticholinergic properties
    e. Phenytoin

6. Chorea gravidarum

7. Senile orafacial dyskinesia

The pathophysiology of TD remains an open question as well. Due to the frequently irreversible nature of TD, some have suggested structural changes in the brain. However, neuropathological studies have not demonstrated localizing structural changes (Roisin et al., 1959). Certain features of TD suggest that the neuronal dopamine systems in the brain have become hyperactive or oversensitive. As an example, the abnormal movements seen in TD will worsen when drugs which antagonize dopamine, such as chlorpromazine or haloperidol, are withdrawn. If brain dopamine levels are increased, such as with the administration of L-dopa, the movements are made worse. On the other hand, drugs which deplete stores of dopamine in brain neurons, such as reserpine, or block its effects, such as haloperidol, tend to suppress TD movements (Gerlach et al., 1974). Acetylcholine may also play a role in TD pathophysiology. It could be that deficiency or hypofunction of acetylcholine is present with a relative dopamine excess. For instance, anticholinergic agents tend to worsen TD and any commonly used antiparkinson drug can markedly worsen abnormal movements secondary to TD. Drugs which increase the availability of brain acetylcholine, such as physostigmine (Antilirium) have benefited some patients with TD where others have shown variable effects (Granacher et al., 1975). These data suggest that the prolonged and often irreversible nature of TD may be subsequent to toxic or pathologic changes in the basal ganglia of the brain. These changes may involve dopamine and acetylcholine neurons or their interactions in the extrapyramidal system.

The present management of TD presents significant problems to the physician. The literature is confusing, anecdotal, and not very helpful. **The essential approach to TD management at this time should focus on removing the offending agent, early case finding, or, if this is not helpful, reducing the intensity of the movements with an additional drug.** Quitkin et al. (1977) suggest that early signs of TD may be reversible. Therefore, at the first sign of TD, if the patient is taking antipsychotic drugs, every effort should be made to discontinue the medication. Obviously, for many chronically psychotic patients this is not practical. In those patients where medication is discontinued, the physician must be prepared for an initial worsening of the movements. In some patients, the abnormal movements will then decrease over time and in many patients will cease entirely. The prime candidates for a trial of antipsychotic medication withdrawal are younger patients in whom there is a greater likelihood of reversibility and in whom tardive dyskinesia may reach incapacitating proportions (Tarsy et al., 1977). **Those patients with neuroses and personality disorders who show signs of TD should be immediately withdrawn from antipsychotic agents unless valid reasons for their continuance can be demonstrated and are documented in their clinical records.**

For patients not capable of being withdrawn from antipsychotic agents, an attempt at suppressing the movements may be tried. Table 23 lists the medications that have been tried in the management of TD. For most of the chronically institutionalized patients, the movements of TD seem of little concern. If these individuals are behaviorly stable, attempted treatment of TD is probably not warranted. If suppression is needed, one can try raising the dose of antipsychotic agent. The movements may diminish but may reappear in their original form with the patient then on higher doses of the offending agent. This is not recommended unless the abnormal movements interfere with eating, ambulation or the respiratory rate problem of diaphragmatic dyskinesia with resultant hypoxemia (Weiner et al., 1978). Usually patients will show suppression of movements when the dosage of antipsychotic drug is raised by 25 to 50%.

Numerous other treatments have been tried with limited success. Deanol (2-dimethylaminoethanol, Deaner) is reported to increase brain acetylcholine levels. In limited uncontrolled trials it was felt to be effective at dosages up to 3 grams per day. The major side effect seems to be excess saliva. However, in controlled studies, it seems little better than placebo (Simpson et al., 1977). Likewise, lithium given to elderly patients until a blood level of 0.6 to 1.2 mEq./liter was achieved gave negative results in one controlled study (Simpson et al., 1976). On the other hand, a 3-week controlled evaluation of lithium in TD gave slight but significant reduction of movements (Gerlach et al., 1975). Papvarine, a dopamine-blocking agent used in vascular brain disease, has shown a modest ability to diminish movements of TD at dosages of 300 mg. b.i.d. However, the clinical results were not as striking as the statistical results (Gardos et al., 1976) and parkinsonism can superimpose upon TD. Choline and lecithin have been used in an attempt to load patients with an acetylcholine precursor and theoretically raise acetylcholine levels in a anner similar to L-dopa's use in Parkinson's disease for raising brain dopamine. At dosages of 16 grams daily, improvement in some patients with TD has been noted (Davis et al., 1975). Unfortunately, the gut metabolizes choline to trimethylamine and makes the patient smell "fishy." The long-term effects of such elevated dosages of choline or its precursor, lecithin, are unknown and caution is advised.

Recently, newer treatments have been reported. Jus (1978) followed chronic schizophrenic patients for 3 years. He simultaneously placed these individuals on reserpine 0.25 mg. to 1.0 mg. daily or haloperidol 0.5 mg. to 2.0 mg. daily. The patient's current dosage of antipsychotic was reduced to its lowest effective level and antiparkinson agents were discontinued. Piperazine phenothiazines were replaced with a piperidine phenothiazine such as mesoridazine (Serentil) or thioridazine (Mellaril). Of 108 patients with TD, 22 showed complete improvement, 43 had considerable improvement and 43 remained unchanged. With further discontinuation of the reserpine or haloperidol, 25 remained improved. Jus stresses that this regimen must be used for months or years to maximize results. Thus, it seems potentially applicable to chronically institutionalized patients.

A more experimental but possible treatment is the combination of reserpine and alpha-methyltyrosine (AMT). The physician would have to secure a personal Investigational New Drug (IND) permit by applying to the FDA. These are available to individual practitioners. AMT reduces dopamine levels by interfering with the enzyme tyrosine hydroxylase. Fahn (1978) has

TABLE 23
Drugs That May Suppress, Modify, or Exacerbate Tardive Dyskinesia

A. Possible suppressors
   1. Dopamine blocking agents
      a. Phenothiazines (e.g. chlorpromazine, Thorazine)
      b. Butyrophenones (e.g. haloperidol, Haldol)
      c. Thioxanthenes (e.g., thiothixene, Navane)
      d. Dibenzoxazepines (e.g. loxapine, Loxitane)
      e. Dihydroindolones (e.g. molindone, Lidone)
      f. Papaverine

   2. Amine depletors
      a. Reserpine

   3. Catecholamine synthesis blocker
      a. Alpha-methyltyrosine (AMT)

   4. Catecholamine release blockers
      a. Lithium carbonate

B. Agents with variable effects
   1. Amantadine (Symmetrel)
   2. Sodium Valproate (Depakene)
   3. Clonazepam (Clonopin)
   4. Benzodiazepines (e.g. Valium, Librium)
   5. Methylphenidate (Ritalin)
   6. 2-dimethlyaminoethanol, deanol (Deaner)
   7. Choline-Lecithin

C. Agents that exacerbate
   1. Anticholinergic agents
      a. Antiparkinson agents (e.g. Artane, Cogentin)
      b. Antihistamines
      c. Tricyclic antidepressants (e.g. Elavil, Tofranil)
      d. Atropine-like antispasmodics

   2. Dopamine-like agents
      a. L-dopa
      b. Amphetamines

started patients on reserpine with a gradual increase of up to 6 mg. daily. Blood pressure must be closely monitored. If reserpine alone is not effective, AMT 250 mg. every other day is added. Patients have to be individually titrated and some require as much as 3 mg. reserpine and 1.5 gm. AMT in combination daily.

Many drug combinations have theoretical utility in the management of TD but none has shown a clear superiority in controlled studies (Jeste and Wyatt, 1979). Table 24 suggests a strategy for approaching this syndrome until more reliable treatment methods are found or until the pathophysiology of this syndrome is more fully understood. At the present time no single agent or treatment seems satisfactory for TD.

In spite of the controversial and conflicting reports involving the question of etiology, prevalence and outcome of TD, a great many authorities tend to agree that it is a "real" entity and that it is related to the use of antipsychotic

TABLE 24
Strategy for Management of Tardive Dyskinesia

- Take a thorough psychiatric, medical and medication history to rule out other causes for abnormal movements as noted in Table 22.

- Observe and record abnormal movements as noted in Table 21. Note in the patient's record whether these individual movements are none = 0, minimal = 1, mild = 2, moderate = 3, or severe = 4.

- Reduce antipsychotic medication to the lowest level necessary to prevent relapse. Observe patient for 3 months as relapse of psychosis may not appear immediately. Discontinue antiparkinson agents.

- If movements persist or psychosis worsens, switch patient to a piperidine phenothiazine (mesoridazine or thioridazine) and titrate to lowest level necessary to control psychosis. Observe for 3 months and record individual movements at intervals.

- If movements persist, slowly add reserpine in 0.25 mg. increments with close observation of blood pressure. If improvement occurs, it should be seen at total dosages below 5 mg. daily.

- If movements persist and limit the patient's function, consider obtaining an IND and adding alpha-methyltyrosine to reserpine in 250 mg. increments up to 1.5 grams daily.

- If movements persist, continue piperidine antipsychotic, discontinue reserpine and AMT. Give 2-3 month trials of lithium carbonate up to 1.2 mEq/l. blood level.

- If movements persist, discontinue lithium and pursue 2-3 month trials of clonazepam (Clonopin) up to 6 gm/day, valproic acid (Depakene) 20 mg./Kg./day, choline up to 15 gm/day, or papavarine (Pavabid) 600 mg./day.

- If movements persist, discontinue all adjunctive medications and continue the patient on the lowest effective antipsychotic maintenance dose.

drugs. However, there is a small group who have been beating a steady drum of alarm that many psychiatrists are practicing antipsychotic drug therapy very defensively and thus often ineffectively for fear of inducing TD in their patients. Others have even advocated that written informed consent be obtained prior to treatment or after 3 months and 1 year of drug therapy (Ayd, 1977b; Sovner et al., 1978). It has been pointed out that a valid consent is often an "illusion," "an impossible dream" and "in practice it is fraught with difficulty and too often impossible to obtain," that "few patients can completely comprehend and utilize the detailed data that must be assimilated for a valid choice to be made" (Feldman, 1978). Out-of-court settlements have been reported for TD (Trent and Muhl, 1976), but no consent form can afford absolute protection from legal suits (Alfidi, 1975). Another writer states that, for the present, patients should be warned of the dangers of tardive dyskinesia so that they can make a choice to avoid irreversible side effects and try "alternative treatments" (Gotbetter, 1978). Such statements display a lack of awareness or ignore the fact that there are no "alternative treatments" and that psychosocial therapies have been shown to be of little or no value in schizophrenia without the addition of antipsychotic drug therapy.

Any measure that restricts the prescribing of antipsychotic drugs would be a tragedy indeed, since the benefits of judicious use of these drugs for psychoses, especially schizophrenia, far outweigh the inherent risk of TD. There are certain antibiotics, anticonvulsants, hormones and cardiovascular preparations, each of which has a higher incidence of permanently disabling side effects (and even deaths) than the entire group of antipsychotics. Still, there is no hue and cry for obtaining written informed consent before prescribing these agents. It appears that success with drug therapy in psychiatry has offended many who, for various reasons or motives, abhor the use of drugs. As a result, a different set of standards is applied to the use of the antipsychotics and other psychotherapeutic drugs than to any other class of drugs (Hollister, 1970). When consideration is given to the hundreds of millions of doses of antipsychotics administered for over decades with the very infrequent development of TD severe enough to be socially or occupationally disabling, the conclusion is inevitable that the antipsychotic agents are among the safest agents in the medical armamentarium. Even if a mild TD develops, it is not a heavy price to pay for relief from the suffering and other disabling symptoms of schizophrenia and other psychoses. Moreover, it is important to note that in a 12-year follow-up study of extensively drug-treated, chronic, hospitalized schizophrenics, not a single case of disabling TD developed in 89 patients (Gardos and Cole, 1979).

Nevertheless, rational psychiatric practice dictates that mental health professionals be alert and routinely scrutinize the patient on antipsychotic drugs to detect the earliest signs of TD. This should be done every 6 months at a minimum. Early lingual dyskinesia can be seen when the mouth is open. There may be a barely perceptible lingual fibrillation, as well as rhythmical forward and backward and, at times, lateral movements of the tongue. Tremor of the tongue alone is a normal finding in many people. Those with early symptoms cannot protrude the tongue for more than a few seconds. Facial tics, particularly eye-blinking, may become apparent. Early digital dyskinesia consists of involuntary movements of the fingers, either extensions or contractions, most often of the index finger (Ayd, 1977b). Discontinuation or lowering the dosage of the antipsychotic as soon as early TD symptoms are discovered will usually result in a complete reversal. However, the risk-benefit ratio must be weighed in each individual case before stopping medication.

Psychiatric nurses and other mental health professionals can be trained to monitor for early signs of TD when the drug orders are written every 30 days for inpatients or during outpatient visits to the office or clinic. It is important that both the positive and negative findings of each examination be specifically covered in the medical records.

In view of the above, the emergence of tardive dyskinetic signs does not necessarily mean that patients must have their antipsychotic therapy stopped or there is no solution for the therapeutic dilemma posed for the clinician by tardive dyskinesia (Gardos and Cole, 1979). On the contrary, there are grounds for optimism that the challenge raised by tardive dyskinesia may be successfully met by the therapist who is innovative, persistent and willing to take legitimate therapeutic risks.

Seizures

Antipsychotic agents reportedly lower the seizure threshold in susceptible individuals. However, in clinical practice this seems to be an infrequent occurrence. Extensive reviews note that these compounds may increase convulsions in epileptic patients or initiate convulsions in previously normal individuals (Shaw et al., 1959). The incidence of this side effect is unknown. The literature may be misleading since in many reports severe dystonic reactions may have been misreported as seizures. There is at present no data to support the claim that any particular antipsychotic is less likely to induce seizures.

The one area where the physician must be careful is alcohol withdrawal. The studies of antipsychotic agents used in alcohol withdrawal document an increase in seizure activity (Greenblatt and Shader, 1975). On the other hand, there does not seem to be direct evidence that patients previously controlled with anticonvulsants will "break through" with seizures if antipsychotics are added. **However, due to possible increased seizure activity, antipsychotic agents should be given cautiously to patients with a history of seizures.**

2. CARDIOVASCULAR EFFECTS

Hypotensive Effects

Orthostatic hypotension is the most common cardiovascular side effect with antipsychotics and is second only to neurologic side effects in frequency. Orthostatic hypotension is hypotension which is made worse upon assuming an upright posture. It is not possible to get an accurate incidence of antipsychotic drug-induced hypotension as the literature is sparse and does not adequately document a standard technique of blood pressure measurement. For instance, those studies that have been cited do not distinguish between sitting and standing blood pressure readings (Shader and DiMascio, 1970).

Since blood pressure readings in most hospitals are made while the patient is supine or sitting, the diagnosis of orthostatic hypotension may be suggested by clinical signs only. The patient may complain of dizziness, unsteady gait, or syncope. Such items as intermittent blurred vision, rapid pulse and sweating with pallor may be present. However, the cardinal feature is the presentation of these signs and symptoms when the patient arises to an erect posture after quiet sitting or lying. Such features may be especially troublesome when the patient arises in the morning, gets out of a chair after watching television, or rises from the toilet. Generally a drop of 15 to 20 mm Hg in systolic pressure will cause clinical signs when the patient arises. However, some patients may show an opposite phenomenon. The patient may be slightly symptomatic when standing or walking but on sitting down for a period of time may become somnolent and appear to fall asleep. Sitting blood pressure in these individuals may be as low as 50/0 mm Hg. Large inpatient wards with open dayrooms probably have far more hypotensive individuals sitting somnolently in chairs than is realized. Since the patient is supported by the chair, he can be literally unconscious due to hypotension but not fall over (Jefferson, 1972).

Sudden and severe drops in blood pressure can reach shock-like proportions, especially following the parenteral use of antipsychotic agents. This shock syndrome, which is comparatively rare, can appear as a sudden motor weakness, pallor, cold sweating, thready pulse, and disorientation or unconsciousness.

Usually the diagnosis of orthostatic hypotension following the use of antipsychotic drugs is relatively easy. The patient has normally been exposed to the medication for only a short period of time and is likely to be on an aliphatic or piperidine phenothiazine, although all currently used antipsychotic agents have caused hypotension in at least some people. **If the patient seems unusually sensitive and manifests severe hypotension on many different chemical classes of antipsychotic drugs, other causes for the hypotension should be sought.** The most confusing entity which could be made worse with antipsychotic agents is idiopathic autonomic insufficiency (idiopathic orthostatic hypotension). This is an uncommon neurologic disorder with features of orthostatic hypotension and symptoms such as impotence, constipation, heat intolerance and lack of sweating. As the disease progresses, a parkinson-like illness (Shy-Drager syndrome) may develop with bradykinesia, a rhythmic postural tremor and mild to moderate muscular rigidity. Some individuals may develop a cerebellar type of incoordination and a gross rhythmic tremor in the lower extremities. The key differentiating features of this illness are that victims are not psychotic and have no signs of schizophrenia and there is no increase in pulse rate as is expected with hypotension. Other disorders which may produce orthostatic hypotension include: anemia, acute cardiac failure, loss of blood volume, vasodepressant drugs, dehydration, prolonged bed rest, adrenocortical insufficiency. Neurological causes of poor blood pressure control include Wernicke's encephalopathy, tabes dorsalis, syringomyelia, surgical sympathectomy, neuropathies of diabetes, amyloidosis and the Guillian-Barré Syndrome (Spalding and Nelson, 1976). In most cases of orthostatic hypotension during antipsychotic drug therapy, the psychotropic agent will clearly be the cause. However, the careful physician should consider the previous entities in puzzling patients.

TABLE 25
Ability to Induce Hypotension Based on the
Ratio of Alpha-adrenergic Blocking Ability
to Dopamine-Blocking Activity

Drug	Sedative/hypotensive activity	
Promazine	+ + + + +	Most Potent
Thioridazine	+ + + +	
Chlorpromazine	+ + + +	
Droperidol	+ + +	
Thiothixene	+	
Haloperidol	+	
Fluphenazine	+	
Trifluoperazine	+	Least Potent

Modified from Peroutka et al., 1977

The etiology of anti-psychotic drug-induced orthostatic hypotension is not entirely clear. Both sedation and orthostatic hypotension from these agents have been attributed to their ability to block central and peripheral alpha-adrenergic receptors. However, the ability to measure blockade of these receptors in the brain has only recently become available. It has been hypothesized that the sedating and hypotensive potential of antipsychotic agents is related to the ratio of alpha-adrenergic blocking ability to dopamine-blocking activity. In other words, drugs with low ratios (e.g., thioridazine or chlorpromazine) will be anticipated to cause hypotension far more frequently than those with high ratios. Table 25 lists these ratios (Peroutka et al., 1977) and shows that those at the bottom of the list (e.g., haloperidol, trifluoperazine or fluphenazine) are much less likely to produce orthostatic hypotension. From these data, the physician can make alternative rational drug choices in the psychotic patient with an orthostatic blood pressure response to a given drug.

The treatment of mild orthostatic hypotension is relatively simple. Most patients will have become tolerant to this effect over time. Sletten et al. (1965) have shown that patients given oral chlorpromazine will have a significant decrease in supine systolic blood pressure at day 10 but not at the 30th or 90th day of treatment. Again, controlled studies of standing and supine blood pressures following antipsychotic agents are not available (Shader and DiMascio, 1970). For those patients who are symptomatic, bed rest, rising from a bed or chair slowly, and elastic stockings should bring relief.

The rare individual who develops severe hypotension and shock must be treated quickly and vigorously. **The cardinal rule in this situation is to never use epinephrine as a pressor agent.** Epinephrine has both alpha- and beta-adrenergic stimulating properties. As antipsychotic agents are alpha-adrenergic blocking agents, the unopposed beta-adrenergic activity of epinephrine will further lower the blood pressure with potentially fatal results.

The management of a severe shock syndrome is best accomplished in a general medical setting. However, many psychiatric hospitals may be too far removed from general medical support and transporting an untreated patient in shock is dangerous. Table 26 outlines an emergency approach to antipsychotic drug-induced shock where medical support is not quickly available.

The patient should be positioned with the head and trunk in a horizontal position and the legs elevated 30 degrees. The first and foremost consideration is to insure that the patient has an adequate airway. The mouth should be quickly checked and any vomitus, dental prostheses, or other objects quickly removed. Suction should be readily available. The patient must have adequate pulmonary ventilation and an Ambu bag or mouth-to-

TABLE 26
Treatment of Hypotension Secondary to Antipsychotic Drugs

Mild	Supine position. Dangle legs over side of bed before arising. Elastic support stockings. Wait for tolerance to develop to hypotension.
Shock	Head and trunk horizontal, feet elevated 30 degrees. Adequate airway, Ambu if needed, oxygen as necessary. Volume replacement with Ringer's solution or dextrose in water or saline. Maintain urine output greater than 50 ml/hr, monitor with Foley catheter. Pressor agents if necessary, *never use epinephrine*. Blanket to preserve body heat, avoid direct external heat. Transfer to a medical ward.

mouth respiration may be necessary. If the patient is cyanotic, start oxygen immediately. Where blood gases are available, maintain the patient's arterial oxygen saturation above 60 mm Hg. The patient should be kept warm with a blanket or heat cradle but do not apply direct external heat as this may dilate peripheral vessels and drop blood pressure further. Ringer's solution, normal saline or 5% dextrose in saline should be infused to increase volume. To prevent fluid overload, this is best monitored by a central venous pressure (CVP) line, not allowing the CVP to exceed 15 cm H_2O. If CVP monitoring is unavailable, the patient should be observed for jugular venous distension and/or dependent pulmonary rales indicative of fluid overload. Usually 500-2000 cc of fluid over a 1-hour period will not cause pulmonary edema in patients with previously normal cardiac function. After airway and IV fluid needs are established and controlled, a Foley catheter should be placed in the urinary bladder. Urine output volume should be maintained above 50 ml/hour to prevent renal tubular necrosis.

If the above measures are inadequate, a pressor agent may be necessary. Levarternol bitartrate (Levophed, sometimes referred to as l-norepinephrine or l-arternol) can be given as 4 ml of 0.2% solution in 500 ml of 5% dextrose and water intravenously. Extravasation should be avoided or tissue necrosis and gangrene may result.

Some clinicians add phentolamine (Regitine) directly to the infusion flask in a 5 to 10 mg. dose. It is believed that, used in this manner, this is an effective antidote to tissue sloughing and does not impair the systemic vasopressor activity of levarterenol (Zucker et al., 1960). Metaraminol (Aramine) bitartrate can be given in one of three possible ways: as 2-10 mg. IM; 0.5-5 mg. very cautiously; or 200 mg. by slow infusion in 500 ml of 5% dextrose in water IV. The latter is recommended. Phenylephrine (Neosynephrine) 10 mg. in 500 ml 5% dextrose in water or saline is also useful.

In all cases the blood pressure should be frequently checked and the pressor infusion regulated to keep systolic BP at 100 to 110. The patient should be transferred to a general medical setting as soon as vital signs are stable.

Congestive Heart Failure

Phenothiazines and other classes of antipsychotic drugs are felt to have a negative inotropic effect (decrease cardiac muscle contractility) upon the heart (Goodman and Gilman, 1975). Some observers feel that chlorpromazine is capable of producing a "toxic cardiomyopathy" and can produce cardiomegaly and heart failure in individuals chronically exposed to antipsychotic agents. One patient with evidence of an old myocardial infarction reportedly developed an acute myocardial infarction during treatment with chlorpromazine alone (Alexander and Nino, 1969). On the other hand, Samet and Surawicz (1974) have studied cardiac output in patients maintained on antipsychotic drugs for periods ranging from 2 months to 20 years. They were unable to demonstrate clinical depression of cardiac output in humans chronically exposed to antipsychotic agents. However, Carlsson et al. (1976) report that both chlorpromazine and thiothixene reduce stroke volume in schizophrenics during exercise, with thiothixene causing the least effect. Other studies by their group have shown that chlorpromazine has a greater adverse effect than haloperidol on exercise response in the heart. At this point in time, it is not clear whether antipsychotic medications will induce heart failure in humans. However, extra caution is probably advisable when using antipsychotic agents in patients with known cardiac disease or history of congestive heart failure.

EKG Effects

Changes in the electrocardiogram have been widely recognized to result from exposure to antipsychotic drugs. For the most part, these changes do not affect cardiac function. Most reports of EKG changes in the literature implicate the phenothiazines, possibly due to their longer history of clinical use. Incidence figures are scanty. Jeeva Raj and Benson (1975) have reported abnormal electrocardiograms in 55% of 20 patients treated with thioridazine, 50% of 49 patients taking chlorpromazine, 37% of 27 patients receiving trifluoperazine, and 30% of 33 patients exposed to fluphenazine decanoate. These disorders of the electrocardiogram seem to worsen as the antipsychotic dosage increases and are probably reversible abnormalities of ventricular repolarization. Thioridazine is the antipsychotic agent most often noted to cause EKG changes. These same changes are less pronounced with chlorpromazine and seem even further less likely with the other antipsychotic medications. The earliest abnormal change noted in the EKG following antipsychotic drugs is a lengthening of the QT interval. Usually widening, blunting and notching of the T wave accompany the QT interval change. At higher dosages of antipsychotic drug, the T wave may become lower and invert. These effects are often more pronounced in the right than in the left chest leads. In some individuals, the QT interval may lengthen without apparent T wave changes. Frequently, the U wave amplitude will also increase. Changes in the S-T segment are usually absent and P wave and QRS changes rarely occur with antipsychotic drugs alone.

Dosage effects are best documented with thioridazine. As little as 200 mg. daily will often cause detectable EKG changes and nearly always at doses around 800 mg. daily. These repolarization changes have often been compared with the effects of quinidine. Phenothiazines may affect the slope and duration of phase 3 of the ventricular action potential. However, they do not seem to have any effect upon depolarization.

Sudden Death

Unexpected and sudden deaths have been reported numerous times since the advent of antipsychotic drugs. However, sudden death was reported in psychotic patients long before chlorpromazine. Controversy remains and it is presently not clear what role antipsychotic agents play in sudden death (death occurring unexpectedly within 1 hour). Leestma and Koenig (1968) reviewed the world's literature and reported an average age of sudden death in phenothiazine-exposed patients to be 41 years of age. Only one patient was under 23. However, a review by Peele and Van Loetzen (1973) found 7 patients under age 21 in 65 such cases. A recent case describes sudden unexplained death in a woman age 20 (Goodson and Litkenhous, 1976).

Arrhythmias, as a potential cause of sudden death, have been most extensively reported in association with thioridazine or chlorpromazine. In most cases, thioridazine seems implicated at a greater frequency than other antipsychotic agents. However, a direct causal relationship between the ability of thioridazine to induce cardiac rhythm disturbances and the incidence of sudden unexplained death has not been shown. Both thioridazine and chlorpromazine have been used in the United States since 1965; therefore, the total number of patients exposed to these agents is greater than those exposed to the butyrophenones and newer agents such as molindone HCl or loxapine succinate.

Attempts have been made to find pathologic lesions in the myocardium of patients who died suddenly and unexpectedly while on antipsychotic agents. Richardson et al. (1966) found pigmentary deposits in the heart muscle of patients who died unexpectedly, but these were not pathologically different fron controls. On the other hand, in 12 sudden deaths who received either chlorpromazine, prochlorperazine, or thioridazine, they found unusual degenerative changes in intramyocardial arterioles. Eight of these patients had abnormal EKGs before death. As the lesions were in the right and left atrioventricular conduction bundle and papillary muscles, it is speculated that the conduction system might well be involved. Electron microscopy has further found nonspecific mitochondrial damage in patients receiving phenothiazines. However, these changes have also been described in other types of heart disease (Guillan et al., 1970). The question of the role of antipsychotic agents in sudden death remains unanswered. A recent survey of 1,932 psychiatric inpatients found cardiac side effects in 1.3% of patients without cardiac disease, while 18.8% of patients with cardiac disease had side effects. This survey included primarily tricyclic antidepressants and antipsychotic agents with 1,854 receiving antipsychotic drugs (Swett and Shader, 1977). **Based on the confusing literature on sudden death and antipsychotic agents, it seems prudent to use lower doses in patients with known or suspected cardiac disease and possibly to avoid chlorpromazine or thioridazine in patients with dysrhythmias.**

3. GASTROINTESTINAL EFFECTS

Side effects found in the GI system seem rather common, especially in inpatient settings, yet exact incidence figures are not available. Judging from the number of orders for antacids or laxitives in patients taking antipsychotic agents, the incidence may well be very significant. **Dry mouth is probably the most frequent side effect reported in patients taking antipsychotic agents and certainly is the most common gastrointestinal complaint.** It occurs secondary to the anticholinergic properties of these agents and the more anticholinergic the antipsychotic, the more likely is dry mouth to occur. If the patient wears dentures, a chronically dry mouth can become a serious problem. This may lead to denture pain, poor eating habits, and adverse nutritional effects (Fann and Shannon, 1978).

The intensity of dry mouth, like most antipsychotic side effects, usually diminishes with time. However, it can persist as a troublesome side effect long after other side effects have become unnoticed. Bethanechol (Urecholine) 25 mg. t.i.d. has been reported to be of benefit with complaints of dry mouth (Everett, 1975). Moreover, it will not cross the blood-brain barrier to exert central effects.

Recently, the Houston Veterans Administration Hospital has reported on a saliva substitute for use in severe dry mouth conditions following head and neck irradiation. Its application in psychiatric patients with drug-induced dry mouth seems successful and no adverse effects are reported (Fann and Shannon, 1978). It is commercially available as Orex (King's Specialty Company, Fort Wayne, Ind.) and Xerolube (First Texas Pharmaceuticals, Dallas Texas). Most patients apply this preparation on average of 5 times daily.

Nausea and vomiting have been reported with most psychotropic agents and the antipsychotics are no exception. This seems quite paradoxical, as chlorpromazine and all agents other than thioridazine have well-documented antiemetic properties. Moreover, symptoms of nausea and vomiting seem to occur with a similar frequency in patients who receive placebo rather than an antipsychotic. Only thioridazine seems to have poor antiemetic properties when compared with chlorpromazine (Shader and DiMascio, 1970). Thus, it is not clear whether antipsychotic agents induce nausea in some patients or whether nausea is merely an unexplained symptom in psychotic agents. However, nausea and vomiting also occur upon the abrupt withdrawal of antipsychotic agents and may represent supersensitivity of dopamine receptors in the chemoreceptor trigger zone of the medulla that were previously blocked by the antipsychotic agent (Yepes and Winsberg, 1977).

Dysphagia is another seemingly common symptom which may be grossly underrecognized. A walk through the dining rooms of a large psychiatric hospital will reveal many patients with milk pouring out of their mouths and upon the front of their clothing. Likewise, every large psychiatric facility has its horror story to relate about a patient choking to death in the dining room. It is often forgotten that dysphagia is an uncommon but potentially disastrous consequence of antipsychotic-induced parkinsonism. This type of dysphagia is almost always hypopharyngeal in nature or, more exactly, cricopharyngeal achalasia (failure of the cricopharyngeal muscles to relax). As a form of hypopharyngeal neuromuscular incoordination, the cricopharyngeus muscle either does not open quickly enough or as the bolus of food descends through the pharynx it closes before all of the food has passed (Palmer, 1974; Solomon, 1977b).

These dysphagic symptoms are likely to occur abruptly and once they begin are not likely to remit spontaneously. Solids are easier to swallow than liquids since liquids cause more aspiration and coughing. However, solids are more likely to obstruct the airway. The main complaints of chronic parkinsonian dysphagia are chronic laryngitis, acute and chronic tracheobronchitis and mild spotty aspiration pneumonia. The differential diagnosis of extrapyramidal dysphagia would include such items as myasthenia gravis, polyneuropathies such as diabetes, tumors, laryngitis, scleroderma, and very rarely tuberculosis of the larynx. It should be remembered that prior to the advent of antipsychotic drugs, psychotic patients bolted their food and had swallowing problems, especially if edentulous.

Due to the difficulty with swallowing in many patients receiving anti-psychotic agents, dining room personnel in psychiatric institutions should be thoroughly trained in emergency treatment of the choking patient. It may be advisable to have parenteral antiparkinson agents readily available along with routine airway resuscitation equipment. If a patient continues to have difficulty in swallowing liquids, it may be advisable to switch the patient to a drug with a lessened neurological side-effect profile, such as mesori-dazine or thioridazine.

Heartburn (pyrosis) seems to occur at a greater than expected frequency in patients on antipsychotic drugs. The anticholinergic properties of many antipsychotics decrease the lower esophageal muscular tone. This in turn drops the intraluminal pressure of the distal esophagus and allows gastric contents to reflux into the lower third of the esophagus (Van Thiel, 1977). Raising the head of the patient's bed 6-7 inches may offer relief, as may the use of an antacid which floats on top of the gastric contents (e.g., Gaviscon). Of course, antacids used chronically may add to constipation problems that often accompany antipsychotic drug usage.

Constipation is a frequent complaint in any hospitalized patient, regardless of the medical nature. Thus, it is often difficult to show clear-cut drug-related constipation. However, the increased occurrence of paralytic ileus and megacolon in patients on long-term antipsychotic therapy would tend to demonstrate that antipsychotic drugs probably decrease bowel function. **In fact, due to their anticholinergic activity, they can potentially mask a surgical abdomen and special care should be used in evaluating abdominal complaints in patients taking high dosages of antipsychotic medications.** Also, fecal impaction should be ruled out in patients with vague abdominal complaints, vomiting or unexplained fever if they are receiving antipsy-chotics. Management of intestinal ileus may require using antipsychotic agents that are very low in their anticholinergic activity such as trifluoper-azine, fluphenazine, or haloperidol.

4. HEMATOPOIETIC EFFECTS

Of the drug-induced blood dyscrasias, antipsychotic drugs are consis-tently associated only with leukopenia and agranulocytosis. Leukopenia generally means that the patient's white blood count (WBC) is below the normal range for a particular laboratory. On the other hand, agranulocytosis has been defined as a combination of a WBC below 3,700/cu mm with a decrease in neutrophils to less than one-third of their normal percentage and with secondary symptoms such as ulceration of mucous membrane and fever from the lowered resistance to infection (Mandel and Gross, 1968). Agranulocytosis secondary to antipsychotic agents is very rare, even though reported incidence varies from 1 per 100 to 1 per 250,000. One of the largest retrospective studies found an agranulocytosis incidence of 0.05% or 1 per 2,000 patients who took phenothiazines and an incidence of leukopenia of 0.8% or 1 per 125 patients (Litvak and Kaebling, 1971). Moreover, the Boston Collaborative Drug Surveillance Program found only 1 or 2 cases of bone marrow depression in 44,430 medical and psychiatric outpatients. However, the number of patients actually exposed to phenothiazines is not clearly stated (Swett, 1975).

Some clinicians feel that patients chronically exposed to antipsychotic medications should have routine laboratory determinations of complete blood counts. Most research studies to date will not support this notion. In fact, routine CBCs are rarely helpful in predicting agranulocytosis; however, they might be useful in spotting leukopenia in large populations of patients. Agranulocytosis is probably of allergic origin and usually occurs within a well-defined time span (between the fifth and tenth weeks of medication), regardless of the dose administered.

The most important factor in recognizing agranulocytosis from psychotropic drugs is clinical observation of the patient. Questioning for the occurrence of mucous membrane sores or fever will provide important clues. With the occurrence of polypharmacy, particular care must be exercised. Each time a new agent is introduced into the treatment of a patient, a new period of risk of bone marrow suppression begins for that patient (Ducomb and Baldessarini, 1977). **One must therefore be alert to the possibility of bone marrow suppression for several weeks following the initiation of treatment with antipsychotic agents, as well as after a change to a new agent or the addition of a second agent (which is not recommended—see Polypharmacy section in Chapter II).**

Table 27 gives the essentials of the diagnosis of agranulocytosis and its management. The differential diagnosis of a patient who demonstrates a severely depressed WBC while taking antipsychotic drugs includes aplastic anemia and acute aleukemic leukemia. Management centers on first stopping the offending agent. Blood samples should be taken for bacterial culture and sensitivity testing. Supportive measures include good oral hygiene, adequate fluid intake and reduction of fever. Patients may need to be isolated to reduce risk of infection. Antibiotics may be necessary. Carbenicillin 20 gm/sq m/day given every 4 hours IV plus cephalothin, 20-80 mg./Kg/day given every 6 hours IV is recommended (Wallerstein, 1975). Prophylactic use of penicillin or other antibiotics is to be avoided. Broad spectrum antibiotics should not be used unless specifically indicated by sensitivity testing of bacterial cultures. Mortality can approach 80% in untreated cases but is much lower with antibiotics. When recovery occurs it is complete, but the offending agent should not be reused. If the patient is highly psychotic,

TABLE 27
Diagnosis and Management of Antipsychotic Drug-Induced Agranulocytosis

Diagnosis	Careful routine evaluation of temperature, oral mucosa, and throat. Chills, fever, sore throat. Ulceration of oral mucosa and throat. Granulocytopenia with relative lymphocytosis. Increased sedimentation rate.
Treatment	Discontinue antipsychotic agent. Blood culture and sensitivity. Good oral hygiene, fluid intake and fever reduction. Isolation. Carbenicillin 10 gm/sq m/day q 4 hours IV plus cephalothin 20-80 mg/ Kg./day q 6 hours IV, if severe. Do not use prophylactic penicillin. Broad spectrum antibiotics if culture and sensitivity indicates.

treatment with an entirely different chemical entity will be necessary. For instance, if the patient develops agranulocytosis to a phenothiazine, a cautious trial of loxapine succinate, molindone hydrochloride or haloperidol may prove successful. However, closer monitoring of the patient's CBC is indicated for the first 4-6 weeks.

For the patient with chronic leukopenia, a different management is necessary. Despite leukopenia, patients can often safely continue on the present antipsychotic. In fact, almost as many patients may develop leukopenia without treatment with psychotropic drugs as with treatment (incidence 0.6% vs. 0.8%). Some patients may even show a return to a normal WBC while continuing to take the offending agent. This has caused investigators to assume that some patients have spontaneous leukopenia which occurs cyclically and is unrelated to drugs (Litvak and Kaebling, 1971). The risk of leukopenia developing into a full-blown agranulocytosis is not presently known. **But, again, it is stressed that careful observation for signs of fever, mouth sores, and malaise in patients receiving antipsychotic drugs by nurses and physicians is the best practical approach to discovery of agranulocytosis at the present time.**

5. HEPATIC EFFECTS

All texts which deal with the side effects of antipsychotic agents include jaundice as a potential uptoward effect. The literature on hepatotoxicity of antipsychotics is almost entirely devoted to chlorpromazine. However, prochlorperazine, trifluoperazine and promazine have been implicated and rarely other psychotics. In actuality, jaundice is seen with far less frequency than in the past but the cause for this decline is unknown. Exact rates of occurrence are not readily available but an overall rate of less than 0.5% for all antipsychotic agents with a frequency of 1-2% for chlorpromazine has been reported (Caldwell, 1976).

If antipsychotic-induced jaundice occurs, it is most likely during the second to fourth week of drug exposure. After the fifth week this complication is rare. Aliphatic phenothiazines (e.g., chlorpromazine, promazine) may have a higher probability of causation. Occurrence and severity of jaundice are unrelated to total dosage and seem idiosyncratic. A prodrome of fever, abdominal discomfort, anorexia, vomiting, diarrhea and an enlarged tender liver may appear but is by no means always present. When jaundice develops, it is of the intrahepatic obstructive type. Biochemical testing will show elevated plasma bilirubin which rarely exceeds 15 mg./100 ml. Direct bilirubin is greater than indirect, bile is present in the urine and serum alkaline phosphatase will be abnormally elevated. The stools will be pale and eosinophilia may be present. In some cases, jaundice may be subclinical with only findings of fever, eosinophilia, and elevated serum alkaline phosphatase.

The duration of jaundice is reversible upon withdrawal of the offending antipsychotic but may take up to 4 weeks to subside. Complete recovery is the general rule; however, 10% of patients may require more than 3 months to improve clinically and in a rare minority as long a period as 3 years has been needed. Some patients have recovered spontaneously even while administration of the offending drug continues. Desensitation to chlorpromazine may occur in some individuals over time. Chronic alcoholism, pregnancy, hypoproteinemia, malnutrition and exposure to known hepatotoxins reportedly predispose individuals to phenothiazine-induced jaundice (Ban, 1969; Caldwell, 1976).

The pathophysiology of antipsychotic-induced jaundice remains equivocal. Liver biopsy has confirmed that when chlorpromazine jaundice is present biopsy specimens show centrilobular cholestasis with a mild inflammatory response but little or no parenchymatous damage. Many clinicians feel that this jaundice is due to a hypersensitivity reaction since eosinophilic infiltration of the liver has been shown with liver biopsy. Recently, it has been suggested that antipsychotic agents alter the physiochemical properties of bile and induce precipitation of bile within liver canaliculi.

The differential diagnosis of jaundice can be quite complex and includes prehepatic or hemolytic causes, congenital hepatic dysfunction such as glucuronyl transferase deficiency or Dubin-Johnson syndrome, acquired cholestatic causes from drugs or viral hepatitis, acquired non-cholestatic causes from drugs such as isoniazid, or viral and spirochetal infections, and post hepatic causes such as lithiasis or carcinoma (Zimmerman, 1968). **In patients** receiving antipsychotic drugs who remain icteric for more than a month following discontinuation of the drug, medical evaluation is advised.

Management of antipsychotic-induced jaundice is usually uncomplicated as in most cases the illness is self-limited and prognosis is favorable. A very small number of fatalities have been reported with chlorpromazine-induced hepatitis but none within the period 1958-1970 (Shader and DiMascio, 1970).

Treatment consists of stopping the offending drug and following the patient with liver-function studies. If the patient is psychotic and requires further treatment, a different chemical class of antipsychotic should be chosen (e.g., switching from chlorpromazine to haloperidol). If chlorpromazine has caused jaundice, it is probably wise to avoid using another phenothiazine as cross-sensitivity with other phenothiazines has been reported on rare occasions (Klatskin, 1963).

6. URINARY TRACT EFFECTS

Difficulty with urination is the most frequent side effect in the urinary tract. Hesitancy, or difficulty initiating micturation, is rather common, especially in older men. Those men with a compromised prostatic gland are more sensitive to the anticholinergic effects of the antipsychotic drugs and may progress to frank urinary retention. Other effects, such as increased urgency, increased flow and incontinence, have been described in both men and women. These effects seem to have complex autonomic nervous system causes and are not simply related to anticholinergic functions of the antipsychotics (Shader and DiMascio, 1970).

When urinary hesitancy or retention occurs, successful treatment can often be accomplished with bethanechol (Urecholine). The dosage needed varies from 10 mg orally q.i.d. to 25 mg. t.i.d. The lower dosages should be used in elderly patients. Generally, bladder difficulty improves with time and is self-limited. The higher anticholinergic antipsychotics such as chlorpromazine and especially thioridazine are the worst offenders. For chronic bladder dysfunction, especially in the elderly, low anticholinergic agents such as trifluoperazine, fluphenazine, or haloperidol are preferable.

7. ENDOCRINOLOGICAL EFFECTS

Breast Changes

Antipsychotic drugs, especially the phenothiazines, have been noted to cause both gynecomastia and galactorrhea. Gynecomastia is seen very rarely in males but without galactorrhea. On the other hand, women may show gynecomastia with or withoug galactorrhea. Up to 10-15% of females may show lactation or secretion of colostrum alone. Generally, lactation is associated with amenorrhea or markedly decreased menstrual flow. Reports of abnormal lactation have appeared with the phenothiazine group, as well as with haloperidol and the thioxanthenes. Since patients receiving antipsychotic agents often receive other psychotropic agents simultaneously, it is important to note that galactorrhea has also been reported with imipramine, amitryptyline, meprobamate, and chlordiazepoxide (Shader and DiMascio, 1970). Thus, if galactorrhea occurs in a woman receiving more than 1 psychotropic, it may be difficult to pinpoint a single causal drug.

As with any medical entity, an etiology for unexplained breast changes should be sought. The differential diagnosis of abnormal lactation includes numerous endocrine and non-endocrine causes and these should be considered in women with galactorrhea (Table 28). Most causes can be quickly ruled out by pregnancy evaluation, laboratory testing, or medical-surgical history. On the other hand, gynecomastia is seen in both men and women, albeit far more often in women. The differential diagnosis includes consideration of endocrine and non-endocrine disorders, as well as careful history, laboratory study, and physical diagnosis to rule out other possible causes of gynecomastia in patients receiving antipsychotics.

The management of galactorrhea and/or gynecomastia is usually uncomplicated. When possible coincident causes have been ruled out, careful counseling of the patient to allay fears is usually sufficient. However, breast

TABLE 28
Differential Diagnosis of Galactorrhea
or Gynecomastia in Patients Receiving
Antipsychotic Agents

Galactorrhea	Gynecomastia
Pregnancy	Puberty (both sexes)
Pseudocyesis	Pregnancy
Oral contraceptives	Male senescence
Acromegaly	Thyrotoxicosis
Thyrotoxicosis	Liver disease
Myxedema	Spinal cord lesions
Pituitary tumors	Adrenal tumors
Post surgery (thyroid, chest, hysterectomy)	Klinefelter's syndrome
Estrogen secreting adrenal tumors	Androgen therapy
Corpus luteum cysts	Estrogen therapy
Chorio-epitheliomas	Heavy marijuana use
	Testicular choriocarcinoma
	Bronchogenic carcinoma
	Following hemodialysis

discharge can be quite distressing to a psychotic or delusional woman. In these cases, clinical judgment may warrant switching to another chemical class of antipsychotic. Likewise, as younger females seem more susceptible to induction of breast discharge and phenothiazines seem more likely than other antipsychotic classes to cause galactorrhea, it may be prudent to use antipsychotics other than phenothiazines in younger floridly psychotic women who may require large doses of medication (greater than 400 mg. chlorpromazine equivalent daily). The young male with gynecomastia will usually respond to concerned counseling about breast enlargement, unless, of course, he is highly delusional or paranoid.

The etiology of breast changes with antipsychotic drugs seems related to the ability of these agents to block the effects of dopamine at its receptors in the brain. These mammotropic changes are associated with the release of prolactin from the pituitary gland. This, in turn, is controlled by prolactin inhibitory factor (PIF) which is released from the hypothalamus. Dopamine stimulates hypothalamic cells to release PIF and thereby controls the release of prolactin. Thus, the dopamine blockade of antipsychotic agents causes a decrease in PIF secretion, which results in an increase in serum prolactin, leading to mammotropic effects (Caldwell, 1976). Elevated serum prolactin has been demonstrated in schizophrenic patients within 72 hours after starting antipsychotic drugs. This effect seems fully reversible and serum prolactin levels return to normal within 48 to 96 hours (Meltzer and Fang, 1976). It seems probable that mammotropic changes can occur with all presently available antipsychotic agents, as all have at least some ability to block brain dopamine function.

Menstrual Changes

Changes in menstrual flow and periodicity are said to occur with antipsychotic drugs. **Amenorrhea is felt to be the most common menstrual change associated with antipsychotic agents.** However, there are no well-controlled studies available to properly delineate this problem. Obviously, these studies are unlikely to be done because of ethical concerns of drug use in women of child-bearing age. Another difficulty in attempting to characterize menstrual dysfunction with antipsychotic agents is ruling out stress-induced anovulatory cycles. Psychosis or hospitalization itself may be a sufficient cause to interrupt the menstrual cycle (Kiritz and Moos, 1974).

Amenorrhea may occur when antipsychotic drugs are started just prior to ovulation and may suppress ovulation for that particular cycle. Normally menstruation will return to normal during the next cycle. In some patients, however, 2 or 3 months may intervene between cycles and a rare number of women will have 1 to 3 periods per year or none at all. Should amenorrhea occur during the course of antipsychotic drug treatment, it is generally no cause for alarm but should alert the physician to consider other causes of menstrual interruption.

Primary amenorrhea implies that the menses have never been established and this can be ruled out in the woman with previously established menstrual cycles. Amenorrhea following antipsychotic agents is of the secondary type. Other causes of secondary amenorrhea include pregnancy, pseudocyesis, menopause, pituitary tumors, adrenal hypo- or hyperfunction, thyroid hypo- or hyperfunction, estrogen medications, ovarian tumors, and anorexia nervosa. An adequate medical evaluation should be done to rule out pregnancy and other medical causes of amenorrhea.

If antipsychotic drugs are established as the cause of menstrual dysfunction, management can often be done simply by reducing the dosage of the antipsychotic drug. In some patients, time itself will allow menstrual periods to return to normal. Others may require a trial of a different chemical class of antipsychotic. The greatest concern to the physician will occur with menstrual absence in sexually active women who have unreliable birth control methods. Should menstrual periods remain highly irregular in these women, it may be necessary to order pregnancy tests. **However, it must be remembered that antipsychotic drugs have been noted to sometimes cause false positive pregnancy tests.** In equivocal cases, gynecologic consultation should be sought.

Changes in Body Weight

Patients who are treated with antipsychotic agents often gain excessive weight. This seems more likely to occur with the use of lower potency drugs like chlorpromazine, thioridazine and mesoridazine and is possibly less likely to occur with higher potency drugs such as trifluoperazine, haloperidol, and fluphenazine. Whether antipsychotics cause an increase in appetite because of some central or hypothalmic effect is not entirely clear. In fact, many psychotic patients will gain weight early in their hospitalization even if antipsychotic agents are not administered (Gordon et al., 1960). On the other hand, the product literature of most antipsychotic drugs and most texts of antipsychotic drug pharmacology cite weight gain early in treatment as a potential untoward effect.

Recently, at least 4 studies have claimed that molindone may be singularly different from other available antipsychotic agents in terms of weight gain (Gardos and Cole, 1977). Schizophrenics tend to show a net weight loss if they are switched from other antipsychotic to molindone. Most of this loss occurs during the first month of molindone therapy. A majority of patients seem to regain lost weight if they are switched back to their original antipsychotic medication.

Water Disorders

Water intoxication rarely occurs in psychotic patients and is generally caused by a "psychogenic" water habit or inappropriate secretion of antidiuretic hormone following the administration of antipsychotic agents. The water intoxication syndrome consists of irritability, lethargy, confusion and seizures progressing into coma. Death can result. Laboratory findings include hyponatremia, hypo-osmolarity of the serum and hyperosmolar urine.

"Psychogenic" water habit is not well defined (Fowler et al., 1977). However, instisutionalized patients may drink excessive quantities of water to the point of frank water intoxication. It may be that the anticholinergic properties of antipsychotic medications produce a very dry mouth and predispose the patient to stand and gulp at the water fountain. Or the psychotic patient may not be able to differentiate the state of dry mouth from the much different state of thirst. In any event, a progressively deteriorating sensorium in hospitalized psychotic patients should suggest water intoxication. A quick check of serum sodium will determine if serum and urine osmolarities should be obtained.

The syndrome of inappropriate secretion of antidiuretic hormone (SIADH) will appear as water intoxication but the patient will not be consuming inordinate quantities of water. This syndrome has been reported with thioridazine, haloperidol, thiothizene, or fluphenazine (Matuk and Kalyanaraman, 1977; Ajouni et al., 1974) and has also been reported in both inpatients and outpatients. Again, serum sodium values will be very low (e.g., 112-120 mEq./liter) and should suggest further workup for water intoxication.

Other disorders may cause SIADH and in fact are more likely to be the etiology than antipsychotic agents. The most common cause is the oat cell bronchiogenic carcinoma. The physician should also consider pulmonary tuberculosis, porphyria, acute leukemia, myxedma, and CNS tumors or infections. Drugs such as chlorpropamide, vincristine, cyclophosphamide, potassium depleting diuretics, carbamazepine, clofibrate and acetaminophen have also been implicated.

Treatment is easily done by water restriction and will be always successful if the patient has "psychogenic" water habit. For the patient with SIADH due to antipsychotic agents, water restriction again is usually quite sufficient for treatment. It may be wise to choose a different chemical class of antipsychotic if continued drug therapy is needed. If SIADH is secondary to an underlying medical condition, its treatment rests upon appropriate therapy for the primary cause.

The etiology of antipsychotic drug-induced SIADH is not clear. However, chlorpromazine and other phenothiazines have been shown to have an antidiuretic effect. Chlorpromazine has also been shown to cause ADH release from the pituitary gland. However, its action on ADH release is not consistent.

Effects Upon Glucose Metabolism

Antipsychotic drugs may produce a hyperglycemic effect in some patients. This was recognized early in the clinical experience with chlorpromazine. Transient hyperglycemia with glycosuria has been seen but remits when the drug is discontinued. Also, some reports of stable diabetes becoming unstable following chlorpromazine administration have been noted. Abnormal or "pre-diabetic" glucose tolerance curves apparently can be induced by chlorpromazine. Occasionally the first symptoms of diabetes mellitus may occur during phenothiazine therapy (Ban, 1969). Possibly these agents may alter the threshold for the appearance of latent diabetes.

The reason for apparent alterations of glucose metabolism or serum glucose levels remains to be explained. However, there are no data available to suggest that antipsychotic agents are contraindicated in psychotic patients with concomitant diabetes mellitus (Shader and DiMascio, 1970) and no evidence that these drugs can induce a diabetic state.

8. DERMATOLOGICAL EFFECTS

Drug Eruptions

These occurrences are what dermatologists would call dermatitis medicamentosa. They are acute or chronic skin reactions to a drug. Almost any drug known to man, whether taken orally, injected, inhaled or absorbed, may cause almost any type of skin reaction in any given individual at any given time. However, this excludes dermatitis following local action of the skin (contact dermatitis). Antipsychotic drug eruptions will often recur upon exposure to the same drug and with these agents a careful adverse skin reaction history should be sought from the patient, family or friends.

The essentials of diagnosis are the abrupt onset of a widespread, symmetric eruption often with uticaria or pruritus. Usually this occurs on the face, neck, upper chest and extremities and generally appears between 14 and 60 days after initiating the medication. About 5-10% of patients receiving chlorpromazine develop an allergic dermatitis (Prien and Cole, 1968), but accurate data for the other antipsychotics are not readily available. Other diagnostic features may include malaise, arthralgia, headache and fever. Any inflammatory skin condition may be mimicked and angioneurotic edema may be present. Severe reactions, including exfoliative dermatitis, have been reported occasionally.

Treatment consists of discontinuing the offending agent. However, this will prove difficult if the patient is treated with multiple medications since the responsible drug may not be readily apparent. Antihistamines may be of value if urticaria or severe itching is present. With significant angioneurotic edema, topical corticosteriods may be of benefit. In severe eruptions, oral corticosteroids may be necessary.

Photosensitivity

Photosensitivity can occur with antipsychotic agents, particularly chlorpromazine, and is a result of the drug combining with proteins in the malpighian layer of skin and forming substances which then react with light. Chlorpromazine is the worst offender and the incidence of phototoxicity is reported as 3% (Winkleman, 1957). Thiothixene has also been reported to increase the tendency to develop photosensitivity (Shader and DiMascio, 1970). The *Physician's Desk Reference* cautions about this as a possibility for most of the antipsychotics. With many more psychotic patients now in the community, extra caution in advising patients about the avoidance of sun may be needed. For many, chlorpromazine may not be the drug of choice.

If photosensitivity occurs, sun exposure should be avoided for up to 4-6 weeks until the drug stored in the epidermis is discarded. A change to another antipsychotic may be necessary to prevent recurrence. Many commercial sun screens are now available as lotions and creams (e.g., benzophenone lotion) and their application to exposed skin of the hands, face and neck may prevent phototoxicity. These have the ability to block much of the light energy below 3500 angstroms and thus prevent this toxic reaction from occurring. Broad-rimmed hats are often necessary.

Hyperpigmentation

This is a rare side effect which can occur after years of medication exposure. Like photosensitivity, it is usually seen following chlorpromazine usage. The skin tends to assume a slate gray to metallic purplish coloration in the areas exposed to sunlight such as the face, neck, and arms. This condition has been observed in hospitalized mental patients, primarily females, who have received chlorpromazine usually for three years or more in dosages ranging from 500 mg. to 1500 mg. daily. The incidence of this effect is about 1% (Gombos and Yarden, 1967). Patients who develop discolored skin often show corneal and lens deposit of pigment. **Thus, patients with hyperpigmentation following prolonged antipsychotic drug exposure should have a thorough eye examination.**

The mechanism of hyperpigmentation may involve an interaction between pigmentary proteins and a 7-hydroxy metabolite of chlorpromazine (Caldwell, 1976). It has been suggested that sensitive individuals may not be able to properly metabolize this substance by conjugation.

The offending drug should be discontinued. Exposure to sun should be avoided as mild cases have shown the ability to depigment over time (Shader and DiMascio, 1970). The high-potency antipsychotics are preferable for patients who have developed hyperpigmentation while on low-potency agents.

9. OPHTHALMOLOGICAL EFFECTS

Blurred Vision

This is a common side effect with both antipsychotic and tricyclic antidepressant drugs. It is far more likely to occur with tricyclic antidepressants than with antipsychotics. However, agents such as thioridazine, mesoridazine or chlorpromazine may cause a significant blurring of vision during the first week or two of their use. This is probably due to their relatively high anticholinergic activity which impairs the tone of the ciliary muscle.

Blurred vision is rarely a serious problem and most patients will become tolerant to this effect within a week or 2. Patients should be reassured that this visual impairment is likely to be temporary, but they should be cautioned to exercise care in the operation of motor vehicles and machinery until their vision improves. For particularly severe blurring, pilocarpine drops may help. A solution of 1 to 2% applied to each eye q.i.d. or during times of reading often helps until the patient's eyesight improves spontaneously. If the problem persists, a change to an antipsychotic of lesser anticholinergic potency such as trifluoperazine or haloperidol should be considered.

Glaucoma

Any drug capable of mydriasis (e.g., anticholinergic antiparkinson or antipsychotic agents) can precipitate acute glaucoma in patients with narrow anterior chamber angles.

About 1% of persons over age 35 have narrow anterior chamber angles but many of these never develop glaucoma. Patients who develop acute glaucoma seek treatment immediately because of intense eye pain and blurring of vision. Examination will show a red injected sclera, steamy colored cornea and a moderately dilated pupil which does not react to light. Intra-ocular pressure measured by tonometry will be elevated above the normal 10-25 mm Hg. Acute glaucoma must be differentiated from conjunctivitis, acute iritis and corneal abrasion. Any patient suspected to have acute glau-coma following antipsychotics or antiparkinson agents should be referred for immediate ophthalmologic consultation, since untreated acute glaucoma can result in permanent blindness within 2-5 days following onset.

Chronic (open angle) glaucoma is an entirely different entity. In chronic glaucoma the intraocular pressure is constantly elevated. The disease is bilateral and genetically determined, probably as an autosomal recessive trait. It is estimated that 2 million people in the United States have glaucoma and of these 90% are of the chronic open angle type. Clinically, patients with chronic glaucoma have an insidious onset, are usually older (above age 45), have no early symptoms, and have a gradual loss of peripheral vision over the years. There may be a slight cupping of the optic disc (Hetherington, 1974).

The use of antipsychotic agents or antiparkinson drugs in patients with chronic glaucoma is probably not contraindicated in most cases. However, an antipsychotic with very low anticholinergic activity should be chosen. Most patients with chronic glaucoma can have their illness controlled with local application of the acetylcholine-like miotic, pilocarpine, 1-2%, 3-4 times daily. Carbonic anhydrase inhibitors such as acetazolamide (Diamox) and ethoxzolamide (Cardiase) can be used to decrease intraocular aqueous pro-duction. Acetazolamide is generally given 250 mg. every 4 hours while ethoxzolamide is used 125 to 250 mg. 2 to 4 times daily. With the concomitant use of these agents in the eye, psychotic individuals can generally be suc-cessfully treated with low anticholinergic agents such as haloperidol, flu-phenazine or trifluoperazine. In any case, ophthalmologic consultation should be obtained.

Corneal-Lenticular Opacities

Disorders of the cornea have been described following very high doses of chlorpromazine (2,000 mg./day or more). This epithelial keratopathy is characterized by white, gray and brown opacities in the areas of the cornea exposed to light. There is considerable disagreement as to whether it is reversible if chlorpromazine is discontinued (Johnson and Buffaloe, 1966). However, it would seem prudent to switch patients on such high doses of chlorpromazine to a high-potency non-phenothiazine. The *Physicians' Desk Reference* (1978) states that these eye lesions may regress after drug dis-continuation.

Changes in the ocular lens arise first as light dusky pigment which appears on the lens capsule. This becomes a stellate cataract and eventually a polar cataract which will be noted in the anterior portion of the lens. Unlike the epithelial keratopathy of the cornea, these changes seem related to duration of chlorpromazine therapy rather daily dose. Occasionally, this pigmentation can be noted in the posterior cornea and conjunctivae. There seems to be a direct correlation with pigment deposition in the skin and the eye.

The reversibility of pigmentation of the eye structures is not settled by investigators. Some researchers have reported substantial improvement with the chelating agent d-penicillamine (Cuprimine, 250 to 500 mg. 4 times daily), secluding the patient from sunlight, giving a low copper diet, and by injecting melatonin. Other researchers have not had similar success (Shader and DiMascio, 1970).

Pigmentary Retinopathy

This is a toxic reaction causing clumping or rarefaction of retinal pigment. It may manifest itself as night blindness and, if severe, can result in decreased daytime visual acuity. On funduscopic examination, one sees pigment deposits which spread from the middle zone between the equator and the posterior pole in an anterior and posterior direction. Very early in the process one may only see small pigmented spots near the choroid. **However, even before the physician can see funduscopic changes, the patient may report a brownish discoloration of vision**. This is reported to occur between the twentieth and fiftieth day of treatment (Shader and DiMascio, 1970). Most cases are reported following the use of phenothiazines, with the great majority of cases confined to thioridazine. Chlorpromazine has been cited as causing pigmentary retinopathy but this is by no means conclusive. In fact, phenothiazines with alaphatic or piperazine side chains may be devoid of this effect. Melanin in the retina seems involved as albinos do not develop this disorder with antipsychotics. The toxic phenothiazine product is deposited in the melanin of the choroid and passes from the choroid to the retina via portal blood vessels in this area. The deposition of the drug in the retina eventually destroys the rods and disturbs the biochemistry of the Mueller cells (Caldwell, 1976).

Cases reported following the use of thioridazine occurred in patients receiving 1200 mg. or more per day of the drug. No reports of retinopathy have occurred if thioridazine doses do not exceed 800 mg./day. **It should be noted that the product literature for thioridazine explicitly warns against exceeding 800 mg./day due to risk of retinopathy**. If retinopathy occurs, it seems almost completely reversible if the drug is stopped. However, impaired eyesight will linger for some time until all metabolites of thioridazine are cleared from tissue stores (Cerletti and Meier-Ruge, 1971). Patients are probably best managed with a non-phenothiazine antipsychotic following development of pigmentary retinotherapy.

10. SEXUAL DYSFUNCTION

Sexual dysfunction associated with thioridazine use in men is now one of the better documented side effects seen with the use of the antipsychotic medications. However, numerous gaps in knowledge and information remain in this area. For example, practically no data exist on the effects of antipsychotics on female libido or orgasmic functioning and few studies in either sex are prospective or more than anecdotal in nature.

Ejaculation disorders are the most frequent sexual dysfunction noted with thioridazine. Kotin et al. (1976) report that in 57 male patients who had taken thioridazine, fully one-third experienced retrograde ejaculation. Sixty percent reported an adverse change in sexual function while taking thioridazine, while only 25% of the patients taking other antipsychotics reported such changes. Few reports of ejaculation disorders are recorded for antipsychotics other than thioridazine. Disturbances in erection are noted occasionally with all antipsychotics but, again, thioridazine has a significantly higher incidence. The effects of antipsychotic drugs upon ejaculation may be associated with charges in the sympathetic branch of the autonomic nervous system. Why the effects are more pronounced with thioridazine is not entirely clear.

Attempts to determine the effects of antipsychotics upon sexual drive or libido are not as clear as for ejaculatory dysfunction. A specific anti-libido effect in men has been claimed for thioridazine and fluphenazine, while thioridazine has been reported of use as an anti-libido agent in "sexually deviant" men (Litkcy and Feniczy, 1967) and sexually aggressive women (Kamm, 1965). However, these reports are uncontrolled, anecdotal and have not been reproduced. Bartholomew (1968) gave fluphenazine enanthate to a group of mentally ill but sexually normal patients and compared effects on libido with the same dosage of fluphenazine enanthate in a group of sexually deviant individuals. Subjective reports of libido decrease were the same for both groups, but no objective measures were used. Conclusive anti-libido effects remain to be proven for the antipsychotic agents in current use.

The management of ejaculatory disturbance from antipsychotic agents is quite simple: Stop the offending agent, substitute another, and reassure the patient. In most instances, this is sufficient. Of even more important concern to clinicians should be inquiry into a patient's sexual function while taking antipsychotic agents. This is often ignored and some feel that sexuality in the schizophrenic patient is unimportant. In reality, many schizophrenics have continued sexual activity, especially in outpatient settings, and private masturbation for sexual gratification is common. It may be that unreported sexual side effects are responsible for some noncompliance in taking antipsychotic medication. **Thus, tactful questions concerning sexual side effects should be asked of every patient taking antipsychotic drugs.**

If sexual side effects are reported or discovered, these should not be ascribed to antipsychotics without consideration for other causes of sexual dysfunction. Notably, diabetes mellitus, endocrine disorders, peripheral artery disease, organic brain disease, the metabolic effects of certain carcinomas, and multiple sclerosis are well known for sexual impairment. Chronic organ system diseases can alter sexual abilities, as is seen in chronic renal, liver, pulmonary and hematopoietic illness. Certainly spinal cord disorders can alter sexual performance. Other drug influences must be carefully sought. Many antihypertensives can affect sexual desire and performance. Clonidine, ganglonic blockers (e.g., hexamethonium), reserpine, phenoxybenzamine, propranol, and methyldopa have all caused sexual dysfunction. The etiologies differ but most involve changes in sympathetic neurotransmitters. Ethyl alcohol is ubiquitous in use and may cause adverse sexual effects. Anticholinergic agents (e.g., tricyclic antidepressants, antiparkinson agents, and antispasmodics) can cause impotence and ejaculatory failure. Monoamine oxidase inhibitors cause sexual difficulty through adrenergic changes. Estrogenic hormones can alter libido and performance. Since patients on antipsychotic agents often have other concomitant diseases or take other medications, the physician must recognize the multiple causes of sexual difficulty. Likewise, antipsychotic agents potentially can alter an already compromised sexual system in patients having other diseases or may interact with any of the medications described.

Priapism is a rare sexual difficulty reported in some male patients following phenothiazines. This is a persistent abnormal erection of the penis and is unassociated with sexual desire. It may be severe enough to require urologic surgery for intracorporal shunting of venous blood. Chlorpromazine and mesoridazine have both been reportedly associated with severe priapism. The cause of this phenomenon is not clear but phenothiazines may block sympathetic control of penile detumescence (Gottlieb and Lustberg, 1977).

Management of this disorder requires expert urologic consultation. However, in patients having excessively prolonged erections, it may be wise to avoid phenothiazines and switch the patient to a thioxanthene, butyrophenone, or other non-phenothiazine.

11. DRUG INTERACTIONS

Drug-drug interactions must always be kept in mind whenever more than one drug is used in a patient. This becomes a more critical consideration with the aging schizophrenic patient who develops disease in other bodily systems and requires concomitant medications. It is a well-recognized fact that the occurrences of drug interactions increase as the number of drugs increases (Smith et al., 1966). In fact, theoretical probabilities of drug-drug interactions can be predicted from the permutations and combinations of numbers of drugs used in any given patient. For example, a patient taking 5 drugs has 120 potential interactions ($5! = 1 \times 2 \times 3 \times 4 \times 5 = 120$). Obviously, these rates do not occur at the theoretical level, which is most fortunate for physicians and patients alike. However, it should forewarn the physician to constantly monitor patients for particular interactions and to evaluate all patient complaints from antipsychotic drugs for the possibility of drug-drug interactions. Table 29 outlines some of the more widely recognized drug interactions with antipsychotic agents that have been reported by Hansten (1975) and others.

12. EFFECTS UPON LABORATORY TESTS

Laboratory testing is now an integral part of modern medical care. Unfortunately, many laboratory tests are modified by drugs. This may lead to both false positive and false negative results. The careful clinician should evaluate all laboratory tests in light of the patient's medication and disease profile. This in itself can become a Herculean task as laboratory procedures often change quickly with new reagents, procedures and automated equipment appearing yearly. For this reason, it is suggested that all physicians have at their disposal a current guide to laboratory testing which will invariably report on those drugs and chemicals known to interfere with laboratory results. Also supervisory personnel in clinical laboratories can usually locate source data which will help identify drugs which may give misleading laboratory results. Table 30 outlines some of the common effects that antipsychotic drugs may have upon laboratory tests (Hansten, 1975).

TABLE 29
Drugs with the Potential for Interactions with Antipsychotics

Drug	Possible Interaction
A. Antacids, Oral	● May inhibit the absorption of oral antipsychotic agents if given together.
B. Anticholinergic Agents 1. Antiparkinson drugs	● Benztropine and trihexyphenidyl have been shown to decrease plasma levels of antipsychotics.
2. Antianxiety	● Atropine-like effects may be enhanced. ● Hydroxyzine may impair therapeutic effect of antipsychotics in a similar fashion to antiparkinson agents.
C. Anticoagulants	● Haloperidol may possibly impair the anticoagulant effect of phenindione.
D. Antidiarrheal	● Attapulgite appears to inhibit the absorption of phenothiazines.
E. Antidepressants	● Phenothiazines may inhibit hepatic metabolism of tricyclic antidepressants.
F. Antihistamines	● Severe hypoglycemia has been reported with orphenadrine and chlorpromazine.
G. Antihelminths	● Caution is advised with using piperazine (for ascariasis) and phenothiazines.
H. Antihypertensives 1. Guanethidine	● Phenothiazines appear to inhibit guanethidine uptake into the adrenergic neuron. Patients may have an exacerbation of blood pressure increase.
2. Clonidine	● Theoretically may potentiate peripheral antihypertensive effects.
3. Methyldopa	● May block alpha-methyl-norepinephrine uptake and cause a paradoxical hypertensive response.
4. Propranolol	● May have an additive hypotensive effect.
I. Antiseizure Agents	● Metabolism of hydantoin may be inhibited.
J. Barbiturates	● Long-term use of barbiturates may increase the metabolism of antipsychotic agents through hepatic enzyme induction.
K. Estrogens	● Estrogens may impair the metabolism of antipsychotic and increase plasma levels.

TABLE 29 (Cont.)

Drug	Possible Interaction
L. Hypoglycemics	● Blood sugars may become unstable when antipsychotics are added to oral hypoglycemics.
M. Levodopa	● May inhibit levodopa response by dopamine blockade.
N. Lithium	● May potentiate the hyperglycemic effects of lithium.
O. Narcotics	● Potentiates the analgesic effects of narcotic agents.
P. Phosphorus Insecticides	● May potentiate the anticholinesterase effects of agents such as parathion and malathion.
Q. Quinidine	● May have an additive quinidine effect upon the heart. Not very likely.
R. Sedative-Hypnotics	● Additive sedative-hypnotic effects.

13. EFFECTS OF ANTIPSYCHOTIC DRUGS IN PREGNANCY, LABOR AND DELIVERY, NEONATAL PERIOD AND BREAST FEEDING

Numerous studies have documented the relatively high intake of prescription and non-prescription drugs during pregnancy. Nelson and Forfar (1971) found retrospectively that 97% of 1,369 mothers in Scotland took prescribed drugs during their pregnancy and 65% of these women self-administered drugs. Earlier studies in the United States found that physicians prescribed at least 1 drug for 92% of more than 3,000 patients and 3.9% received 10 or more drugs during their pregnancy. Between 1958 and 1965 a prospective study of 50,282 pregnancies was conducted under the supervision of the National Institute of Neurological and Communicative Disorders and Stroke. This survey (Heinonen et al., 1977) found that 2.6% of women used phenothiazines during gestational months 1 to 4 and 7.31% used phenothiazines at some time during the pregnancy. Data were not reported for other antipsychotic agents in different chemical classes such as haloperidol, thiothixene, loxapine or molidone. Fifty percent of the phenothiazine prescriptions were for prochlorperazine (Compazine).

Physicians must recognize how incredibly difficult it is to prove a causal relationship between a drug and fetal malformation. Ethical considerations do not allow us to test human fetuses for toxic reactions to drugs. Statistically, it is very difficult to prove a relationship. For instance, if a malformation

TABLE 30
Effects of Antipsychotic Agents upon Clinical Laboratory Tests

A. Serum Tests

  1. Cholesterol
- Phenothiazines seem to increase serum cholesterol in a dose-related fashion.

  2. Cholinesterase
- Scant reports in the French and German literature claim that phenothiazines can decrease cholinesterase levels.

  3. Creatinine Phosphokinase
- Elevations of CPK are non-specific and seem related to intramuscular injections with local muscle injury or intrinsic to the muscular activity of psychotic patients.

  4. Glucose
- May elevate serum glucose.

  5. Thyroid
- Large doses of antipsychotics have been reported to diminish QBI. Data for serum thyroxine not available.

  6. Uric Acid
- May elevate uric acid. Equivocal.

B. Urine Tests

  1. Bilirubin
- Very high doses of chlorpromazine may result in false positives with Bili-Labstix. Icotest sticks seem unaffected.

  2. Catecholamines
- Chlorpromazine interferes with the Pisano test for urinary metanephrines. Other phenothiazines may have a similar effect. Fluorometric catecholamine determination is unaffected.

  3. Color
- The urine of patients on phenothiazines has been reported to turn pink to red or red brown upon standing.

  4. Glucose
- Glycosuria may be seen with hyperglycemia.

  5. 5-Hydroxyindoleacetic Acid
- May get a false decrease with nitrosonaphthol reagent.

  6. Ketones
- An atypical color may appear with the Gerhardt ferric chloride test for acetoacetic acid.

  7. Pregnancy Tests
- Immunologic tests may give either false positive or false negative results. Individual test literature should be consulted.

  8. Steroids
- 17-KS and 17-OHCS tests may be impaired.

  9. Urobilinogen
- Values may appear increased due to reactions with Ehrlich's reagent.

  10. VMA
- Urinary VMA may be decreased in patients receiving antipsychotics.

has a frequency of 1%, 2 populations of at least 3,000 pregnancies are needed to show that 1 incidence rate is twice another ($p < .01$). At the height of the thalidomide tragedy, the annual limb malformation rate in Birmingham, England, rose from 2 to 11. This is in a city of 1,000,000 people with a birth rate of 20,000 per year. Thus, it is estimated that the smallest suitable study size for abnormalities with frequency of 0.1% is a birth population of at least 20,000. Obviously, many malformations might not even be detected by most current sampling methods for drugs in pregnancy.

Other important sources of error lie in the assumption that there is a relationship between laboratory animals and man in teratogenetic effects from psychotropic or any other drugs. There is a significant species difference between an animal's and a human's embryotoxic sensitivity to phenothiazines; further, mice, rats and rabbits show different malformation rates for the same drug. This has serious implications, as the public wants animal pretesting of drugs for embryotoxic effects but animal data may be of dubious value anyway. Thus, the setting of minimal standards against a background of limited or spurious knowledge can result in a false sense of security and was partially responsible for the thalidomide disaster.

The use of antipsychotic agents in pregnant females has not been viewed with any significant concern until the last 2 years. However, the product literature for antipsychotic agents has always carried a disclaimer for their cautioned use during pregnancy. The following statement is a consensus of the pharmaceutical drug industry derived from the *Physician's Desk Reference.*

> Safety for the use of antipsychotics during pregnancy has not been established; therefore, it is recommended that the drug be given to pregnant patients only when, in the judgement of the physician, it is essential. The potential benefits should clearly outweigh possible hazards. Reproductive studies in rodents have demonstrated a potential for embryotoxicity, increased neonatal mortality and nursing transfer of the drug. Tests in the offspring of the drug-treated rodents demonstrate decreased performance. The possibility of permanent neurologic damage cannot be excluded.

Placental Transport of Antipsychotic Drugs

Phenothiazines easily cross the placental barrier and both the original drug and its metabolites have been identified in maternal plasma, fetal plasma, amniotic fluid and in the urine of neonates (O'Donoghue, 1971). As the human liver, the placenta is able to metabolize drugs using a similar microsomal cytochrome P-450 enzyme system. However, these enzyme systems are about a 40- to 50-fold smaller quantity than found in the liver

(Netter and Bergheim, 1975). Likewise, the human fetal liver and adrenal gland have drug metabolizing capabilities. The fetal hepatic metabolizing system is detectable as early as 6 to 7 weeks of gestational age. In fact, the fetal liver may respond to the induction of enzyme systems from drugs passed across the placenta from the maternal circulation. It has been suggested that these early fetal metabolic systems may cause the accumulation of metabolites on the fetal side or produce fetal metabolites which are in themselves toxic (Pelkonen et al., 1975). However, there are insufficient data to demonstrate that this actually occurs with antipsychotic drugs at the present time.

Teratology of Antipsychotics

All phenothiazines and most of the other antipsychotic agents seem capable of causing cogential malformations in laboratory animals if given in sufficient quantity. As noted, there are species differences and statistical pitfalls which make the extrapolation of these animal data to humans less than ideal. Yet, presently there are only 2 ways of determining tetratogenic potential from pharmaceutical agents. We can give drugs to animals and watch for malformations in their offspring or we can wait for the ultimate test—the widespread use in human beings (Mellin, 1964). With our present knowledge, it appears that the interpretation of animal studies can be used only to develop hypotheses for further observations in human beings.

The paucity of literature in this area is frightening. Moreover, many large systemic reviews of the available medical literature have not found convincing evidence to implicate antipsychotic drugs in fetal malformations. This is in contrast to the recent findings of fetal risk from exposure to antiseizure medications, benzodiazepines, meprobamate and lithium ion. However, some recent large-scale studies indicate that phenothiazines, at least, may not be as safe as previously thought. The French National Institute of Health and Medical Research (INSERM) carried out a prospective study of 12 university hospitals in Paris. From 1963 to 1969, 12,764 women were followed and medication exposure during the first trimester was determined. Phenothiazines were subdivided according to chemical structure (aliphatic, piperidine, piperazine). A statistically significant increase in malformation rate was associated with the intake of aliphatic type phenothiazines (Rumeau-Roquette et al., 1977). Likewise, the Boston study has shown a slight statistical association of fetal malformation with trifluoperazine usage and a heterogenous group called "other phenothiazines." They found no association when all phenothiazines as a group were examined (Heinonen et al., 1977). These data from large populations suggest that there may be individual diferences in fetal risk from exposure to different phenothiazines. **Until more** is known about antipsychotics and pregnancy, it seems wise to avoid the use of antipsychotic drugs during the first trimester of pregnancy. However, in grossly psychotic women, the risk of fetal wastage from untreated psychosis may outweigh fetal malformation risk from exposure to antipsychotic drugs. On the other hand, most large-scale studies involve the use of antipsychotic drugs in non-psychotic women. The primary clinical reason for use is control of pregnancy-related emesis. Therefore, we still have no reliable data of fetal exposure to the high doses of antipsychotics necessary to treat psychosis. Unfortunately, the psychiatrist and obstetrician still must make a risk benefit decision in the psychotic female who is pregnant and requires antipsychotic drug therapy.

Labor and Delivery

Antipsychotic agents have been used in obstetrics for neuroleptanalgesia, to potentiate narcotic analgesia, to block autonomic reflexes and for post-delivery antiemetic activity. The major difficulties to the mother are their known side effects, such as orthostatic hypotension, akathisia or occasional extrapyramidal reactions. In general, short-term exposure during labor and delivery seems to cause little maternal difficulty (Dripps et al., 1968).

In the mother who has been exposed to antipsychotics throughout her pregnancy, some post-delivery neonatal difficulty can occur. Some babies will show athetoid posturing of the hands, attacks of opisthotonos, increased muscle tone, motor restlessness, and tremors. Hypothermia and hypotension have not been described as neonatal problems (Tamer et al., 1969). In the cases of neonatal extrapyramidal dysfunction reported to date, some have persisted for 3-10 months (Green and Zelson, 1976). It is important to rule out intracranial bleeding, sepsis, hypocalcemia, hypomagnesemia and meningitis as other potential causes of neurologic difficulty in the immediate neonatal period.

Persistent Neonatal Effects

Animal studies have recently raised concern about long-term behavioral effects in children born to mothers who have received antipsychotic agents during pregnancy. Chlorpromazine has been found to affect the long-term behavior of mice offspring whose mothers were exposed to this antipsychotic during pregnancy (Ordy et al., 1966). Other animal studies have shown long-term changes in neonatal behavior (Thornburg and Moore, 1976).

However, even with data from animal studies, there is a paucity of material on human neonates exposed prenatally to psychotropic agents. No long-term studies are available for humans. Kris (1965) followed 52 children born to mothers maintained on pharmacotherapy during pregnancy because of psychosis. However, these children were not adequately screened or repeatedly tested by standard neuropsychological means. These reports give no concrete findings. Thus, we really have no idea of the impact of antipsychotic drugs on the behavior and development of children exposed to these chemicals in utero.

Other scattered studies have found that promethazine (Phenergan), a week phenothiazine used as an antihistimine, can suppress human neonatal immulogic function (Rubinstein et al., 1976) and its ability to assist in treating erythroblastosis fetalis in utero has raised concerns (Gusdon and Herbst, 1976). This documented immunosuppressive action of promethazine raises questions about its long-term effects on mother and fetus, as well as about the other more potent phenothiazines.

Some studies have suggested that the use of promazine (Sparine), chlorpromazine or other phenothiazines might increase neonatal jaundice in infants born prematurely to mothers receiving these agents. Scokel and Jones (1962) reported that promazine and promethazine increased the incidence of neonatal jaundice. However, careful subsequent studies have not confirmed this and suggest that risk of hyperbilirubinemia is not increased by using phenothiazines (de Lamerens et al., 1964). Likewise, due to the predilection of certain phenothiazines for melanin pigments (e.g., chlorpromazine and thioridazine), it has been recommended that all children born to mothers given antipsychotic drugs during pregnancy be longitudinally examined for possible retinal complications (Drugs and the fetal eye, 1971). However, to date no occurrences of visual difficulty have been noted in such children.

Brazelton (1970) has studied the long-term effects of prenatal drugs on subsequent child behavior. He has stressed that tranquilizers and premedications administered during delivery appear to affect the neonates' initial weight gain and response to nursing and early learning tasks. However, no follow-up studies have progressed beyond the immediate postnatal period in humans, and the knowledge of possible long-lasting effects should be sought. This is especially critical due to the deinstitutionalization if schizophrenic men and women and the increased likelihood of pregnancy in this ambulatory psychotic population.

Breast Feeding

When one looks for data on concentrations of antipsychotic drugs in the milk of human mothers, practically no data are available. Blacker et al. (1962) have measured the amount of chlorpromazine in the milk of a psychotic woman receiving 1200 mg. daily. Milk samples were taken at 60, 120, and 180 minutes. They calculated that the child would receive 10 micrograms (.01 mg.) in a 124 ml breast sample. It was reported that on 600 mg. of chlorpromazine daily, detectable levels of drug could not be found in the milk. However, the sensitivity and specificity of their assay techniques are not reported. Presently there are no good data on the excretion of antipsychotic drugs into human breast milk. However, animal data have demonstrated that chlorpromazine, prochlorpromazine, trifluoperazine and haloperidol are present in the milk of nursing dogs and rabbits (Ayd, 1973). Likewise, infant rabbits who have nursed from mothers chronically dosed with haloperidol have been found to have increased brain levels of homovanillic acid. This demonstrates that significant amounts of the drug not only reach the brain through nursing but apparently change dopamine turnover. Nearly all drugs ingested by the mother are excreted into her milk either in unchanged form or as metabolites. Compounds such as atropine, anticoagulants, antithyroid drugs, antimetabolites, cathartics, dihydrotachysterol, iodides, narcotics, radioactive preparations, ergot, tetracyclines, and metronidazole have resulted in adverse effects in the nursing infants. **Breast feeding should be contraindicated in any mother whose illness requires high doses of any drug (Yaffe and Stern, 1976), including antipsychotic agents.**

14. POISONING AND OVERDOSAGE

Accidental or intended overdosage with antipsychotic agents can occur for numerous reasons. Children may accidentally take their parents' medications or the young schizophrenic patient might purposely overdose with suicidal intent. Fortunately, these agents have a wide margin of safety and most overdoses are nonfatal. Doses as high as 17 grams of chlorpromazine have been reported without death. However, people have died as the result of excessive doses of chlorpromazine, thioridazine and trifluoperazine (Davis, et al., 1968). Therefore, physicians should have skill in the recognition and management of antipsychotic poisoning.

Recognition of the signs of overdosage depends on the chemical class of antipsychotic ingested. This is by no means pathognomonic and the physician must assume that other concomitant medications may have been taken as well. Many patients taking antipsychotic agents are also receiving antiparkinson drugs, tricyclic antidepressants and benzodiazepines. The aliphatic and piperidine phenothiazines (chlorpromazine, thioridazine, mesoridazine, piperacetazine) and tend to central nervous system (CNS) depression. Coma and unresponsiveness predominate and signs of anticholinergic toxicity are frequent (Table 31). The piperazine phenothiazines (e.g., trifluoperazine, fluphenazine) and haloperidol, or thiothizene can produce CNS excitation. Neuromuscular or parkinsonian signs will usually predominate. The toxic picture for loxapine and molindone is not clear due to limited clinical experience, but probably lies between the aliphatic and piperazine signs.

Other frequent signs of poisoning (Table 31) which may be seen with any antipsychotic are severe postural hypotension, loss of temperature-regulating ability, seizures, and respiratory depression. Hypotension results from alpha-adrenergic blockade. Usually the patient will have lowered body temperature but elevated temperature is sometimes seen, especially with anticholinergic toxicity, resulting from thioridazine poisoning. The antipsychotics in high doses are known to lower seizure thresholds.

Treatment can vary slightly according to clinical presentation. The comatose patient must be approached in a standard fashion as many causes are responsible for coma and the diagnosis of antipsychotic overdosage may not be readily apparent. Table 31 provides an approach to the comatose patient. Should antipsychotic overdosage be proven, other treatment steps may be taken. Attempts at emesis are usually futile as all antipsychotics (except thioridazine) have strong antiemetic properties. Gastric lavage may remove significant portions of drug as antipsychotics have some water solubility and their anticholinergic properties often delay gastric emptying. Continuous EKG monitoring should be maintained to recognize and treat potential arrhythmias. This should be undertaken in a general medical setting where possible. Atrial tachyarrhythmias are usually benign and may not require treatment unless cardiac output is impaired. However, ventricular tachyarrhythmias (ventricular tachycardia or fibrillation) should be treated. Bradyarrhythmias may require stimulation or pacing.

General supportive measures should be instituted in the conscious patient. First order of priority is to maintain an open airway and provide ventilatory assistance if needed (Ambu bag or respirator). Gastric lavage will be useful. Antipsychotic agents are strongly protein-bound and peritoneal dialysis or hemodialysis is probably worthless. Forced diuresis is likewise of little value. Hypotension should be initially treated with volume expansion. If pressors are needed, only alpha-adrenergic stimulators should be used (norepinephrine, metaraminol or dopamine, see Cardiovascular Effects section or Table 31). Seizures are usually self-limiting but if repetitive they should be treated with short-acting barbiturates. Dystonic reactions are treated by intravenous diphenhydramine (Benadryl) 25 mg. per minute not to exceed 100 mg. total dosage. If hypothermia is a problem, maintain body warmth with blankets or heat cradles. Hypothermia can be missed if thermometers are not fully shaken down. The use of external heat should be avoided as it may aggravate

TABLE 31
Diagnosis and Treatment of Antipsychotic Drug Overdosage

Diagnosis	• Somnolence, coma or excitation. • Peripheral and central signs of anticholinergic toxicity (Table 32). • Extrapyramidal signs. • Orthostatic hypotension. • Seizures. • Temperature regulation disturbance. • Respiratory depression. • Shock. • Forrest urine test for phenothiazines.
Approach to Coma	• Vital signs immediately. Airway and blood pressure support if needed. • Place large bore intravenous catheter or CVP line. Start cardiac monitor. • Draw blood samples for glucose, BUN, and electrolytes. Urine or blood drug screen. • Push 25 to 50 ml of 50% glucose solution IV unless blood sugar can be determined immediately. • Get thorough history, do complete physical and neurological examination. • Accurate diagnosis is essential to plan further treatment steps.

Approach to Treating Adverse Side Effects from Overdosage	• Maintain ventilatory support
	• Gastric lavage if conscious.
	• Volume expansion for hypotension.
	• If pressors needed: Add the following to 500 ml of 5% dextrose in water.
	    Norepinephrine, 4 mg.
	    Metaraminol, 200 mg.
	    Phenylephrine, 1 mg.
	    Dopamine, 400 mg.
	    Infuse at sufficient rate to maintain systolic BP at 100 to 110.
	• *Do not use epinephrine.*
	• Repetitive seizures should respond to 50-100 mg/min of IV amobarbital. Avoid respiratory depression. *Do not exceed 1 gm.*
	• Diphenhydramine 25 mg/min IV for dystonic reactions. *Do not exceed 100 mg.*
	• Blankets or heat cradles for hypothermia. *Avoid external heat.*
	• Cooling blankets or alcohol baths for hyperthermia. If due to anticholinergic toxicity, use physostigmine (Table 32).
	• Record fluid intake and output. Indwelling urinary catheter if needed.

shock through peripheral vasodilatation. Hyperthermia may require cooling blankets or alcohol sponge baths. This may be an indication of anticholinergic poisoning. Fluid intake and output must be recorded in a flow sheet fashion and an indwelling urinary catheter may be required to properly monitor hydration and renal function.

It is possible that toxicity from excessive intake of antipsychotics can present the signs of an anticholinergic intoxication. Thioridazine is the most highly anticholinergic agent of antipsychotics available in the U.S. and is the most likely to produce anticholinergic toxicity at excessive doses. The only other antipsychotic drugs which have any probability of causing excessive anticholinergic activity are chlorpromazine, mesoridazine and triflupromazine (Vesprin). The physician who diagnoses anticholinergic toxicity in a patient taking an antipsychotic must remember that other highly anticholinergic agents such as antiparkinson drugs or tricyclic antidepressants may have been ingested as well.

Table 32 outlines the key diagnostic features of anticholinergic toxicity. Diagnosis rests upon finding the central signs of acetylcholine blockade paired with the peripheral findings of parasympathetic block. These features are identical to those that would be produced from excessive atropine intake. The old medical school adage, "dry as a bone, red as a beet, hot as a furnace, mad as a hatter and blind as a bat," makes the diagnosis easy to remember. This refers to the key findings of dry skin and mucous membranes, flushed skin, hyperthermia, confusion, disorientation and blurred vision.

A special antidote now exists for anticholinergic toxicity (Granacher and Baldessarini, 1976). Physostigmine (Antilirium), unlike neostigmine or pyridostigmine, crosses the blood-brain barrier. Being a reversible anticholinesterase, it will increase peripheral and central levels of acetylcholine and reverse the anticholinergic toxicity. Its use and signs of excess are outlined in Table 32. If a diagnosis of anticholinergic poisoning is made, physostigmine administration will both confirm the diagnosis and treat the disorder. An initial test dose of 1 to 2 mg. is given slowly IV (rapid injection may cause seizures) or IM. It may have to be repeated at 15 to 30 minute intervals due to its short duration of action. This requires close monitoring of the patient. An easy way to follow a patient receiving physostigmine is by a flow chart. This would include the items most likely to show rapid clinical change such as vital signs, pupillary size and responsiveness to light, bowel sounds, urinary output, moistness of skin and mental status, especially agitation, orientation and short-term memory. These clinical signs should be recorded every 15 minutes and thereby will indicate improvement or worsening and the need for further physostigmine. **Physostigmine should not be used in severely poisoned patients with EKG signs of conduction disturbance.**

When physostigmine is given to a patient with anticholinergic toxicity,

TABLE 32
Clinical Syndromes Induced by Anticholinergic and Cholinergic Drugs

Anticholinergic Syndrome

1. Central:
   Anxiety, agitation, restless purposeless overactivity, delirium, disorientation, impairment of immediate and recent memory, dysarthria, hallucinations, myoclonus, seizures.

2. Peripheral:
   Tachycardia and arrhythmias, large sluggish pupils, scleral injection, flushed warm dry skin, increased temperature, decreased mucosal secretions.
   Urinary retention, reduced bowel motility.

3. Treatment:
   Adults: Initial or test dose: 1-2 mg. physostigmine salicylate i.m. or slowly i.v. Repeat as needed after at least 15-30 minutes.

   Children: 0.5-1.0 physostigmine salicylate, as for adults.

Physostigmine-induced Cholinergic Excess

1. Central:
   Confusion, seizures, nausea and vomiting, myoclonus, hallucinations often after a period of initial improvement of CNS status when given to treat the anticholinergic syndrome.

2. Peripheral:
   Bradycardia, miosis, increases mucosal secretions, copious bronchial secretions, dyspnea, tears, sweating, diarrhea, abdominal colic, biliary colic, urinary frequency or urgency.

3. Treatment or prevention:
   Atropine sulfate (central and peripheral): 0.5 mg./mg. physostigmine, i.m. or s.c.
   Methscopolamine bromide (Pamine, peripheral): 0.25-0.50 mg./mg. physostigmine, i.m. (but extremes of 0.1-0.75 mg./mg. physostigmine have been used.)
   Glycopyrrolate (Robinul, peripheral): 0.25-0.50 mg./mg. physostigmine, i.m.

the response is dramatically rapid. Within 5-10 minutes following an IV dose, pulse will diminish, agitation and disorientation will improve, recent memory will return, sweating will be noticed and bowel sounds can be heard. Some patients may develop urinary urgency. If the physician has erred in the diagnosis, a state of cholinergic excess will result from the use of physostigmine. Patients will drop their pulse to 50 or 60/min., get small pupils, hypersalivate, sweat profusely and develop excessive bronchial secretions. Severe diarrhea may result or urinary incontinence can occur. Should this develop, atropine, methscopolamine, or glycopyrrolate will quickly reverse this toxicity (Table 32).

Depending on the amount and character of the anticholinergic ingested, the patient may lapse back to the toxic state in 30 minutes to an hour and then repeated injections may be needed. The patient should be treated with physostigmine until clinical signs improve or signs of cholinergic toxicity appear (Table 32). To stop short of this may undertreat the patient. For cases of mild anticholinergic toxicity, the patient is best managed by observation, fluids, and mild sedation with a benzodiazepine (e.g. diazepam, Valium). Severely poisoned cases should be followed in an intensive care unit where cardiac monitoring is available. Cases in between can sometimes be treated and released straight from the emergency room.

VI

Lithium Therapy

1. HISTORY

Lithium is not properly classified as an antipsychotic agent but is, rather, antimanic. However, it is frequently combined with antipsychotic drugs. This is particularly likely to occur in the management of acute manic psychosis and in certain schizoaffective states. Thus, lithium is discussed in a thorough manner to aid the physician in its rational use, particularly when it is combined with antipsychotic agents.

The clinical properties of lithium ion in manic-depressive illness were first evaluated by Cade in Australia on March 29, 1948. There was a little wizened man of 51 who had been in a state of chronic manic excitement for 5 years. He had lived on a back ward during that time and was restless, dirty, destructive, mischievous and interfering. He was started on lithium citrate 1200 mg. t.i.d. On the fourth day of treatment, his therapist noted a change but the nursing staff did not agree. However, on the fifth day he appeared quieter, tidier, less disinhibited and less distractible. His progress was rapid and at the end of 3 weeks he was on a convalescent ward. He remained well and left the hospital on July 9, 1948. He was on a maintenance dose of lithium carbonate 600 mg. daily and returned to his old job. The carbonate salt had been substituted for the citrate because of nausea. He was readmitted 6 months later after stopping his lithium due to overconfidence in his recovery. He was again stabilized on lithium and discharged 1 month later to return to his work (Cade, 1970).

How Cade came to consider lithium in the treatment of manic psychoses is worth noting. He felt that mania might be due to a state of intoxication produced by the circulating success of some metabolite. This led to the injection of urine from manic patients into guinea pigs. These intraperitoneal injections showed that the manic urine was far more toxic to these animals than urine from non-manics. Further study demonstrated that this toxicity was due to the presence of urea. Since urea from manics was in no higher concentration than from non-manics, it was speculated that uric acid might be the culprit. To test this hypothesis, urea and a soluble uric acid salt were given. This uric acid salt happened to be lithium urate. The lithium urate seemed to protect the guinea pigs from toxicity. Even more importantly, the guinea pigs lost their natural timidity and frantic righting reflex; instead, they became placid, tranquilized and unresponsive to stimulation. Further tests showed the calming action was due to lithium and not urate (Johnson and Cade, 1975).

However, about the same time in the United States the death knell rang for lithium's use in American medicine. Three articles and a letter in the *Journal of the American Medical Association* in March, 1949, reported deaths from lithium intoxication using lithium chloride salt substitutes. Subsequently, lithium was not approved for use in this country until the 1970s. Fortunately, Schou in Demnark saw Cade's obscure report in the *Medical Journal of Australia* and proceeded with successful clinical trials in humans.

2. BIOLOGY

Lithium belongs to the alkali metal group which includes sodium, potassium, rubidium, and cesium. It has the lowest atomic weight of all the known metals (6.94) and is the third lightest of all elements. Of all the alkali metals, lithium ion has the largest hydrated diameter, is the least lipid soluble, and has the lowest diffusion coefficient (Prockop and Marcus, 1972). Lithium colors a flame red and its emission line is at 670 .7 nm. It is found naturally in mineral waters and in trace amounts in sea water, plants and animal tissues (Schou, 1968).

Lithium is readily abosrbed from the gastrointestinal tract. The most widely used form in the United States is lithium carbonate, which is the only lithium salt in clinical use in this country. Lithium cloride seems too hygroscopic to be manufactured into tablets, but citrate and acetate salts have been used in other countries.

The peak serum concentration of lithium is reached in roughly 30 minutes, while the plateau concentration is achieved in 12 to 24 hours. Lithium crosses cell boundaries at a relatively slow rate and this transport lag probably accounts for the delay of 6 to 10 days in achieving a therapeutic response (Singer and Rotenberg, 1973). Lithium does not bind to plasma proteins (Talso and Clarke, 1951) and it appears that different areas of the brain transport and store lithium in an unequal manner. Postmortem examinations of humans have shown lithium concentrations to be highest in the pons (Francis and Traill, 1970). Other studies have demonstrated by EEG that the orbito-frontal cortex is the first brain area to be affected by lithium administration (Barratt et al., 1970). How lithium enters and leaves the central nervous system remains a mystery. It seems to be a passive process without active transport and no studies are presently available to quantitate the influx of lithium into brain or nervous tissue.

The distribution of lithium ion seems determined by genetic factors. Dorus et al (1975) have shown that the in vivo distribution of lithium ion across red blood cell membranes varies far more in dizygotic twin pairs than in monozygotic twin pairs. These studies indicate that both plasma and red blood cell lithium responders have an association with a family history of bipolar illness, whereas no such association can be demonstrated in families with a history of unipolar illness (Mendlewicz et al., 1973). These findings suggest that bipolar illness is a genetically determined membrane disease.

Lithium has about 70 to 80% reabsorption in the proximal tubular system of the kidney (Table 33). Here it is competitive with sodium reabsorption. Thus, as sodium reabsorption decreases, lithium reabsorption increases. likewise, by increasing the concentration of sodium appearing at the proximal tubule, one can induce lithium diuresis. The renal lithium clearance is about 20% of the glomerular filtration rate or roughly 20-25 ml/min. After lithium tablets are swallowed, lithium is quickly absorbed and serum levels peak at about 30 minutes. Should lithium be discontinued, a very rapid drop occurs in the first 24 hours and continues rapidly for 5 or 6 days. The remaining lithium is slowly excreted over a roughly 2-week period.

At the present time, a unified theory of the mechanism of action of lithium upon recurrent mood disorders is not fully developed. Lithium ion has been shown to antagonize the synaptic transmission of catecholamines as well as interfere with the activity of the hormonal cell messenger adenylate cyclase. Lithium may bring about changes in intracellular sodium concentrations during recurrent mania or depression. Other effects of lithium have been described such as changes in carbohydrate metabolism and cerebral glucose metabolism, alterations in acetylcholine synthesis, and influences upon cerebral amines and aminoacids. However, none of these observations sufficiently demonstrates lithium's mode of action.

TABLE 33
Metabolism, Distribution and Excretion of Lithium Ion

Reabsorption	• 99% of filtered sodium is reabsorbed, 70 to 80% is reabsorbed in the proximal tubule, 15 to 20% is reabsorbed distally.
	• For lithium, the fraction reabsorbed is only 70 to 80%, all in the proximal tubular system.
Competition with Sodium	• Proximal reabsorption of sodium and lithium is competitive.
	• A deficiency of sodium increases lithium retention and risk of lithium toxicity.
	• Likewise, excessive sodium intake causes lithium diuresis.
Clearance	• In man, the glomerular filtration rate is about 125 ml/min.
	• The renal lithium clearance in healthy persons is about 20 ml/min.
Distribution	• Peak serum concentration occurs about 30 minutes after intake.
	• Plateau concentrations occur in 12-24 hours.
Excretion	• If lithium is discontinued following steady state levels, lithium is excreted rapidly for the first 5 to 6 days and then slowly for the next 10-14 days.

3. INDICATIONS FOR USE

Presently, lithium's use is recommended in three general circumstances. (1) It is used as an adjunct to antipsychotic agents in acute mania and may be used in acute recurrent depressions but is presently not the treatment of choice. (2) It is the drug of choice for the prophylaxis of bipolar mania and depression. (3) It is occasionally used empirically in other psychiatric conditions as described below (Kerry, 1975). Lithium's major role has been shown to be in the treatment of mania. Controlled studies generally report a 70-80% improvement rate in manic patients. The outcome from these studies supports lithium as superior to placebo in acute mania but inferior to chlorpromazine in highly agitated patients (Peet, 1975).

Lithium's ability to improve depression is not as clearly supported as its ability to treat mania. However, some patients with a diagnosis of manic-depressive illness, depressed type, will respond positively. Paradoxically, some patients with this diagnosis will get no positive benefit from lithium. Also, a few unipolar depressions have shown favorable response to lithium but data are too unclear to be presently definitive (Mendels, 1975). It may be that unipolar depressives who respond to covert bipolar patients who may have a manic episode later in their life. In any event, depressed patients are more likely to respond to lithium if there is a positive family history of bipolar affective illness (Mendlewicz et al., 1972).

Lithium has shown a positive response in some cases of schizophrenia, schizoaffective type, but seems markedly inferior to antipsychotic agents in the treatment of the schizophrenias. The literature is not clear on lithium's positive benefit in schizoaffective states. There are no standardized criteria to assist in the differentiation of this syndrome from schizophrenia or affective illness. Some studies suggest that the addition of lithium to antipsychotic agents improves treatment results in excited schizoaffective patients. However, this has not been demonstrated under controlled conditions (Prien, 1975).

4. INITIATION OF LITHIUM THERAPY

Lithium should not be started for an initial mood swing (Cade, 1975). Since lithium is generally taken for life, to do so may needlessly expose the patient to continuous medication. Patients who experience the first manic episode in their early 20s usually have a 6 to 10 year interval before the next episode. As one is dealing with a recurrent illness, it is wisest to wait and see if a second mood swing occurs later in life and then initiate a lithium trial. This is an especially good practice in patients who display a single mood swing but have no family history of affective illness.

As with any form of medical therapy, lithium treatment begins with a thorough historical, physical, and laboratory evaluation (Table 34). Careful attention to detail must be performed during history-taking. The patient's history should be probed for evidence of renal, thyroid, or cardiovascular disease. Particular attention should be paid to classical signs and symptoms of manic-depressive psychosis in the family history, as these features identify those likely to respond to lithium. Taylor and Abrams (1975) have shown that positive lithium responders frequently exhibit euphoric moods and grandiose delusions, and tend to have cyclothymic premorbid personality styles. On the other hand, nonresponders are rarely euphoric, frequently show incomplete auditory hallucinations, tend to have formal thought disorders and withdrawn, depressive premorbid personality styles.

Family history requires careful examination. It may be necessary to speak

TABLE 34
Evaluation of the Patient for Lithium Therapy

Caveat:	• Is this the patient's first mood swing?
Indicators of potential positive lithium response:	• Euphoria, grandiose delusions, flight of ideas, pressure and push of speech, motor hyperactivity, increased energy, premorbid cyclothymic personality style, recurrent depressions, and positive family history of affective illness. Also, atypical manic features of irritability and hostility.
Indicators of potential negative lithium response:	• Lack of euphoria, auditory hallucinations, formal thought disorder, delusions without relation to mood, gross hysterical symptoms, difficulty with contact, prolonged depressions, withdrawn-depressive premorbid personality styles, and negative family history of affective illness.
Target organs for specific physical examination:	• Central nervous system, cardiovascular system, renal system and thyroid gland.
Recommended baseline laboratory evaluations:	• Electrocardiogram, complete blood count, routine urinalysis including specific gravity, serum creatinine, creatinine clearance, thyroid functions, thyroid antibodies.

with relatives of the patient in order to get accurate history. In the United States, history of affective disorders prior to lithium introduction (around 1971) may be spurious. The clinician should ask about suicide, recurrent hospitalizations, grandiose behavior, and other relevant symptomatology. Careful physical examination should exclude significant disease, especially of the heart, kidneys, or thyroid gland. Mental status and neurological examinations should carefully look for organic impairment of the central nervous system. An electrocardiogram should be obtained for screening and to rule out sinus abnormalities which might be aggravated by lithium. A complete blood count assists with baseline data and gives a pre-lithium white blood cell count in case of lithium-induced leukocytosis. A routine urinalysis and serum creatinine should be used as a screen of renal function. Patients with renal abnormalities should have a 24-hour creatinine clearance performed. However, this may be impractical in the highly manic patient who will not assist with accurate urine collection and may require postponement to a more cooperative time. Baseline thyroid studies are a must in order to evaluate those patients who may later develop goiters. Patients with past episodes or family history of thyroiditis are at risk and thyroid antibody determinations may be of assistance.

The treatment of acute mania is smoother for both patient and staff if antipsychotic drugs are used to quell excitement until lithium approaches therapeutic levels. All antipsychotic agents will have a specific quieting action upon manic excitement. However, it is probably wisest to choose haloperidol. Recent reports of lithium-phenothiazine toxicity have emerged. Apparently, phenothiazines can increase intracellular lithium to levels far higher than that measured in the plasma. For instance, patients have developed organic brain syndromes with non-toxic plasma levels of lithium. However, these patients were also receiving thioridazine or fluphenazine. Recent laboratory work confirms that phenothiazines will force lithium into cells whereas haloperidol does not. These data refute the claims that haloperidol and lithium may cause irreversible brain damage (Pandey et al, 1979). Table 35 outlines the management of acute mania.

TABLE 35
Basic Principles in the Pharmacologic Management of Acute Mania

Antipsychotic Agents	• Use a high potency antipsychotic agent such as haloperidol.
	• If agitation is quite high, use an intramuscular form the first 24 hours, e.g. haloperidol 5-10 mg. hourly until quiet.
	• As agitation diminishes switch to concentration or tablet/capsule. Give ⅓ in a.m., ⅔ h.s., e.g. haloperidol 10 mg. a.m., 20 mg. h.s.
	• Remember that intramuscular antipsychotic agents are 2-4 times as potent as oral forms.
	• Taper off medication as patient responds to lithium carbonate.
	• Phenothiazines may increase the likelihood of lithium toxicity.
Lithium Carbonate	• Start lithium only when patient is cooperative enough to take oral medication.
	• Begin with t.i.d. or q.i.d. dosage regimens to minimize side effects.
	• Generally 600-900 mg. per day is an adequate starting dose.
	• Titrate dose upward based upon serum levels of lithium.
	• Attain a serum level of 1.2-1.6 mEq./L. and reduce to 0.8-1.2 mEq./L. for maintenance.
	• Remember to use lower doses in the elderly or those with impaired kidney function.

Lithium is generally started in divided oral dosages at a dose range of 600 to 900 mg. on the first day, rising to 1200 to 1800 mg. on the next day, with adjustment thereafter depending upon serum lithium levels. This is done while the patient is being quieted with antipsychotic agents, if necessary, or may be given alone if agitation is minimal. In the United States, the carbonate salt of lithium is available in 300 mg. tablets or capsules which contain 8.1 mEq. of lithium ion. Lithium carbonate is well tolerated but may cause slight gastric distress in some. Should this occur, giving the medication after meals generally alleviates the problem.

The starting dosage of lithium is generally determined empirically as above. However, it is now possible to determine a rough index of an individual patient's lithium clearance and from these data arrive at the dosage regimen that will result in a steady state therapeutic level of 0.6-1.2 mEq./L. of lithium. The procedure is quite simple. One merely gives the patient 600 mg. of lithium carbonate at 8:00 a.m. on day 1. On day 2, a serum sample is taken at precisely 8:00 a.m. (24 hours later) and the lithium level determined in the laboratory. **The morning dose of lithium must be held before blood is drawn!** The serum level at 24 hours following a 600 mg. loading dose of lithium carbonate will then predict the dosage regimen necessary to maintain a steady state blood level of 0.6-1.2 mEq./L. of lithium. Table 36 outlines this procedure and gives the predicted dosage regimens for various lithium serum levels. This technique can be quite successful and reproducible if certain factors are kept in mind. The most important factor of success is that the patient must take the medication. Secondly, blood samples must be collected at exactly 24 hours following the loading dose. Thirdly, the laboratory must be capable of accurate serum lithium analyses to the second decimal place. Finally, the limitations of any predictive technique must be kept in mind.

For example, suppose a manic patient was given 600 mg. of lithium carbonate precisely at 8:00 a.m. on day 1. The following morning the patient is sent to the lab. and blood is drawn. The laboratory reports that afternoon that the serum lithium is 0.17 mEq./L. By looking at Table 36, one can see that 0.17 mEq./L. is between 0.15 and 0.19 mEq./L. This corresponds to 300 mg. q.i.d. The patient would be started on 300 mg. q.i.d. and the physician could then expect this patient's serum lithium to be between 0.6 and 1.2 mEq./L. witin a few days. Further determinations of lithium should be made and the dose adjusted up or down accordingly. If the laboratory reported a 24-hour value greater than 0.30 mEq./L., kidney disease, sodium depletion, or diuretic use should be suspected. Further evaluation of the patient should be done before starting lithium in this situation.

Once lithium is started, careful monitoring of serum lithium on a Monday-Wednesday-Friday basis is usually advised for the first 1 or 2 weeks or until

TABLE 36
Method of Predicting Initial Dosage Regimen of Lithium Therapy

Procedure:

The patient is given a loading dose of lithium carbonate 600 mg. by mouth at 8:00 a.m. on day 1.

Precisely at 8:00 a.m. (or exactly 24 hours following the loading dose) on day 2, blood is drawn and a serum lithium determination made. The morning dose of lithium must be held until blood is drawn!

The resulting serum lithium value is entered into the table below to predict the dosage regimen.

Determination of Dosage Regimen:

Serum lithium (mEq./L.) 24 hours following 600 mg. loading dose	Dosage regimen to maintain 0.6-1.2 mEq./L. lithium level
0.24-0.30*	300 mg. b.i.d.
0.20-0.23	300 mg. t.i.d.
0.15-0.19	300 mg. q.i.d.
0.10-0.14	600 mg. t.i.d.
0.05-0.09	900 mg. t.i.d.
0.05	1200 mg. t.i.d.

*For serum levels above 0.30 mEq./L. administer lithium with caution and further patient evaluation advised.

From Cooper, T. B. and Simpson, G. M.: The 24-hour lithium level as a prognosticator of dosage requirements, *Am. J. Psychiatry* 133: 440-443, 1976.

the patient is stable. Blood levels should be raised to 1.2-1.6 mEq./L. to insure a therapeutic effect. Some authors have advised going as high as 2.0 mEq./L., but this is generally unnecessary and increases the likelihood of toxicity in most individuals. Table 35 outlines some of the salient points of lithium administration in acute mania. In general, the manic patient will show a positive response to lithium within 5 to 10 days.

It must be remembered that the manic patient can tolerate higher doses of lithium and a reduction in dosage may be necessary as the mood approaches normal. Close monitoring of serum lithium is required at this time. Also, for the highly disturbed patient who is also receiving antipsychotic agents, as the manic behavior quiets, a reduction in dosage of these agents will likely be necessary. Once control of the patient's behavior is attained, the patient is ready for discharge. Weekly lithium levels should probably be obtained the first month of outpatient follow-up; thereafter monthly estimations will probably suffice for the first year. Likewise thyroid, cardiac and renal status should be checked at the same time.

5. MAINTENANCE THERAPY AND PROPHYLAXIS

The most important use of lithium in psychiatry is the prophylaxis of bipolar manic illness. The term "prophylaxis" as used in most lithium studies refers only to the prevention of attacks severe enough to require hospitalization or adjunctive medication. Controlled studies demonstrate that lithium clearly reduces or prevents the recurrence of mania in the majority of bipolar patients. Quitkin et al. (1976) reviewed the 8 reported controlled studies of bipolar manic-depressive illness through 1974. In all, 438 patients were studied and it was concluded that lithium carbonate specifically prevents manic recurrence in bipolar patients. Some patients do relapse and may have a manic breakthrough even while being maintained on lithium with blood levels in the therapeutic range. However, data indicate that manic breakthroughs are probably less common than depressive breakthroughs but mania is far more likely to result in a hospitalization. One controlled study (Prien et al., 1974) suggests that patients who have one manic breakthrough while receiving lithium carbonate may do no better than placebo patients once their mood stabilizes. Presently there are insufficient studies to further evaluate this finding. Dunner et al. (1976) have found that 25% of their patients fail on lithium prophylaxis in the first 3 months. A low but persistent percentage will fail thereafter. Patients who have early failures (within first 3 months) tend to have subsequent early failures even if treated and maintained on lithium carbonate. In summary, patients maintained on lithium carbonate will show a considerable relapse rate if they are followed for sufficient time. On the other hand, manic bipolar patients very clearly have improved function and fewer recurrences on prophylactic lithium carbonate when compared with placebo controls.

Some data are suggestive that lithium ion is prophylactic for recurrent depression in both bipolar and unipolar patients. However, this evidence is not conclusive at this time. There appear to be some serious methodological problems in the studies to date which will not allow the same conclusions about lithium's effects upon mania to be drawn for depression (Quitkin et al., 1976). It appears that the recurrence of depression in bipolar patients is probably more common than mania. On the other hand, the social consequences of mania are more severe. Manic patients are far more likely to be hospitalized, lose their jobs, or become divorced than depressed patients.

A recent study by Fieve et al. (1976) indicated that lithium is highly effective in the prophylaxis of the depressive state for bipolar I patients. Bipolar I is defined as previous hospitalizations for mania and mild to severe depressions. They further found lithium to be possibly prophylactic for depression in bipolar II patients. These are defined as patients with previous hospitalizations for depression and with a history of hypomania not requiring hospitalization. Data for unipolar depression indicates that depressions in this population were modified by lithium to fewer episodes with less severe pathology. However, the response was not as clear-cut as for the bipolar I and II groups.

Lithium for prophylaxis may be started during mania or during a disease-free interval. It may be started either on an inpatient or outpatient basis; however, inpatient initiation is more efficient. The general guidelines for workup and serum lithium level estimation in prophylaxis will be the same as previously described in Tables 34 and 35. The use of lithium with tricyclic antidepressants for prophylaxis has been examined in a few studies. However, presently no clear guidelines are available for this combination. On the other hand, there is no evidence to date that the combination of lithium with a tricyclic antidepressant has any undo drug interaction hazards for the patient. However, for the bipolar patient, imipramine has been shown to cause a higher incidence of manic episodes (Prien et al., 1973b).

For full prophylactic effect, serum lithium levels should be maintained at or above 0.8 mEq./L. Schou (1968) has contended that levels below 0.8 mEq./L. may not insure the full prophylactic effect of lithium. Prien et al. (1974) have evaluated the effectiveness of lithium prophylaxis in recurrent depression and found that serum levels between 0.5 and 0.7 mEq./L. or doses below 1000 mg./day were relatively ineffective in preventing occurrences. This is clinically significant as there is a disparity in the published prescribing information for lithium carbonate in the United States. The manufacturer's package insert recommends levels of 0.6-1.2 mEq./L., while the American Society of Hospital Pharmacists suggests levels of 0.5-1.5 mEq./L. The lower ranges of these recommendations are probably too low for adequate prophylaxis.

It has been suggested that lithium has prophylactic benefit for schizophrenia, schizo-affective type; however, data are presently insufficient to draw this conclusion. One large study does demonstrate a prophylactic effect in schizoaffective illness, but it was uncontrolled (Angst et al., 1970). The only controlled studies noted thus far have been all diagnostic categories. When treatment results are statistically analyzed separately, schizoaffectives do poorly on lithium alone. However, due to the small sample size, it is impossible to draw valid conclusions and further research must be done in order to evaluate the potential benefit of lithium as a prophylactic agent in schizoaffective illness.

Psychosocial management is important to a successful lithium maintenance program. Lithium is still a "new" agent in American psychiatry. For this reason, many people suddenly find their life changes from frequent mood swings to relatively stable moods for months or years at a time. This may well have a major impact upon patients and their families. Often a peculiar psychosocial pattern develops in which patient, spouse, children, friends and associates all play a part. The patient who was formerly buffered by others in order to deal with his incessant mood swings may suddenly be returned to a useful and functional role. Moreover, manic patients, especially, often become estranged from others due to their intolerable behavior. When prophylactic lithium brings stability to their lives, they may have extreme difficulty reestablishing former interpersonal relationships. A major affect of lithium treatment upon marital relations has been noted. The radical reshuffling of roles and responsibilities can alter previously established marital balances. A spouse who was once responsible for holding the home together may suddenly be displaced by the reemergence of the manic patient's normality (Demers and Davis, 1971).

Another problem may well be that the patient does not like the way lithium makes him feel. Many complain it makes them feel flat or removes their spontaneity. Often, some patients feel that the most productive or creative periods in their lives occurred during hypomania. Generally, if the patient stays symptom free for an extended period of time, he will readjust and find that actually the productivity and creativity are as good as or even better than before the initiation of lithium.

6. USE IN PREGNANCY

Women seem slightly more likely than men to develop manic depressive illness (Spiegel and Bell, 1959). Unfortunately, the peak incidence of manic-depressive illness is during the reproductive years of the woman. The prophylactic benefits of lithium ion are now clearly documented. Thus, this almost insures that the fetus and lithium will meet during at least some pregnancies.

Following the Federal Drug Administration approval for lithium use in the United States, a register of babies born to mothers receiving lithium during pregnancy was established. This was in conjunction with registers in Canada and Denmark. This International Register of Lithium Babies* attempts to compile data on all babies exposed to lithium in utero. Warnings of possible teratogenic potential of lithium have been issued (Weinstein and

---

*American Register of Lithium Babies (M. Weinstein, M.D., and M. Goldfield, M.D.), 401 Parnassus Ave., San Francisco, California 94122; Scandinavian Register of Lithium Babies (M. Schou, M.D.), Arrhus University-Department Psychiatry, Psychiatric Hospital, 8240 Risskov, Denmark; Canadian Register of Lithium Babies (A. Villeneuve, M.D.), Hospital St. Michael, Archange, Quebec, Canada.

Goldfield, 1975). At that time 143 cases of lithium use had been collected by the Register of Lithium Babies. Later data (Schou, 1976) suggest a higher than expected ratio of cardiovascular anomalies. Obviously, the numbers are still too small to make conclusive statements. However, Ebstein's anomaly is appearing at a far greater rate than expected. Since insufficient data exist to fully answer the question, guidelines for decreasing fetal risk from lithium exposure are discussed below.

The major areas of concern for the physician will be the usage of lithium during pregnancy, maternal toxicity during labor and delivery, neonatal toxicity, and breast feeding. The risk of lithium use during pregnancy can be reduced by proper patient selection. Women with the potential for conception should be treated with lithium only for the management and prophylaxis of mania and depression. Current data probably do not justify its use in other conditions (Weinstein and Goldfield, 1975). An effective form of contraception should be provided for women requiring lithium. If a woman becomes pregnant during lithium prophylaxis she should be immediately withdrawn from lithium treatment. It is recommended that physicians following fertile women on lithium prophylaxis advise their patients to notify them of the first missed or changed menstrual period. Immediate laboratory testing for pregnancy should be done. Unfortunately, a woman may be as much as six weeks pregnant before she notices menstrual changes. A woman should remain on lithium during her first trimester of pregnancy only if there is historical evidence that discontinuation would seriously endanger the woman or the pregnancy. The following statement is a consensus of the pharmaceutical history (*PDR*, 1978):

> Adverse effects on implantation in rats, embryo viability in mice and metabolism *in vitro* of rat testes and human spermatozoa have been attributed to lithium, as have been embryo malformations in submammalian species and cleft palates in mice. Studies in rats, rabbits and monkeys have shown no embryo malformations.
>
> There are insufficient data at the present time to determine the effects of lithium carbonate on human fetuses. At this point, lithium should not be used in the first trimester, unless in the opinion of the physician, the potential benefits outweigh possible hazards.

Electroconvulsive therapy is the safest treatment for the pregnant manic or depressed patient.

If it is necessary to use lithium in a pregnant woman, the smallest possible dose should be used to achieve the minimum serum level compatible with prophylaxis (roughly 0.8 mEq.L.), as no placental barrier to lithium exists. The lithium concentration in umbilical cord blood is essentially the same as the maternal circulation and closely reflects the mother's serum lithium levels (MacKay et al., 1976). **Thus, it is highly important to avoid fluctua-**

tions in serum lithium concentrations in the mother. Since lithium is so readily transmitted to the fetus, "pulses" of high lithium concentration should be avoided (Weinstein and Goldfield, 1975). Two major factors will increase the likelihood of exposing the fetus to high lithium concentrations: (1) sodium loss (e.g., low salt diet, excessive sweating) or the use of sodium-losing diuretics, (2) giving more than 300 mg. of lithium carbonate in a single dose. In the pregnant woman receiving lithium carbonate, the use of diuretics for ankle edema, weight reduction diets, or low sodium diets should be avoided. Secondly, the dosing of daily lithium should be done much more frequently. Instead of the routine 600 mg. b.i.d. or t.i.d. schedule, a schedule of 300 mg. of lithium carbonate at 9:00 a.m., 1:00 p.m., 5:00 p.m., and 10:00 p.m. or the like should be used. A maximum of 300 mg. should be given at any 1 dose. Since maternal lithium concentrations are highest at 1 to 4 hours after an oral dose, a minimum of 4 hours between doses should be maintained. This is, of course, assuming that the woman is stabilized on a prophylactic regimen and does not require acute treatment. For the acutely manic woman, in her second or third trimester of pregnancy, lithium can be used with care. Antipsychotics (e.g., haloperidol) should be used to quell excitement and lithium slowly added to the regimen. A suggested starting dose of 300 mg. b.i.d. may be used with the addition of 300 mg. every other day. **It must be remembered that the renal clearance of lithium increases 50-100% during pregnancy so lithium levels should be determined more frequently.** In general, daily to every other day lithium determinations are advised in the hospital and determinations every 2 weeks are recommended for outpatients. Lithium determinations should be more frequent during the last half of pregnancy.

As the woman approaches labor and delivery, special considerations for lithium usage are required. The increased renal lithium clearance during pregnancy may cause the pregnant woman to have declining serum lithium levels while the lithium dose remains stable. It is advised that during the last half of pregnancy, serum lithium be determined weekly at a minimum. Should more lithium be required to maintain a therapeutic level, one can add 150 mg. increments to the daily regimen as needed by using scored lithium carbonate tablets (J. B. Roerig Division, Charles Pfizer Company, Inc.). These scored 300 mg. tablets can be broken into roughly 150 mg. halves.

Tremendous changes in fluid balance occur at the time of labor and delivery. Therefore, special care must be taken in lithium management at this time. It has been noted that women can begin labor with serum levels well within the therapeutic range and become severely lithium toxic during and immediately following delivery. Serum lithium levels may become as high as 4.4 mEq./Liter (Vacaflor et al., 1970; Wilbanks et al., 1970). In those

TABLE 37
The Use of Lithium During Pregnancy

Teratology	May cause a greater than expected number of major cardio-vascular anomalies. Avoid the use of lithium during the first trimester. Use reliable contraception, discontinue lithium at first missed period.
Maintenance During Second and Third Trimester	Do not "pulse" fetus, give no more than 300 mg. in any one dose. Keep serum level at around 0.8 mEq./Liter. Do not use diuretics or sodium restricted diets. Remember that renal lithium clearance is 50% to 100% higher during pregnancy. Check serum levels weekly if necessary.
Labor and Delivery	Reduce daily lithium dose 50% in last week of pregnancy. Stop lithium entirely at onset of labor. Restart lithium at pre-pregnancy dosage level day after delivery.
Neonatal Lithium Toxicity	"Floppy" infant, low Apgar score. Low or fast heart rate, hypothermia, cyanosis Absent Moro reflex, poor suck, poor respiratory effect.
Breast Feeding	Avoid

cases reported the mothers had been salt restricted and treated with sodium depleting diuretics prior to delivery. Because of risks of unsuspected lithium intoxication at delivery, it is advised to reduce the daily lithium dose 50% during the last week of pregnancy and to discontinue it entirely at the onset of labor. Lithium may then be safely reinstituted at the pre-pregnancy dosage requirements immediately following delivery (Weinstein and Gold-field, 1975). However, breast feeding must be avoided. Table 37 gives management guidelines for the usage of lithium during pregnancy.

Because the lithium concentration in the fetal circulation closely approximates maternal serum concentrations, neonatal lithium toxicity is a possibility. Reports of neonatal lithium toxicity have included mothers with toxic lithium levels at delivery and mothers with no signs of maternal lithium toxicity (Silverman et al., 1971; Strothers et al., 1973). Neonatal lithium toxicity presents with hypotonia or "floppiness," low Apgar scores during the first half-hour of life, either bradycardia or tachycardia, hypothermia, dusky color, absent Moro reflex, poor suck response, and poor respiratory effect. The serum lithium levels steadily drop over a 1 to 2 week period and to date no deaths or permanent sequelae in these children have been reported. The larger questions on long-term neonatal effects or interference with childhood development have not been answered and further collection of data is required.

Infants who breast feed from mothers maintained on prophylactic lithium will have serum lithium concentrations that approximate the concentrations in breast milk. It has been determined that the lithium concentration in human breast milk varies from 30% to 100% of that in the maternal serum (Catz and Giacoia, 1972). Thus, breast feeding during mother's use of lithium could potentially cause neonatal lithium toxicity. Infants commonly develop vomiting and diarrhea with subsequent alterations in fluid balance and would be more likely to respond adversely to lithium. These factors plus lack of knowledge about renal lithium clearance in neonates increase the likelihood of possible lithium toxicity. Moreover, there is a complete lack of information about the long-term effects of lithium ion upon the developing human nervous system. Therefore, breast feeding by mothers maintained on lithium should be avoided.

7. USE IN CHILDREN

Manic-depressive illness, until very recently, has been considered a disorder of adulthood. In fact, it is classically described as beginning in the third decade. However, it was reported in 1973 (Feinstein and Wolpert) that rapidly shifting emotional states in children which do not seem appropriate to environmental stress should be carefully evaluated as possible manifestations of manic-depressive illness. They stressed the importance of emotional states that tend to remain prolonged or refractory to therapeutic intervention.

Previous authors have stressed that precipitating events are not a conspicuous causal factor in childhood affective illness (Redlich and Freedman, 1966). This is disputed and childhood episodes often seem to begin with a subtle elevation of affect as a response to some environmental influence. A change in environmental conditions will not relieve the emotional states that tend to remain prolonged or refractory to therapeutic intervention.

Previous authors have stressed that precipitating events are not a conspicuous causal factor in childhood affective illness (Redlich and Freedman, 1966). This is disputed and childhood episodes often seem to begin with a subtle elevation of affect as a response to some environmental influence. A change in environmental conditions will not relieve the behavioral disturbance of true affective illness and it continues endogenously. The presence of affective disorders in close relatives of these children is an important diagnostic aid.

It must be stressed that the diagnosis of juvenile manic-depressive illness is extremely difficult and should be done by a qualified child psychiatrist. As with the manic adult, juveniles who are treated with lithium can tolerate higher starting doses of lithium carbonate during the acute phase of their illness. The starting dose of lithium in the adolescent is 900-1200 mg. per day. The serum level should be gradually increased to roughly 1.0 mEq./L. by adding 300 mg. every 2 days. Initial blood levels should be obtained 2 days following the first dose and at 2 day intervals until the therapeutic level is achieved. The usual maintenance dose is 300 mg. t.i.d. or q.i.d. and lithium blood levels should be determined weekly until levels remain stable. The profile of adverse effects and the recognition and management of toxicity are the same as for adults. The initiation of lithium therapy in juveniles should be done in the hospital. Parental consent is recommended (White, 1977). Table 38 outline guidelines for usage of lithium in children.

Lithium carbonate has been tried in other behavior disturbances of childhood, including aggressive disorders of adolescence. A positive response is noted for most studies but in general they were uncontrolled (Kline and Simpson, 1975). The diagnostic groups were so heterogenous that further work must be done before conclusions can be drawn. Likewise, lithium has been tried in the hyperkinetic syndrome of childhood but was judged not as effective as stimulants (Greenhill et al., 1973).

Presently, the only proven effective use of lithium in children is in adolescents exhibiting symptoms of manic episodes. Its use in depression is not clear. **Physicians should note that lithium carbonate is not approved for use in children under 12 years of age. Information on the safety and**

TABLE 38
The Use of Lithium Carbonate in Children

Patient Selection:	Age over 12 years Positive family history Written parental consent Child psychiatrist evaluation if possible Hospitalize
Initial Therapy:	900-1200 mg. per day Blood levels every 2 days until therapeutic level of 1.0 mEq./L. attained Same initial workup as for adults
Maintenance:	300 mg. t.i.d. or q.i.d., usually Blood levels weekly until stable, then monthly Maintain 0.8-1.2 mEq./L.

efficacy in children under 12 years of age is not available and the use of lithium in this age group cannot be recommended at this time.

8. SIDE EFFECTS AND THEIR TREATMENT

Effects Upon Normal Subjects

Since so many diagnostic categories are presently being treated with lithium, the effects of lithium in normal individuals should be noted. Schou et al. (1968a) reported that normal subjects taking an average of 925 mg. of lithium carbonate daily experienced tiredness and muscular weakness. He also reported that when he and his colleagues took roughly 1,800 mg./day for 3 to 6 weeks, they suffered increased irritability, emotional lability, indifference, malaise, and feelings of derealization. Linnoila et al. (1974) found that lithium decreases reaction time during simulated driving tasks. Judd et al. (1977) assessed 23 normal men on affect, mood and personality factors in a controlled trial of lithium carbonate. The average attained serum level of lithium was 0.91 mEq./Liter. Their findings showed substantial amounts of lethargy, dysphoria, loss of interest in interpersonal relations and the environment. Increased mental confusion was also noted. No changes were noted with personality inventory responses. **Therefore, it seems that lithium carbonate is able to induce affect and mood changes in normal subjects but does not alter basic personality traits**.

Many feel that lithium slows a person's thoughts. Obviously, the clinical effect of lithium upon manic patients is to modulate racing thoughts to a more normal rate. Schou et al. (1968a) have reported that lithium impairs a person's subjectively experienced ability to concentrate, comprehend, and memorize. Judd et al. (1977) evaluated cognitive function in 24 normal male subjects and found performance deficits on 3 or 5 tasks that measured cognitive and motor function. Apparently, lithium slows performance in these areas. **Based on these data, there is presently evidence that lithium causes changes in cognitive performance of normal persons**. Therefore, these factors should be kept in mind when assessing subjective complaints or mental status changes in patients who are maintained on lithium.

Gastrointestinal Effects

The most common minor side effect of lithium therapy is probably gastrointestinal distress. All patients will generally give gastric complaints to some degree, especially during the period that serum lithium levels are rapidly rising. The incidence of complaints is about 33% and subsides to roughly 0% over a 1 to 2 year treatment period (Schou, et al., 1970).

The major symptoms of the gastrointestinal system include nausea, vomiting, anorexia, and diarrhea. This group of side effects is also part of the lithium toxicity picture (see below) and the patient with GI complaints will require careful assessment to insure that these are not early manifestations of lithium toxicity. **The most serious GI side effect is diarrhea**. Lithium may have to be readjusted as diarrhea can impair a patient's general condition by contributing to excess sodium and water loss, and excessive sodium loss enhances lithium toxicity.

The management of mild GI side effects is simple. One may give lithium immediately following meals to lessen gastric irritation. Also, the doses may be given 4 or 5 times daily with food in order to decrease the bolus of lithium that the patient takes at any one time. Eating soda crackers before taking the lithium dose may be beneficial. Anti-diarrhea agents such as diphenoxylate HCl (Lomotil 2.5 mg. prn) may be useful.

Neuromuscular Effects

Muscular weakness is often reported by the patient in the early phases of starting lithium therapy. It is fairly common but seems to occur less often than tremor or gastrointestinal complaints. Weakness tends to slowly disappear or improve after the first few weeks of therapy. Other neuromuscular effects that have been rarely reported are fasicultations, facial spasms, tendon jerks, trembling, twitchings, transient facial paralysis, and headaches (Vacaflor, 1975). Neuromuscular symptoms often seem dose-related and in most instances no treatment is needed as they are self-limiting.

However, the emergence of myasthenia gravis during lithium treatment (Neil et al., 1976) and severe muscular weekness with eyelid ptosis (Granacher, 1977) have been reported. It is proposed that lithium may induce neuromuscular cholinergic insufficiency in some susceptible individuals. Moreover, lithium has been shown to potentiate both depolarizing and nondepolarizing neuromuscular blockers (Hill et al., 1976). Therefore, caution is advised with the use of neuromuscular blockers in individuals on chronic lithium maintenance. *The use of succinylcholine during electroconvulsive treatment of a depressive phase of manic-depressive illness could conceivably prolong respiratory paralysis if the patient had positive serum lithium levels.*

Other reports of neuromuscular difficulty secondary to lithium have included muscular rigidity including cogwheel type. Shopsin and Gershon (1975) contend that muscular rigidity is a common side effect in patients receiving lithium maintenance. However, Simpson's group disagrees that this is related to lithium treatment and suggest that careful evaluation will reveal that the patient has been recently exposed to or is concomitantly taking antipsychotic agents (Branchey et al., 1976).

Tremor

Tremor is a common side effect that is seen early in lithium therapy and is usually self-limiting. However, it can appear later in lithium treatment and may interfere with fine motor performance of the individual. Hand tremor is also embarrassing to many people and as a consequence may cause them to withdraw socially.

The management of lithium-induced tremor can be difficult. A reduction of dosage may be helpful in some, remembering not to go below 0.8 mEq./Liter serum lithium level so as to avoid losing the prophylactic effect. Some persons have responded by taking most of the lithium dosge at bedtime; however, this may cause nighttime dyspepsia. Small dosages of diazepam may be helpful. Although propanolol, a beta-adrenergic blocker, has been reported useful in dosages of 40 to 120 mg. per day, a controlled study failed to demonstrate its usefulness in lithium-induced tremor (Kellett et al., 1975). However, their maximum dosage of 40 mg. per day of propranolol may have been insufficient. It must be remembered that propranolol can induce its own gastrointestinal distress such as nausea and diarrhea and, should this occur, the clinician must evaluate between a cause secondary to propranolol or lithium (Brown, 1976).

Kidney Function

The major renal disturbance noted by patients taking lithium is polyuria and polydipsia. It has been reported (Forrest et al., 1974) that 40% of patients experience polydipsia and 12% will have confirmed polyuria of greater than 3 liters per day. Results were suggestive of mildly impaired renal concentrating ability. Generally, these renal side effects are of no clinical significance and cause only mild discomfort for most patients. However, if the polyuria exceeds 4 liters per day, it may be necessary to make some clinical adjustments.

Polyuria can become so severe (4 liters or more of dilute urine daily) that it resembles nephrogenic diabetes insipidus. This syndrome is thought to result from lithium ion's ability to interfere with antidiuretic hormone (ADH) activity. This may be through preventing its access to the appropriate renal tubular membrane site or by blocking the response of ADH-sensitive adenylate cyclase within the renal tubular cell.

The essential features of lithium-induced diabetes insipidus are polyuria interfering with daytime patient activity and sleep, and urine with a very low specific gravity that will become concentrated following water deprivation of 18 hours. If the polyuria is secondary to diabetes insipidus of pituitary origin, vasopressin 5 to 10 units will correct the inability to concentrate urine. On the other hand, lithium-induced nephrogenic diabetes insipidus will show little or no change in urine concentrating ability 1 to 2 hours following vasopressin.

Until recently, little could be done for patients who had severe urine loss with the use of lithium. However, the thiazine diuretics have been shown to be quite useful even though their mechanism of action is unknown. One generally starts with 25 to 50 mg. of hydrochlorthiazide or an equivalent dose of another thiazine diuretic. The dose of diuretic is then titrated until urine output returns to a normal level. **Serum lithium must be monitored daily with appropriate reduction in daily intake. The addition of thiazides produces initial sodium diuresis with resulting lithium retention and possible lithium toxicity.** Some individuals may require as much as a 50% reduction in daily lithium intake while taking thiazides. Table 39 outlines principles of treatment for lithium-induced diabetes insipidus.

The long-term use of lithium has led to questions about its effects upon kidney function. Ramsey et al. (1972) reported that lithium induced a defect in renal concentrating ability in 3 of their patients. However, others (MacNeil and Jenner, 1975; Viol et al., 1976) point out that these effects are often transient and are, moreover, fully reversible if lithiun is discontinued. They cite no evidence of permanent structural damage to the kidney following the chronic use of lithium.

A recent study reports on 14 patients receiving long-term lithium therapy and cites the development of chronic renal lesions in some. Eight patients had at least one episode of lithium intoxication and 6 had lithium-induced decrease in renal concentrating ability. All 14 patients had renal biopsies. In 13 specimens, a pronounced degree of focal nephron atrophy or intestinal fibrosis, or both, was present. An age-matched control sample was used and the number of sclerotic glomeruli in the lithium group was 5 times as great. There was no correlation between age, length of treatment or other factors and the degree of fibrosis. Features known to be associated with acute toxic changes were no different in the 2 groups (Hestbech et al., 1977).

The authors concluded that kidneys from patient receiving long-term lithium treatment may undergo focal atrophy and fibrosis. They also speculated that it is possible that chronic renal disease may only develop in patients in whom the renal concentration of lithium periodically or continually reaches toxic values. They warn that their clinical studies and histological findings suggest that long-term lithium treatment may be a potential health hazard. **The possibility of these hazards should forewarn psychiatrists to reserve chronic lithium treatment for those patients who are truly candidates for its benefits** (Ayd, 1977c).

The elderly patient can be safely treated with lithium but requires significantly lower dosages due to decreased renal function. Elderly subjects

TABLE 39
Lithium Side Effects and Their Management

Side Effect	Management
Gastrointestinal Distress	• Give lithium following meals. • Give lower doses more often.
Muscular Weakness	• Generally requires no treatment. • Use caution with neuromuscular blockers.
Tremor	• Reduce dosage (Keep serum level at 0.8 mEq./Liter, however). • Propranolol 40-80 mg./day might be beneficial. • Valium may improve tremor.
Polyuria Nephrogenic Diabetes Insipidus	• Hydrochlorthiazide 25-50 mg. daily or more. • Decrease lithium intake 40% with 50 mg., 60% with 75 mg. or 70% with 100 mg.
Hypothyroidism	• 1-thyroxine 0.05 to 0.2 mg. daily. • Follow serum thyroxine levels.
QRS Widening and T-Wave Depression	• No management required.
Atrial or Ventricular Dysrhythmia	• May require discontinuation of lithium and management with antipsychotic agents.
Leukocytosis	• No treatment needed.
Maculopapular Rash	• 50:50 zinc ointment with 0.5 percent menthol if pruritis is present.
Uriticaria	• Antihistamines, topical steroids.
Edema	• If severe, spironolactone 50 mg. may benefit.
Weight Gain	• Diet with normal sodium intake.

will show about a 30% decrease in glomerular filtration rate due to renal aging. This in turn may increase the half-life of lithium to 36-48 hours (vs. 24 hours in younger adults). Thus it is best to start the older person on 300 to 600 mg. of lithium daily and slowly increase the dosage by 150 mg. daily increments. Blood levels should generally remain in the neighborhood of 0.6-0.6 mEq./L. and not be allowed to exceed 1.0 mEq./L. The maximum daily dosage in most elderly patients will be around 900 mg. daily.

Thyroid Gland

There is now clear evidence that lithium can depress thyroid function and produce clinical hypothyroidism with or without goiter, or goiter without hypothyroidism. This risk of abnormal thyroid function appears to be much higher in women than in men. This fact is unexplained. The cause for lithium's interference with thyroid function is not clear at this time. It has been speculated that thyroid stimulating hormone (TSH) dependent adenyl cyclase is somehow affected by lithium. Lithium is known to be concentrated within the thyroid gland. This in turn interferes with secretion of iodine, T3 and T4. This produces a lowering of circulating thyroid hormone which in turn stimulates TSH secretion by negative feedback. If a sufficient amount of TSH is secreted, the gland is stimulated to hypertrophy and a diffuse, non-tender enlargement of the gland develops. If preexisting thyroid damage or disease is present (e.g., thyroiditis), the effects are less likely to be transient and clinical hypothyroidism is more likely (Berens and Wolff, 1975)

Most patients treated with lithium will remain euthyroid or slightly hypothyroid even if a goiter develops. However, recent studies indicate that the prevalence of hypothyroidism can be as high as 20% in women (Lindstedt et al., 1977) and the incidence in both men and women is roughly 3% (Berens and Wolff, 1975).

It is very important that the clinician observe patients on lithium carefully as signs of hypothyroidism can be easily confused with signs of depression and thereby overlooked. The essentials of diagnosis of lithium-induced hypothyroidism include weakness, fatigue, cold intolerance, constipation, menorrhagia, and hoarseness. This may be accompanied by dry skin, coarse hair, puffy skin, and bradycardia. Serum thyroxine (T4) will be below normal and serum TSH will be elevated. Anemia (often macrocytic) may be present. These signs of lithium-induced hypothyroidism are no different than those seen with primary thyroid deficiency.

Discontinuation of lithium will reverse the clinical state of hypothyroidism. However, this is unnecessary as both goiter and hypothyroid signs will respond to thyroxine. It is recommended that hypothyroid patients be started on 0.05 mg. of l-thyroxine daily and gradually raised to 0.2 mg. or the dose necessary to maintain serum T4 within the normal range. With this addition of supplemental thyroxine (T4), hypothyroid patients may be safely continued on lithium therapy. There have been no cases recorded thus far in which thyroid dysfunction secondary to lithium treatment was permanent or related to thyroid malignancy.

Cardiovascular Effects

The major effects of lithium relating to the cardiovascular system have generally been reported as EKG changes. Depression of T-waves is the most common finding (Demers and Heninger, 1971). In summary, EKG changes are almost always mild, are similar in appearance to hyperkalemia (QRS widening and T-wave depression), are not noticeably dose-related, and the frequency of occurrence varies according to the number of leads monitored on the EKG (Vacaflor, 1975).

As experience with lithium increases, isolated reports of dysrhythmia are emerging. Symptomatic sinus node abnormalities may be seen with dizziness, lightheadedness and syncope. Atrial activity is usually very irregular but the normal rhythm cannot always be classified as a specific type of sinoatrial block. Carotid sinus massage and Valsalva maneuvers will not affect the dysrhythmia. Discontinuation of lithium returns sinus rhythm to normal and the administration of a test dose of 1 mg. atropine intravenously results in an increase in sinus rate with regularization of rhythm. It appears that intrinsic cardiac disease may increase the likelihood of this disorder. **Physicians are advised to evaluate a patient's EKG status carefully during lithium administration and not ascribe complaints of dizziness or lightheadedness to psychopathology** (Wellens et al., 1975; Wilson et al., 1976).

Ventricular irritability also seems possible (Tangedahl and Gau, 1972) and first degree atrioventricular block has been reported (Jaffe, 1977). Myocarditis with or without heart failure has also been seen during lithium therapy (Tseng, 1971; Swedberg and Winblad, 1974).

The management of these disorders is not simple, since cardiovascular drugs have not been shown to be of benefit. In most cases it has been necessary to discontinue lithium to reverse the dysrhythmia. In cases of myocardial dysfunction the physician may be forced to manage mania symptomatically with antipsychotic medications rather than lithium over the long-term, as the use of lithium in the face of symptomatic dysrhythmia or myocarditis is unwise.

Hematopoietic Effects

Lithium has been shown to increase the white blood cell count (leukocytosis) in patients receiving lithium therapy (O'Connell, 1970). This leukocytosis is relatively common and may occur in the majority of patients receiving lithium carbonate. The actual white blood cell count varies from 10,000/mm^3 to 14,000 mm^3 but has been reported as high as 20,000 mm^3. The majority increase in white blood cells is neutrophilic and is reversible and not related either to dose or serum concentration of lithium (Vacaflor,

1975). Apparently lithium has the ability to induce granulocyte production and recently it was shown that patients with neutropenia secondary to cancer chemotherapy will show an increase in leukocytes if given lithium carbonate during their chemotherapy (Stein et al., 1977). Clinically, the physician must remain aware that leukocytosis can be a normal finding with lithium therapy. On the one hand, leukocytosis is not a cause for concern during lithium treatment; however, it could confuse the clinical picture in patients with medical or surgical illness that produce leukocytosis.

Cutaneous Effects

Skin lesions do occur with lithium therapy but are relatively uncommon. Most cutaneous side effects are maculopapular in character. Various conditions such as acne, alopecia areata and exacerbation of psoriasis have been described. Most skin reactions will occur in the first 3 to 4 weeks of treatment. These effects do not seem to be dose-related and are shown to be reversible if lithium is discontinued (Vacaflor, 1975).

The erythematous, maculopapular lesions may be treated with 50:50 zinc ointment, with 0.5% menthol added if pruritis is a problem. Topical steroids have been found helpful and antihistamines are useful if an urticarial component is present. Accompanying local infections generally respond to neosporin-polymyxin-bacitracin topical antibiotic preparations. Should the skin condition persist or worsen following the above suggestions, dermatologic consultation is advised.

Edema

The frequency of edema during lithium therapy has not been established. In most cases the edema is pretibial but is also seen in the ankles and face. It is usually transitory and generally does not require active treatment. However, some cases have been severe enough to require discontinuation of lithium. The reinitiation of lithium in those patients who developed edema does not necessarily lead to edema again.

The development of edema does not seem related to either dose or serum level of lithium (Vacaflor, 1975). In very severe cases of pretibial edema, spironolactone may be useful. Spironolactone is a competitive antagonist of aldosterone, a potent mineral-corticoid which increases renal tubular reabsorption of sodium and chloride and facilitates the excretion of potassium. There are no long-term follow-up studies on the use of spironolactone in lithium induced-induced pretibial edema.

Excessive Weight Gain

The gaining of excessive weight during lithium maintenance therapy seems to be a common problem. The magnitude of this problem is not well documented. However, a recent report shows that of 70 patients maintained on lithium therapy for 2 to 10 years, 45 patients gained an average of about 22 pounds (10 Kg.). Their weight after lithium treatment was about 20% higher than their ideal body weight. An important finding was that all patients who gained weight during lithium treatment were overweight before lithium therapy was started (Vendsborg et al., 1973).

Some authors have speculated that increased weight gain during lithium treatment is related to changes in glucose utilization. In fact, glucose tolerance does dramatically increase in the first few days of lithium treatment (Vendsborg and Rafaelsen, 1973). However, this seems to be a transient and expected finding. A 12-month controlled study upon normal volunteers failed to show that lithium significantly changed glucose tolerance or serum lipids (Vendsborg and Prytz, 1976). In the light of present studies, increased glucose tolerance does not seem to be likely as an explanation for weight gain in lithium therapy.

Management of patients who gain weight on lithium maintenance can be especially troublesome to the physician as patients vehemently complain about this distressing side effect. Research data indicates patients on lithium maintenance experiencing excessive weight gain can safely diet as long as normal sodium intake (100 mEq./day) is maintained. **The physician should emphasize that weight loss can and will occur if calories are restricted and sodium intake is normal** (Dempsey et al., 1976).

The Interaction of Lithium with Other Drugs

As with any pharmacologic agent, the possibility of drug-drug interactions must be kept in mind when 2 or more drugs are taken concurrently. Lithium is no exception and there are several established interactions of lithium with other medicinal agents (Hansten, 1975). These agents with potential for adverse interaction can be grouped as diuretics, antipsychotic agents, aminophylline-like agents, amphetamines, various potassium and sodium salts, urea and neuromuscular blockers. Table 40 describes these potential interactions. The potential interactions with neuromuscular blockers have been previously discussed. Tricyclic antidepressants are included as some data suggests that lithium may enhance their antidepressant effects.

TABLE 40
Drugs with the Potential for Interactions with Lithium

Drug	Possible Interaction
A. Diuretics	
1. Acetazolamide (Diamox)	● May impair proximal tubular reabsorption of lithium ions and increase lithium excretion.
2. Ethacrynic Acid (Edecrin)	● Enhances sodium excretion which may in turn cause lithium retention and produce toxicity.
3. Furosemide (Lasix)	● Same as for ethacrynic acid. However, it seems to cause less lithium retention than thiazides.
4. Thiazide Diuretics	● Same as for ethacrynic acid.
B. Antipsychotics	
1. Phenothiazines	● Could potentially enhance the hyperglycemic effect of lithium. In contrast to haloperidol, phenothiazines increase cellular uptake of lithium and may increase the likelihood of toxicity.
2. Haloperidol	● Has been reported to enhance irreversible brain damage following lithium toxicity. Has not been reported in patients whose serum lithium levels are within the therapeutic range. Has the same potential for additive hyperglycemia as the phenothiazines.
C. Aminophylline Agents	● Appears to increase the renal excretion of lithium.
D. Amphetamines	● Apparently can suppress amphetamine highs. Also reported to block amphetamine induced anorexia.
E. Salts	
1. Potassium Iodide	● Reported to act synergistically with lithium in inducing hypothyroidism.
2. Sodium Bicarbonate	● Increased sodium probably increases lithium excretion.
3. Sodium Chloride	● Same as for sodium bicarbonate.
F. Urea	● Appears to increase the renal excretion of lithium.
G. Neuromuscular Blockers	
1. Succinylcholine (Depolarizing)	● Prolongs neuromuscular blockade.
2. Pancurronium Bromide (Non-depolarizing)	● Same as for succinylcholine.
H. Tricyclic Antidepressants	● May enhance antidepressant effect.

Lithium Effects Upon Clinical Laboratory Tests

Lithium has been noted to alter the results of clinical laboratory tests on both serum and urine (Hansten, 1975). The ability to induce leukocytosis and spuriously elevate white blood cell counts has been previously discussed. Table 41 describes the laboratory test alterations that have been reported following the use of lithium.

9. LITHIUM INTOXICATION

The most important method of detecting lithium toxicity is observation for clinical signs. Laboratory assessment of serum lithium values should only be considered as confirmatory. In general, toxicity of clinical importance is not seen until serum values reach 1.5 mEq./L. However, very severe intoxication has been reported in elderly patients at blood levels of 1.6 to 2.2 mEq./Liter (Van der Velde, 1971) and less serious toxicity even at normal therapeutic levels (0.8-1.2 mEq./L.), particularly in the presence of phenothiazines. Severe toxicity in all age groups can be expected at serum lithium levels greater than 2.0 mEq./Liter and levels about 5 mEq./Liter can be fatal (Schou, 1969).

The earliest and most revealing signs of toxicity to lithium salts are nausea and vomiting, diarrhea, a fine resting tremor of the hands, muscular weakness, diuresis, polydipsia, and slight ataxia. The most important organ systems involved are the central nervous system, neuromuscular system, cardiovascular system, gastrointestinal system, and renal system. Table 42 outlines the most common signs of toxicity referable to each system.

TABLE 41
Effects of Lithium Upon Clinical Laboratory Tests

A. Serum	
1. Serum Cortisol	● May slightly depress morning serum cortisol levels.
2. Serum Glucose	● May cause elevation in early phases of therapy.
3. Serum Magnesium	● Has been shown to increase serum levels.
4. Serum Potassium	● Serum potassium may decrease in depressed patients.
5. Serum Thyroxine	● May be reduced.
6. Serum Uric Acid	● May have a decrease due to possible lithium uricosuric effect in manic patients.
B. Urine	
1. Urine Glucose	● Urine glucose may be elevated.
2. Urine Protein	● Proteinuria may be produced or exacerbated.
3. Urinary VMA (Vanillyl-mandelic Acid)	● May increase VMA excretion but probably not enough to interfere with differential diagnosis of hypertension.

TABLE 42
Common Early Signs of Lithium Toxicity in Specific Organ Systems

Central Nervous System	Fine tremor of the hands
	Headaches
	Ataxia
	Dizziness
	Impaired coordination
	Tinnitus
	Somnolence
	Blurred vision
	Organic brain syndrome
Neuromuscular System	Muscular weakness
	Trembling
	Fasciculations
	Hyperactive tendon reflexes
	Parkinson-like symptoms
	Dysphagia
Cardiovascular System	Dysrhythmia
Gastrointestinal System	Nausea
	Vomiting
	Anorexia
Renal System	Polyuria
	Polydipsia
	Proteinuria

It is important that lithium toxicity be diagnosed as soon as possible. Toxicity is often insidious in its development and the early signs are often so undramatic that they are often overlooked by patients, treatment staff or physicians. The early signs noted above may gradually progress to coma. Intoxication of a severe nature will progress to coarse tremor, muscular twitchings, hypotonia of muscles, asymmetric deep tendon reflexes, seizures, hyperextension of the arms and legs and grayish hue of the skin (Schou et al., 1968b). EEG changes show high voltage slow waves, decreased alpha activity with increased delta and theta waves, and an increased likelihood of focal abnormalities in individuals who have previously demonstrated baseline focal EEG disorders (Shopsin et al., 1970).

The treatment of severe lithium toxicity rests upon general medical supportive care of vital functions, discontinuation of lithium salts, and removal of lithium through the kidneys or by either peritoneal or hemodialysis. Standard treatment for shock, coma, respiratory difficulty and fluid or electrolyte imbalance should be rapidly instituted. As soon as lithium intoxication is suspected, lithium administration should be discontinued.

This in itself will be sufficient to avoid severe intoxication in most instances. In general, most cases of moderate lithium toxicity (2.0-4.0 mEq./Liter) can be treated by increasing the renal clearance of lithium. For most individuals, renal lithium clearance is about 20% of the glomerular filtration rate or 15-30 ml/min (Thomsen and Schou, 1968). **It should be remembered that lithium clearance is lowered by four major possibilities: (1) high serum lithium concentration, (2) low sodium intake, (3) administration of sodium depleting diuretics, and (4) preexisting glomerular disease.** To raise the renal clearance of lithium it is necessary to correct the negative sodium balance for the first 3 conditions. In preexisting glomerular disease, it may be necessary to use dialysis as lithium clearance will normalize only if the glomerular filtration rate becomes normal. Therefore, it is recommended that saline infusion be started on all lithium poisonings (Table 43).

Dialysis should be used in those patients whose serum lithium is greater than 4.0 mEq./Liter. Where serum lithium is between 2.0 and 4.0 mEq./Liter, a plot of serum lithiums at 3-hour intervals should be kept on semilogarithmic paper (Thomsen and Schou, 1975). If the plot of serum lithium values intersects the horizontal line later than 36 hours at any time during forced diureses, institute dialysis (Figure 6). Dialysis is independent of renal function in its effect upon serum lithium and supplements the renal elimination of lithium ion.

Peritoneal dialysis seems capable of clearing 15 ml/min. of lithium (Wilson et al., 1976) and hemodialysis can obtain a lithium clearance of as high as 50 ml/min. (Amdisen and Skjoldborg, 1969). When dialysis is discontinued, lithium will pass from tissues into the blood with a subsequent rise in serum lithium values. Lithium is extensively tissue bound. Only the plasma fraction of lithium is available for removal by dialysis. If dialysis is discontinued too early because the patient's serum values are normal, a rebound effect may

TABLE 43
Suggested Treatment Regimen for a Patient with Lithium Intoxication

(1) Evaluate general physical and neurological status.
(2) Determine serum lithium.
(3) If clinical status warrants or serum values of lithium are quite high, transfer patient to an intensive care service.
(4) Start saline infusion as negative sodium balance and lowered lithium clearance often cannot be recognized in advance.
(5) Monitor central venous pressure, serum electrolytes, fluid input and output, and urinary sodium excretion continuously.
(6) If serum lithium is greater than 4.0 mEq./Liter, begin peritoneal or hemodialysis.
(7) If serum lithium is between 2.0 and 4.0 mEq./L., follow the serum lithium every 3 hours and plot on semilogarithmic paper as demonstrated in Figure 6.

occur and cause the serum lithium to return to the toxic range within hours. Long and frequent dialysis may be necessary. Thus, some authorities prefer peritoneal dialysis, despite its lower lithium clearance, because of its ease at round the clock duration. Therefore, dialysis may have to be repeated depending upon the patient's clinical state and serum levels should be followed by continued semilogarithmic plotting of serum lithium values (Figure 6).

After the first 6 hours, draw a line which passes through the plotted serum lithium value for 3 hours and 6 hours, respectively, until it intersects with the hours after the first serum lithium line corresponding with 0.6 mEq./Liter, Figure 6. If the line intersects before 36 hours, continue supportive care (airway control, positional changes, x-ray surveillance of the lungs, etc.). Continue to determine serum lithium every 3 hours. Plot new values on the semilogarithmic graph. Draw a line through each successive 3-hour plot, continuing it to intersect with the horizontal line. If at any time the intersection occurs later than 36 hours, begin dialysis.

Acute overdosage with lithium salts is managed in a similar manner as for slowly developing lithium toxicity; however, it should be remembered that clinical signs of toxicity appear about 48 hours after the acute drug ingestion. As with any acute drug overdose, airway and cardiovascular support should be given if needed. Conscious patients can be induced to vomit and gastric lavage should be performed with physiologic saline or tap water. Oral potassium chloride is *not* effective in reducing serum lithium levels, and aminophylline, urea, acetazolamide or sodium bicarbonate are not con-

FIGURE 6

DETERMINING NEED FOR
RENAL DIALYSIS IN LITHIUM POISONING

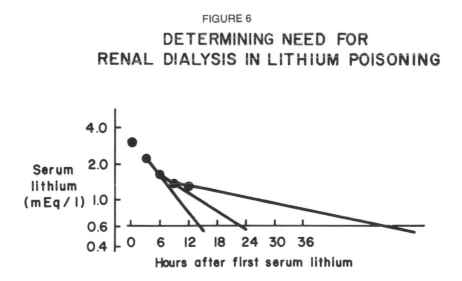

sidered superior to sodium chloride diureses. The use of sodium chloride diuresis is recommended for patients with reversible lithium toxicity and dialysis preferable for other patients requiring active treatment (Thomsen and Schou, 1975).

This concludes the use of antipsychotic agents and lithium ion. Roughly 25 years have lapsed since the modern chemical treatment of psychosis began. As we have seen, these drugs have not brought utopia to the mentally disabled. Yet, their thoughtful use has moved us dramatically from Bedlam and for many has at least loosened the bonds of psychotic illness. Much remains to be done. Even as this book is printed, increased knowledge of antipsychotic pharmacokinetics, plasma drug levels and the epidemiology of tardive dyskinesia is developing. Potential hazards of lithium use may modify therapeutic approaches with this agent. However, knowledge is power to change and hopefully exciting approaches to the treatment of psychosis will appear in future editions of this text.

References

Abrams, R.: Drugs in combination with ECT. In: Greenblatt, M. (Ed.) *Drugs in Combination With Other Therapies*. New York: Grune & Stratton, Inc., 1975.

Abuzzahab, F.S.: Considerations in antipsychotic chemotherapy: The role of drugs in crisis intervention. *An Interview, No. 3, McNeil Laboratories, Inc.* 1976.

Adamson, L., Curry, S.H., Bridges, P.K., Firestone, A.F., Lavin, N.I., Lewis, D.M., Watson, R.D., Xavier, C.M., and Anderson, J.A.: Fluphenazine decanoate trial in chronic inpatient schizophrenia failing to absorb oral chlorpromazine. *Dis. Nerv. Syst.* 34: 181-191, 1973.

Ajouni, K., Kern, M.W., Tures, J.F., Thiel, G.B., and Hagan, T.C.: Thiothixene-induced hyponatremia. *Arch. Intern. Med.* 134: 1103-1105, 1974.

Alfidi, R.J.: Controversy, alternatives and decisions in complying with the legal doctrine of informed consent. *Radiology* 114: 231-241, 1975.

Alexander, C.S. and Nino, A.: Cardiovascular complications in young patients taking psychotropic drugs. *Am. Heart J.* 78: 757-769, 1969.

Alexander, L.: *Treatment of Mental Disorders*. Philadelphia: W.B. Saunders Co., 1953.

Altman, H., Evenson, R.C., Sletter, I.W., and Cho, D.W.: Patterns of psychotropic drug prescription in four midwestern state hospitals. *Curr. Ther. Res.* 14: 667-672, 1972.

Amdisen, A. and Skjoldborg, H.: Haemodialysis for lithium poisoning. *Lancet* 2: 213, 1969.

287

Amdur, M.A.: Acute psychosis. *J.A.M.A.* 230: 1634, 1974.
Amdur, M.A.: Confirming a side effect. *Am. J. Psychiatry* 133: 864, 1976.
Amdur, M.A.: Frequent questions about long-acting injectable fluphenazines. *Illinois Medical Journal* 7: 193-196, 1978.
Anderson, W.H. and Kuehnle, J.C.: Strategies for the treatment of acute schizophrenics. *J.A.M.A.* 229: 1884-1889, 1974.
Anderson, W.: Ambulatory treatment of acute psychosis. *Panel Discussion at Annual Meeting of American Psychiatric Association*, Miami Beach, Fla. May 10-14, 1976.
Anderson, W.H. and Kuehnle, J.C.: Dosage of antipsychotic drugs. *New Engl. J. Med.* 294: 670, 1976.
Anderson, W.H., Kuehnle, J.C., and Catanzano, D.M.: Rapid treatment of acute psychosis. *Amer. J. Psychiatry* 133: 1076-1078, 1976.
Angst, J., Weis, P., Grof, P., Baastrup, P.C., and Schou, M.: Lithium prophylaxis in recurrent affective disorders. *Br. J. Psychiatry* 116: 604-614, 1970.
Appleton, W.S.: The snow phenomenon: tranquilizing the assaultive. *Psychiatry* 28: 88-93, 1965.
Asnis, G.M., Leopold, M.A., Duvoisin, R.C., and Schwartz, H.A.: A survey of tardive dyskinesia in psychiatric outpatients. *Am. J. Psychiatry* 134: 1367-1370, 1977.
Asnis, G.M.: Asnis replies. *Am. J. Psychiatry* 135: 1248-1249, 1978.
Astrachan, B.M., and Detre, T.P.: Post hospital treatment of the psychotic patient. *Compr. Psychiat.* 9: 71-80, 1968.
Ayd, F.J.: A survey of drug induced extrapyramidal reactions. *J.A.M.A.* 175: 1054-1060, 1961.
Ayd, F.J., Jr.: Drug Holidays—Intermittent pharmacotherapy for psychiatric patients. *Int. Drug Ther. Newsletter* 1: 26-28, 1966.
Ayd, F.J., Jr.: Prevention of recurrence (Maintenance Therapy). In: DiMascio, A., and Shader, R.I. (Eds.) *Clinical Handbook of Psychopharmacology.* New York: Jason Aronson, 1970.
Ayd, F.J., Jr.: Neuroleptic therapy for chronic schizophrenia. *Int. Drug Ther. Newsletter* 6: 12-13, 1971.
Ayd, F.J., Jr.: Once-a-day neuroleptic and tricyclic antidepressant therapy. *Int. Drug Ther. Newsletter* 7: 33-49, 1972a.
Ayd, F.J., Jr.: Haloperidol: Fifteen years of clinical experience. *Dis. Nerv. Syst.* 33: 459-469, 1972.
Ayd, F.J. Jr.: Rational pharmacotherapy: Once-a-day drug dosage. *Dis. Nerv. Syst.* 34: 371-378, 1973a.
Ayd, F.J.: Excretion of Psychotropic drugs in human breast milk. *Int. Drug Therapy Newsletter* 8: 33-35, 1973b.
Ayd, F.J., Jr.: Rules for neuroleptic therapy. *Int. Drug Ther. Newsletter* 9: 33-36, 1974a.
Ayd, F.J., Jr.: Do antiparkinson drugs interfere with the therapeutic effects of neuroleptics: *Int. Drug Ther. Newsletter* 9: 29-30, 1974b.
Ayd, F.J., Jr.: Treatment-resistant patients: A moral, legal and therapeutic challenge. In: Ayd, F.J., Jr. (Ed.) *Rational Pharmacotherapy and the Right to Treatment.* Baltimore: Ayd Medical Communications, Ltd., 1975a.
Ayd, F.J., Jr.: The depot fluphenazines: A reappraisal after 10 years clinical experience. *Am. J. Psychiatry* 132: 491-499, 1975b.
Ayd, F.J., Jr.: The bioequivalency and clinical efficacy of generic and proprietary chlorpromazine. *Int. Drug Ther. Newsletter* 10: 1-2, 1975c.
Ayd, F.J., Jr.: The long-acting injectable fluphenazine: titrating for optimal effect. Informational pamphlet distributed by Squibb & Sons, E.R., 1976a.
Ayd, F.J., Jr.: Phenothiazine prophylaxis of schizophrenic relapse. *Int. Drug Ther. Newsletter* 11: 37-40, 1976b.
Ayd, F.J., Jr.: Haloperidol update: 1975, *Proc. Royal Soc. Med.*, 69: Supplement 1, 1976c.
Ayd, F.J.: Psychotropic drug therapy during pregnancy. *Int. Drug Therapy Newsletter* 11: 5-11, 1976d.
Ayd, F.J., Jr.: Guidelines for using short-acting intramuscular neuroleptics for rapid neuroleptization. *Int. Drug Ther. Newsletter* 12: 5-12, 1977a.
Ayd, F.J., Jr.: Ethical and legal dilemmas posed by tardive dyskinesia. *Int. Drug Ther. Newsletter* 12: 29-34, 1977b.

Ayd, F.J.: Chronic renal lesions: A hazard of long term lithium treatment. *Int. Drug Ther. Newsletter* 12: 37-40, 1977c.

Ayd, F.J.: Amantadine therapy for neuroleptic-induced extrapyramidal reactions. *Int. Drug Ther. Newsletter* 12: 22-24, 1977d.

Ayd, F.J., Jr.: The depot fluphenazines: twelve years' experience—an overview. In: Ayd, F.J., Jr. (Ed.), *Depot Fluphenazines: Twelve Years of Experience*, Baltimore: Ayd Medical Communications, 1978a.

Ayd, F.J., Jr.: A drug-free month for outpatient schizophrenics. *Int. Drug Ther. Newsletter* 13: 30-31, 1978b.

Ayd, F.J., Jr.: Dependence on antiparkinson drugs. *Int. Drug Ther. Newsletter* 13: 11-12, 1978c.

Bacher, N.M., and Lewis, II.A.: Addiction of reserpine to antipsychotic medication in refractory chronic schizophrenic outpatients. *Am. J. Psychiatry* 135: 488-490, 1978.

Bakke, O.: Clinical experience with depot neuroleptics. *Acta Psychiatr. Scand.* (Suppl.) 246: 32-41, 1973.

Baldessarini, R.J., Gelenberg, A.J., and Lipinski, J.F.: Grams of antipsychotics? *New Eng. J. Med.* 294: 113-114, 1976.

Baldessarini, R.J.: *Chemotherapy in Psychiatry*, Cambridge, Mass.: Harvard University Press, 1977.

Ban, T.: *Psychopharmacology*, Baltimore: Williams and Wilkins Co., 1969.

Ban, T. A.: Pharmacotherapy of schizophrenia: Facts, speculations, hypotheses, and theories. *Psychosomatics* 15: 178-187, 1974.

Ban, T.A.: *Psychopharmacology of Thiothixene*, New York: Raven Press, 1978.

Banta, R.C., and Markesbury, W.R.: Elevated manganese levels associated with dementia and extrapyramidal signs. *Neurology* (Minn.) 27: 213-216, 1977.

Barratt, E.S., Russell, G., Creson, D., and Tupin, J.: Neurophysiological and behavioral correlates of lithium. *Dis. Nerv. Syst.* 31: 335-337, 1970.

Bartholomew, A.A.: A long acting phenothiazine as a possible agent to control deviant sexual behavior. *Am. J. Psychiatry* 124: 917-923, 1968.

Berens, S.C., and Wolff, J.: The endocrine effects of lithium. In: F.N. Johnson (Ed.) *Lithium Research and Therapy*, New York: Academic Press, pp. 425-472, 1975.

Blacker, K.H., Weinstein, B.J., and Ellman, G.L.: Mother's milk and chlorpromazine. *Am. J. Psychiatry* 119: 178-179, 1962.

Blackwell, B.: Drug deviation in psychiatric patients. In: F.J. Ayd, Jr. (Ed.) *The Future of Pharmacotherapy, New Drug Delivery Systems*. Baltimore, International Drug Therapy Newsletter, 1973.

Blackwell, B.: Rational drug use in psychiatry. In: Ayd, F.J., Jr. (Ed.) *Rational Psychopharmacotherapy and the Right to Treatment*, Baltimore: Ayd Medical Communications, Ltd., 1975.

Bloch, H.S.: Brief sleep treatment with chlorpromazine. *Compr. Psychiat* 11: 346-355, 1970.

Branchey, M.H., Charles, J., and Simpson, G.M.: Extrapyramidal side effects in lithium maintenance therapy. *Am. J. Psychiatry* 133: 444-445, 1976.

Branchey, M.H., Lee, J.H., Amin, R., and Simpson, G.M.: High- and low-potency neuroleptics in elderly psychiatric patients. *J.A.M.A.* 239: 1860-1862, 1978.

Brauzer, B., and Goldstein, B.J.: Comparative effects of intramuscular thiothixene and trifluoperazine in psychotic patients. *J. Clin. Pharmacol.* 8: 400-403, 1968.

Brauzer, B., and Goldstein, B.J.: The differential response to parenteral chlorpromazine and mesoridazine in psychotic patients. *J. Clin. Pharmacol.* 10: 126-131, 1970.

Brazelton, T.B.: Effects of prenatal drugs on the behavior of the neonate. *Am. J. Psychiatry* 126: 1261-1266, 1970.

Brophy, J.J.: Single daily doses of neuroleptic drugs. *Dis. Nerv. Syst.* 39: 120-123, 1969.

Brown, W.T.: Side effects of lithium therapy and their treatment. *Can. Psychiat. Assoc. J.* 21: 13-21, 1976.

Browning, D.H., Ferry, P.C.: Tardive dyskinesia in a ten-year-old boy. *Clin. Ped.* 15: 955-957, 1976.

Bruun, R.D., Shapiro, A.K., Shapiro, E., Sweet, R., Wayne, H., and Solomon, G.E.: A follow-up of 78 patients with Gilles de la Tourette's Syndrome. *Am. J. Psychiatry* 133: 944-

947, 1976.

Burger, A.: History. In: Usdin, E. and Forrest, I.S. (Eds.) *Psychotherapeutic Drugs Part I*, *Principles*, New York: Marcel Dekker, Inc., 1976.

Burgoyne, R.W.: Effect of drug ritual changes. *Am. J. Psychiatry* 133: 284-289, 1976.

Burke, J.C., High, J.P., Laffan, R.J., and Ravaris, C.L.: Depot action of fluphenazine (Prolixin) enanthate in oil. *Fed. Proc.* 21: 339, 1962.

Bursten, B.: Using mechanical restraints on acutely disturbed psychiatric patients. *Hosp. and Community Psychiatry* 26: 757-759, 1975.

Byck, R.: Drugs and treatment of psychiatric disorders. In: Goodman, L.S., and Gilman, A. (Eds.) *The Pharmacological Basis of Therapeutics.* New York: Macmillan, 1975.

Cade, J.F.J.: The story of lithium. In: Ayd, F.J., Jr. (Ed.) *Discoveries in Biological Psychiatry.* Philadelphia: Blackwell, 1970.

Cade, J.F.J.: Phenothiazines in delirium tremens: Pro and Contra, *Am. J. Psychiatry* 131: 931, 1974.

Cade, J.F.J.: Lithium—when, why and how, *Med. J. Aust.* 1: 684-686, 1975.

Caffey, E.M., Forrest, I.S., Frank, T.V., and Klett, C.J.: Phenothiazine excretion in chronic schizophrenics, *Am. J. Psychiatry* 120: 578-582, 1963.

Caffey, E.M., Diamond, L.S., Frank, T.V., Klett, C.J., Rothstein, C., Grasberger, J.C., Herman, L.: Discontinuation or reduction of chemotherapy in chronic schizophrenics. *J. Chron. Dis.* 17: 347-358, 1964.

Caldwell, A.E.: History of psychopharmacology. In: Clark, W.G., and del Guidice, J. (Eds.) *Principles of Psychopharmacology*, New York: Academic Press, 1978, pp. 9-40.

Caldwell, J.: Toxic effects of psychotherapeutic agents. In: Usdin, E., and Forrest, I.S. (Eds.) *Psychotherapeutic Drugs, Part I, Principles*, New York: Marcel Dekker, Inc., pp. 437-481, 1976.

Callahan, E.J., Alevizos, P.N., Teigne, J.R., Newman, H., and Campbell, H.A.: Behavioral effects of reducing the daily frequency of phenothiazine administration. *Arch. Gen. Psychiat.* 32: 1285-1290, 1975.

Carlsson, A.: Antipsychotic drugs, neurotransmitters and schizophrenia, *Am. J. Psychiatry*, 135: 164-173, 1978.

Carlsson, C., Dencker, S.J., Grimby, G., Haggendal, J., and Johnson, G.: Hemodynamic effects of thiothixene and chlorpromazine in schizophrenic patients at rest and during exercise. *Int. J. Clin. Pharmacol.* 13: 262-268, 1976.

Carpenter, W.T., Jr.: A drug-free month for outpatient schizophrenics, *Schizophrenia Bulletin* 4: 148-149, 1978.

Carter, R.G.: Psychotolysis with haloperidol, rapid control of the acutely disturbed psychotic patient. *Dis. Nerv. Syst.* 38: 13-16, 1977.

Casey, D.E.: Managing tardive dyskinesia. *J. Clin. Psychiatry* 39: 748-753, 1978.

Casey, J.F., Hollister, L.E., Klett, C.J., Lasky, J.J., and Caffey, E.M.: Combined drug therapy of chronic schizophrenics. Controlled evaluation of placebo, dextroamphetamine, imipramine, isocarboxazid and trifluoperazine added to maintenance doses of chlorpromazine. *Am. J. Psychiatry* 117: 997-1003, 1961.

Cassem, N.H., and Sos, J.: Intravenous use of haloperidol for acute delirium in intensive care settings. Presented at the annual meeting of the American Psychiatric Association, Atlanta, May, 1978.

Catz, C.S., and Giacoia, G.P.: Drugs and breast milk. *Ped. Clin. N. Amer.* 19: 151-166, 1972.

Cavenar, J.O., Jr., and Maltbie, A.A.: Another indication for haloperidol. *Psychosomatics*, 17: 128-130, 1976.

Cerletti, A. and Meier-Ruge, W.: Toxicological studies on phenothiazine-induced retinopathy. *Proc. Eur. Soc. Study Drug Tox.* 12: 170-187, 1971.

Chapel, J.L.: Emergency room treatment of the drug-abusing patient. *Amer. J. Psychiatry* 130: 257-259, 1973.

Chien, C.P. and Cole, J.O.: Depot phenothiazine treatment in acute psychosis: a sequential comparative clinical study. *Amer. J. Psychiatry* 130: 13-17, 1973.

Chouinard, G., Annable, L., Serro, M., Albert, J.M., and Charette, R.: Amitriptyline-perphenazine interaction in ambulatory schizophrenic patients. *Arch. Gen. Psychiatry* 32: 1295-1307, 1975.

Claghorn, J.L., Johnstone, E.E., Cook, T.H.: Group therapy and maintenance treatment of schizophrenia. *Arch. Gen. Psychiatry* 31: 361-365, 1974.

Cohen, S.: The major tranquilizers. *Drug Abuse and Alcohol Newsletter* 4: Nov. 1975.

Cole, J.O.: Introduction: Symposia on long-acting phenothiazines in psychiatry. *Dis. Nerv. Syst.* (Suppl.) 31: 5, 1970.

Cole, J.O.: *Pharmacotherapy in the Practice of Medicine*, edited by M.E. Jarvik, New York: Appleton, Century, Crofts, 1977.

Coleman, J.H., and Hayes, P.E.: Drug-induced extrapyramidal effects—a review. *Dis. Nerv. Syst.* 36: 591-593, 1975.

Cooper, T.B., and Simpson, G.M.: The 24-hour lithium level as a prognosticator of dosage requirements: 2-year follow-up study. *Am. J. Psychiatry* 133: 440-443, 1976.

Corbett, L.: Techniques of fluphenazine decanoate therapy in acute schizophrenic illnesses. *Dis. Nerv. Syst.* 36: 573-575, 1975.

Crane, G.E.: Persistent dyskinesia. *Br. J. Psychiatry* 122: 395-405, 1973.

Cressman, W.A., Plostnieks, J., and Johnson, P.C.: Absorption, metabolism and excretion of droperidol by human subjects following intramuscular and intravenous administration. *Anesthesiology* 38: 363-369, 1973.

Curran, J.P.: Tardive dyskinesia: side effect or not? *Am. J. Psychiatry* 130: 406-410, 1973.

Cusano, P.P., May, J., and O'Connell, R.A.: The medical economics of lithium treatment for manic depressives. *Hospital and Community Psychiat.* 28: 169-173, 1977.

Davis, J.M., Blatlett, E., and Termini, B.A.: Overdosage of psychotropic drugs: A review. I. Major and minor tranquilizers. *Dis. Nerv. Syst.* 29: 157-164, 1968.

Davis, J.M.: Dose equivalence of the antipsychotic drugs. *J. Psychiat. Res.* 11: 65-69, 1974.

Davis, J.M., and Cole, J.O.: Antipsychotic drugs. In: Freedman, A., Kaplan, W.I., and Sadack, B.J. (Eds.) *Comprehensive Textbook of Psychiatry II*, Baltimore: Williams & Wilkins, 1975.

Davis, J.M.: Maintenance therapy in psychiatry: 1. Schizophrenia. *Am. J. Psychiatry*, 132: 1237-1245, 1975.

Davis, J.M., 1976: According to an informational pamphlet distributed by the manufacturer, Squibb and Sons, E.R., 1976a

Davis, J.M.: Recent developments in the drug treatment of schizophrenia. *Am. J. Psychiatry* 133: 308-314, 1976b.

Davis, K.L., Berger, P.A. and Hollister, L.F. · Choline for tardive dyskinesia. *New Eng. J. Mod.* 293. 152, 1975.

Demers, R.G., and Davis, L.S.: The influence of prophylactic lithium treatment on the marital adjustment of manic-depressives and their spouses. *Comproh. Psychiatry* 12: 348-353, 1971.

Demers, R.G., and Heninger, G.R.: Electrocardiographic T-wave changes during lithium carbonate treatment. *J.A.M.A.* 218: 381-386, 1971.

Dempsey, G.M., Dunner, D., Fieve, R.R., Tibor, F., and Wond, J.: Treatment of excessive weight gain in patients taking lithium. *Am. J. Psychiatry* 133: 1082-1084, 1976.

Denoker, S.J.: High dose treatment with neuroleptics in the acute phase of mental disease. *Proc. Royal Soc. Med.* 69: Supplement I, 1976.

Detre, T.P., and Jarecki, H.G.: *Modern Psychiatric Treatment*. Philadelphia: J.B. Lippincott, 1971.

Diamond, H., Tislow, R., Snyder, T., and Rickels, K.: Peer review of prescribing patterns in a CMHC. *Am. J. Psychiatry* 133: 697-699, 1976.

Diamond, L.S., and Marks, J.B.: Discontinuance of tranquilizers among chronic schizophrenic patients receiving maintenance dosage. *J. Nerv. Ment. Dis.* 131: 247, 1960.

DiMascio, A., and Shader, R.I.: Drug administration schedules. *Amer. J. Psychiatry* 126: 796-801, 1969.

DiMascio, A., and Demirgian, E.: Antiparkinson drug overdose. *Psychosomatics.* 11: 596-601, 1970.

DiMascio, A., and Shader, R.I.: *Clinical Handbook of Psychopharmacology*. New York: Aronson, 1970.

DiMascio, A.: Toward a more rational use of antiparkinson drugs in psychiatry. *Drug Therapy*, 1: 23-20, 1971.

DiMascio, A.: Psychotropic drug overuse: An examination of prescription practices. *Massachusetts J. of Mental Health*, 2: 25-38, 1972.

DiMascio, A.: Innovative drug administration regimens and the economics of mental health care. In: F.J. Ayd, Jr. (Ed.) *Rational Psychopharmacotherapy and the Right to Treatment*. Baltimore: Ayd Medical Communications, Ltd., 1975.

Donlon, P.T. and Rada, R.T.: High dosage piperacetazine in ambulatory schizophrenic patients. *Dis. Nerv. Syst.* 35: 231-236, 1974.

Donlon, P.T. and Tupin, J.P.: Rapid "Digitalization of decompensated schizophrenic patients with antipsychotic drugs. *Amer. J. Psychiatry* 131: 310-312, 1974.

Donlon, P.T.: Upper dose range initial therapy. According to an informational pamphlet distributed by E.R. Squibb & Son, 1975.

Donlon, P.T., Axelkok, A.D., Tupin, J.P., and Chien, Ching-Piao: Comparison of depot phenothiazines: duration of action and incidence of side effects. *Comp. Psychiatry*, 17: 369-376, 1976.

Dorus, E., Pandey, G.N., and Davis, J.M.: Genetic determinants of lithium ion distribution: In vitro and in vivo monozygotic-dizygotic twin study. *Arch. Gen. Psychiatry* 32: 1097-1102, 1975.

Dripps, R.P., Eckenhoff, J.E., and Vandam, L.D.: *Introduction to Anesthesia*, Third Edition, Philadelphia: W.B. Saunders Co., 1968.

Drugs and the fetal eye, *Lancet* 1: 122, 1971.

Duberstein, L.E.: Pharmacologic management of vertigo, a review. *J. of Vertigo* 3: 1-8, 1977.

Ducomb, L., and Baldessarini, R.J.: Timing and risk of bone marrow depression by psychotropic drugs. *Am. J. Psychiatry* 134: 1294-1295, 1977.

Dudley, D.L., and Rowlett, D.: Emergency use of intravenous haloperidol. Presented at the annual meeting of the American Psychiatric Association, Atlanta, May, 1978.

Dunner, D.L., Fleiss, J.L., and Fieve, R.R.: Lithium carbonate prophylaxis failure. *Br. J. Psychiatry* 129: 40-44, 1976.

Eisenberg, L.: Principles of drug therapy in child psychiatry with special reference to stimulant drugs. In: Chess, S., and Thomas, A. (Eds.) *Annual Progress in Child Psychiatry and Child Development*, Vol. 5, New York: Brunner/Mazel, 1972, pp. 612-632.

Everett, H.C.: The use of bethanechol chloride with tricyclic antidepressants. *Am. J. Psychiatry* 132: 1202-1204, 1975.

Fahn, S.: Paper presented at the annual meeting of the American Neurological Association, 1978.

Fann, W.E. and Linton, P.H.: Use of perphenazine in psychiatric emergencies: the concept of chemical restraint. *Curr. Ther. Res.* 14: 478-482, 1972.

Fann, W.E., and Wheless, J.C.: Effects of psychotherapeutic drugs on geriatric patients. In: Usdin, E., and Forrest, T.S. (Eds.) *Psychotherapeutic Drugs, Part I, Principles*. New York: Marcel Dekker, 1976.

Fann, W.E., and Shannon, I.L.: A treatment for dry mouth in psychiatric patients. *Am. J. Psychiatry* 135: 251-252, 1978.

Farazza, A.R. and Martin, P.: Chemotherapy of delirium tremens. A survey of physicians' references. *Am. J. Psychiatry* 131: 1031-1033, 1974.

FDA Drug Bulletin: Tardive dyskinesia associated with antipsychotic drugs. May, 1973.

Feinstein, S.C., and Wolpert, E.A.: Juvenile manic depressive illness. *J. Am. Acad. Child Psychiatry* 12: 123-136, 1973.

Feldman, P., Bay, A.P., Baser, A.N., Bhasker, K.N. and Kennedy, L.L.: Parenteral haloperidol in controlling patient behavior during acute psychotic episodes. *Curr. Ther. Res.* 11: 362-366, 1969.

Feldman, W.S.: Is informed consent possible in psychiatry? *Legal Aspects of Medical Practice* 6: 29-31, 1978.

Fieve, R.R., Kumbaraci, T., and Dunner, D.L.: Lithium prophylaxis of depression in bipolar I, bipolar II, and unipolar patients. *Am. J. Psychiatry* 133: 925-929, 1976.

Fink, E.B., Longbaugh, R., and Stout, R.: The paradoxical under-utilization of partial hospitalization. *Am. J. Psychiatry* 135: 713-715, 1978.

Fitzgerald, C.H.: A double-blind comparison of haloperidol with perphenazine in acute psychotic episodes. *Curr. Ther. Res.* 11: 515-516, 1969.

Forrest, F.M., Forrest, I.S., and Mason, A.S.: A rapid urinary test for chlorpromazine, pro-
mazine and mepazine (Pacatal). *Am. J. Psychiatry* 114: 931, 1958.
Forrest, F.M. and Forrest, I.S.: Urine color test for the detection of phenothiazine compounds.
Clin. Chem. 6: 11-15, 1960.
Forrest, F.M., Forrest, I.S., and Mason, A.S.: Review of rapid urine tests for phenothiazine
and related drugs. *Am. J. Psychiatry* 118: 300-309, 1961.
Forrest, F.M., Getter, C.W., Snow, H.L., and Steinbach, M.: Drug maintenance problems
of rehabilitated patients: the current drug dosage "merry-go-round." *Am. J. Psychiatry*
121: 33-40, 1964.
Forrest, F.M., Forrest, I.S., and Kanter, S.L.: Elimination of false negative results with the
FPN Forrest Test for phenothiazine derivatives in urine, *Clin. Chem.* 12: 379-384, 1966.
Forrest, F.M., and Forrest, I.S.: Piperacetazine in chronic mental patients; clinical observation
and new urine color test. *Curr. Ther. Res.* 14: 689-695, 1972.
Forrest, J.N., Cohen, A.D., Torreth, J., Himmelhoch, J.M., and Epstein, F.H.: On the
mechanism of lithium induced diabetes insipidus in man and rat. *J. Clin. Invest.* 53:
1115-1123, 1974.
Forsman, A.O.: Individual variability in response to haloperidol. *Proc. Royal Soc. Med.* 69:
Supplement I, 1976.
Fowler, R.C., Kronfol, Z.A., and Perry, P.J.: Water intoxication, psychosis and inappropriate
secretion of antidiuretic hormone. *Arch. Gen. Psychiatry* 34: 1097-1099, 1977.
Francis, R.I., and Traill, M.A.: Lithium distribution in the brains of two manic patients. *Lancet*
2: 523-524, 1970
Francis, V., Korsch, B.M., and Morris, M.J.: Gaps in doctor-patient communication. *New
Eng. J. Med.* 280: 535-540, 1969.
Freeman, H.: The therapeutic value of combinations of psychotropic drugs: A review. *Psy-
chopharm. Bull.* 4: 1-27, 1967.
Gardiner, G.: The need for drug monitoring in psychiatric practice. *Brit. J. Psychiat.* 114: 877-
881, 1968.
Gardos, G., and Cole, J.O.: The importance of dosage in antipsychotic drug administration—a
review of dose-response studies. *Psychopharmacologia* 29: 221-230, 1973.
Gardos, G.: Are antipsychotic drugs interchangeable: *Dis. Nerv. Syst.* 159: 343-348, 1974.
Gardos, G., and Cole, J.O.: Maintenance antipsychotic therapy: Is the cure worse than the
disease? *Am. J. Psychiatry* 133: 32-36, 1976.
Gardos, G., and Cole, J.O.: Weight reduction in schizophrenics by molindone. *Am. J. Psy-
chiatry* 134: 302-304, 1977.
Gardos, G., and Cole, J.O.: Public health issues in tardive dyskinesia. Read at the 132d annual
meeting of the American Psychiatric Association, Chicago, Ill., May 16, 1979.
Gardos, G., Cole, J.O. and Sniffen, C.: An evaluation of papaverine in tardive dyskinesia. *J.
Clin. Pharmacol.* 16: 304-310, 1976.
Gary, N.E. and Saidi, D.: Methamphetamine intoxication. *Amer. J. Med* 64:537-540, 1978.
Gelenberg, A.J. and Mandel, M.R.: Catatonic reactions to high potency neuroleptic drugs.
Arch Gen. Psychiatry 34: 947-950, 1977.
Gerlach, J., Reisby, N. and Randrup, A.: Dopaminergic hypersensitivity and cholinergic hy-
pofunction in the pathophysiology of tardive dyskinesia. *Psychopharmacologia* 34: 21-
35, 1974.
Gerlach, J., Thorsen, K., and Munkvad, I.: Effort of lithium on neuroleptic-induced tardive
dyskinesia compared with a placebo in a double-blind cross over trial. *Pharmakopsy-
chiatric* 8: 51-56, 1975.
Gerle, B.: Clinical observation on the side effects of haloperidol, *Acta Psychiat. Scand.* 40: 65-
67, 1964.
Gerstenzank, M.L., and Krulinsky, E.V.: Parenteral haloperidol in psychiatric emergencies:
double-blind comparison with chlorpromazine. *Dis. Nerv. Syst.* 38:581-583, 1977.
Gittelman-Klein, R., Klein, D., Katz, S., Saraf, K., and Pollack, E.: Comparative effects of
methylphenidate and thioridazine in hyperkinetic children. 1. Clinical results. *Arch
Gen. Psychiatry* 33: 1217-1231, 1976.
Goldberg, H.L.: Initiating therapy with prolixin decanoate. According to an informational
pamphlet distributed by E.R. Squibb & Sons, 1976.

Goldberg, H.L., DiMascio, A. and Chaudhary, B.: A clinical evaluation of prolixin enanthate. *Psychosomatics* 11: 173-177, 1976.

Goldberg, S.C., Frosch, W.A., Drossman, A.K., et al.: Prediction of response to phenothiazines in schizophrenia. *Arch. Gen. Psychiatry* 26: 367-373, 1972.

Gombos, G.M. and Yarden, P.E.: Ocular and cutaneous side effects after prolonged chlorpromazine treatment. *Am. J. Psychiatry* 123: 872-874, 1967.

Good, W.W., Sterling, M., and Holtzman, W.H.: Termination of chlorpromazine with schizophrenic patients. *Am. J. Psychiatry* 115: 443-448, 1959.

Goodman, L.S. and Gilman, A.: *The Pharmacologic Basis of Therapeutics*, Macmillan Co., New York, 1975.

Goodson, W.H. and Litkenhous, E.E.: Sudden and unexplained death in a psychiatric patient taking thioridazine. *South Med. J.* 69: 311-320, 1976.

Gordon, H.L., Law, A., Hohmen, K.E. and Groth, C.: The problem of overweight in hospitalized psychotic patients. *Psychiat. Quart.* 34: 69-82, 1960.

Gotbetter, S.: Tardive dyskinesia: a latent legal concern for psychiatrists. *Legal Aspects of Medical Practice* 6: 39-43, 1978.

Gottlieb, J.I., and Lustberg, J.: Phenothiazine-induced priapism. *Am. J. Psychiatry* 134: 1445-1446, 1977.

Gottschalk, L.A., Dinovo, E., Biener, R., Brich, H., Syben, M., and Noble, E.P.: Plasma levels of mesoridazine and its metabolites and clinical response in acute schizophrenia after a single intramuscular drug dose. In: Gottschalk, L.A., and Merlis, S. (Eds.), *Pharmacokinetics of Psychoactive Drugs: Blood Levels and Clinical Response.* New York: Spectrum Publications, Inc., 1976.

Granacher, R.P., Baldessarini, R.J., and Cole, J.O.: The pharmacologic evaluation of tardive dyskinesia. *New Eng. J. Med.* 292: 326, 1975.

Granacher, R.P. and Baldessarini, R.J.: The usefulness of physostigmine in neurology and psychiatry. In: H.L. Klawans (Ed.) *Clinical Neuropsychopharmacology*, Vol. 1, 1976, pp. 63-80.

Granacher, R.P.: Facial dyskinesia after antihistamines. *N. Engl. J. Med.* 296: 516, 1977.

Granacher, R.P.: Neuromuscular problems associated with lithium. *Am. J. Psychiatry* 134: 702, 1977.

Granacher, R.P.: Titrating intramuscular dosages for elderly patients. *Am. J. Psychiatry* 137: 997, 1979.

Granacher, R.P., and Ruth, D.D.: Droperidol and acute agitation. *Curr. Ther. Res.* 25: 361-365, 1979.

Green, M. and Zelson, C.: The effect of psychotherapeutic drugs on the neonate. In: E. Usdin and I.S. Forrest (Eds.) *Psychotherapeutic Drugs*, Part 1, Marcel Dekker, Inc., New York, 1976, pp. 521-544.

Greenblatt, D.J., and Shader, R.I.: Drug interactions in psychopharmacology. In: R.I. Shader (Ed.) *Manual of Psychiatric Therapeutics*, Boston: Little, Brown & Co., 1975.

Greenberg, L.M., and Roth, J.: Different effects of abrupt vs. gradual withdrawal of chlorpromazine in hospitalized chronic schizophrenic patients. *Am. J. Psychiatry* 123: 226, 1966.

Greenhill, L.L., Reider, R.O., Wender, P.H., et al: Lithium carbonate in the treatment of hyperactive children. *Arch Gen. Psychiatry* 28: 636-640, 1973.

Grinspoon, L., and Shader, R.I.: Psychotherapy and drugs in schizophrenia. In: Greenblatt, M. (Ed.) *Drugs In Combination With Other Therapies.* New York: Grune & Stratton, 1975.

Groves, J.E., and Mandel, M.R.: The long-acting phenothiazines. *Arch. Gen. Psychiatry* 32: 893-900, 1975.

Grozier, M.L.: Useful clinical pointers. In: Ayd, F.J., Jr. (Ed.), *The Future of Pharmacotherapy New Drug Delivery Systems.* Baltimore: International Drug Therapy Newsletter, 1973.

Guillan, R.A., Zleman, S., Reinert, R.E.D., and Smalley, R.L.: Sudden death in patients under phenothiazine therapy. *J. Kan. Med. Soc.* 71: 213-218, 1970.

Gusdon, J.P., and Herbst, G.: The effect of promethazine hydrochloride on fetal and maternal lymphocytes. *Am. J. Obs. Gynec.* 126: 730-731, 1976.

Hamid, T.A., and Wertz, W.J.: Mesoridazine vs. chlorpromazine in acute schizophrenics: A double-blind investigation. *Am. J. Psychiatry* 130: 689-692, 1973.

Hamill, W.T., and Fontana, A.F.: The immediate effects of chlorpromazine in newly admitted schizophrenic patients. *Am. J. Psychiatry* 132: 1023-1027, 1975.

Hamilton, L.D.: Aged brain and the phenothiazines. *Geriatrics* 21: 131-138, 1966.

Hansell, N., and Willis, M.A.: Outpatient treatment of schizophrenia. *Am. J. Psychiatry* 134: 1082-1085, 1977.

Hansten, P.B.: *Drug Interactions*. Philadelphia: Lee and Febiger, 1975.

Hare, E.H., and Wilcox, D.C.: Do psychiatric inpatients take their pills? *Brit. J. Psychiat.* 113: 33-40, 1967.

Heinonen, O.O., Sloane, D. and Shapiro, S.: *Birth Defects and Drugs in Pregnancy*. Littleton, Mass.: Publishing Sciences Group, 1977.

Helper, M., Welcott, R., and Garfield, S.: Effects of chlorpromazine on learning and related processes in emotionally disturbed children. *J. Consult Psychology* 27: 1-9, 1963.

Hestbech, H., Hansen, H.E., Amdisen, A., et al.: Chronic renal lesions following long term treatment with lithium. *Kidney Int.* 12: 205-213, 1977.

Hetherington, J.: Symposium: Glaucoma. *Tr. Am. Acad. Ophth.* 78: 239, 1974.

Hill, G.E., Wang, K.C., and Hodges, M.R.: Potentiation of succinylcholine neuromuscular blockade by lithium carbonate. *Anesthesiology* 44: 439-442, 1976.

Hogarty, G.E., Goldberg, S.C. and the Collaborative Study Group, Baltimore: Drugs and sociotherapy in the aftercare of schizophrenic patients. One year relapse rates, *Arch. Gen. Psychiatry* 28: 54-64, 1973.

Hogarty, G.E., Goldberg, S.C., Schoolar, N.R. et al.: Drugs and sociotherapy in the aftercare of schizophrenic patients: adjustment of nonrelapsed patients. *Arch. Gen. Psychiatry* 31: 609-618, 1974.

Hogarty, G.E., Goldberg, S.C., Schooler, N.R.: Drugs and sociotherapy in the aftercare of schizophrenia: A Review. In: Greenblatt, M. (Ed.) *Drugs in Combination With Other Therapies*. New York: Grune & Stratton, Inc., 1975.

Hogarty, G.E., Ulrich, R.F., Mussare, F. and Artistigueta, N.: Drug discontinuation among long-term successfully maintained schizophrenic outpatients. *Dis. Nerv. Syst.* 37: 494-500, 1976.

Hollister, L.E., Jones, K.P., Brownfield, B., and Johnson, F.: Chlorpromazine alone and with reserpine. Use in the treatment of mental diseases. *California Med.* 83: 218-221, 1955.

Hollister, L.E., Overall, J.E., Johnson, M.H., Shelton, J., Kimbell, I., and Brunse, A.: Amitriptyline alone and combined with perphenazine in newly admitted depressed patients. *J. Nerv. Ment. Dis.* 142: 460-160, 1967.

Hollister, L.E.: Choice of antipsychotic drugs. *Amer. J. Psychiatry* 127: 186-190, 1970.

Hollister, L.E.: Optimum use of antipsychotic drugs. In: Masserman, J.H. (Ed.) *Current Psychiatric Therapies*. New York: Grune & Stratton, Inc., 1972.

Hollister, L.E.: *Clinical Use of Psychotherapeutic Drugs*. Springfield, Ill.: Thomas, 1973.

Hollister, L.E.: Polypharmacy in psychiatry. Is it necessary, good or bad? In: Ayd, F.J., Jr. (Ed.) *Rational Psychopharmacotherapy and The Right to Treatment*. Baltimore: Ayd Medical Communications Ltd., 1975.

Hollister, L.E.: Presidential Address at 11th Congress of the Collegium Internationale Neuro-Psychopharmacologicum in Vienna, Austria, Sept., 1978.

Irwin, D.S., Weitzel, W.D., and Morgan, D.W.: Phenothiazine intake and staff attitudes. *Am. J. Psychiatry* 127: 67-71, 1971.

Itil, T., Keskiner, A., Heinemann, L. et al.: Treatment of resistant schizophrenics with extreme high dosage fluphenazine hydrochloride. *Psychomatics* 11: 456-463, 1970.

Jacobsen, E.: Psychotropic agents. In: Detre, T.P. and Jarecki, H.G. (Eds.) *Modern Psychiatric Treatment*. Philadelphia: Lippincott, 1971.

Jaffe, C.M.: First-degree atrioventricular block during lithium carbonate treatment. *Am. J. Psychiatry* 134: 88-89, 1977.

Janssen, P.A.J., and Van Bever, W.F.M.: Advances in the search for improved neuroleptic drugs. In: Essman, W.B., and Valzelli, L. (Eds.) *Current Developments in Psychopharmacology*, Vol. 2, New York: Spectrum, 1976.

Jefferson, J.W.: Atypical manifestations of postural hypotension. *Arch. Gen. Psychiatry* 27: 250-251, 1972.

Jellinek, T.: Mood elevating effect of trihexyphenidyl and biperiden in individuals taking antipsychotic medication. *Dis. Nerv. Syst.* 38: 353-355, 1977.

Jeste, D.V., Potkin, S., Sinha, S., et al: Tardive dyskinesia: reversible or irreversible? Proceedings of the 131st Annual Meeting of the American Psychiatric Association, Washington, D.C., May, 1977.

Jeste, D.V., and Wyatt, R.J.: In search of treatment for tardive dyskinesia: Review of the literature. *Schiz. Bull.* 5: 251-293, 1979.

Jeeva Raj, M.V., and Benson, R.: Phenothiazines and the electrocardiagram. *Postgrad. Med. J.* 51: 65-68, 1975.

Jobe, P.C.: Pharmacotherapy of schizophrenia. *Curr. Concepts in Psychiatry* 2: 6-11, 1976.

Johnson, A.W., and Buffaloe, W.J.: Chlorpromazine epithelial keratopathy. *Arch. Ophthal.* (Chicago) 76: 664-668, 1966.

Johnson, D.A.W.: Prevalence and treatment of drug-induced extrapyramidal symptoms. *Br. J. Psychiatry* 132: 27-30, 1978.

Johnson, F.N., and Cade, J.F.J.: The historical background to lithium research and therapy. In: Johnson, F.N. (Ed.) *Lithium Research and Therapy*, New York: Academic Press, 1975.

Judd, L.L., Hubbard, B., Janowsky, D.S., Huey, L.Y., and Attewell, P.A.: The effect of lithium carbonate on affect, mood, and personality of normal subjects. *Arch. Gen. Psychiatry* 34: 346-351, 1977.

Jus, A.: Paper presented at the Collegium Internationale Neuro-Psychopharmacologicum, Vienna, Austria, 1978.

Kaim, S.C., Kett, C.J., and Rothfield, B.: Treatment of the acute alcohol withdrawal state: A comparison of four drugs. *Am. J. Psychiatry* 125: 54-60, 1969.

Kalda, R.: Chlorpromazine contraindicated in delirium tremens. *Am. J. Psychiatry* 130: 1042, 1973.

Kamm, I.: Thioridazine for sexual hyperactivity. *Am. J. Psychiatry* 121: 922-923, 1965.

Kellett, J.M., Metcalf, M., Bailey, J., and Coppen, A.J.: Beta blockade in lithium tremor. *J. Neurol. Neurosurg. Psychiat.* 38: 719-721, 1975.

Kerry, R.J.: The management of patients receiving lithium treatment. In: F.N. Johnson (Ed.) *Lithium Research and Therapy*, New York: Academic Press, 143-163, 1975.

Keskiner, A.: According to an informational pamphlet distributed by the manufacturer, E.R. Squibb & Sons, 1976.

Ketai, R.: Psychotropic drugs in the management of psychiatric emergencies. *Postgraduate Medicine* 58: 87-93, 1975.

Ketai, R.: High dosage and versatile drug therapy with treatment-resistant psychotic patients. Hosp. Community Psychiatry, 1: 37-39, 1976.

Kiev, A.: Acute psychosis: a medical emergency. *Drug Therapy*, Oct. 1977.

Kinross-Wright, V.: The intensive chlorpromazine treatment of schizophrenia. *Psychiat. Res. Rep.* 1: 53-62, 1955.

Kiritz, S., and Moos, R.H.: Physiologic effects of social environments. *Psychosom. Med.* 36: 96-114, 1974.

Klatskin, G.: Toxic and drug-induced hepatitis. In: Shiff, L. (Ed.) *Diseases of The Liver*. Montreal: Lippincott, 1963, pp. 453-538.

Klawans, H.L., and Shenker, D.Wm.: Observations on the dopaminergic nature of hyperthyroid chorea. *J. Neural. Trans.* 33: 73-81, 1972.

Klein, D.F. and Davis, J.M.: Diagnosis and Drug Treatment of Psychiatric Disorders. Baltimore: Williams and Wilkins, 1969.

Klein, D.F.: Who should not be treated with neuroleptics but often are. In: Ayd, F.J., Jr. (Ed.) *Rational Psychopharmacotherapy and the Right To Treatment*. Baltimore: Ayd Medical Communications, Ltd., 1975.

Klerman, G.L.: Pharmacotherapy of schizophrenia. *Ann. Rev. Med.* 25: 199-217, 1974.

Kline, N.S., and Simpson, G.M.: Lithium in the treatment of conditions other than the affective disorders. In: Johnson, F.N. (Ed.) *Lithium Research and Therapy*. New York: Academic

Press, pp. 85-97, 1975.

Kobayashi, R.M.: Tardive dyskinesia. *New Eng. J. Med.* 296: 257-260, 1977.

Kotin, J., Wilbert, D.E., Verberg, D., and Soldinger, S.M.: Thioridazine and sexual dysfunction. *Am. J. Psychiatry* 133: 82-85, 1976.

Kris, E.: Children of mothers maintained on pharmacotherapy during pregnancy and postpartum. *Curr. Ther. Res.* 7: 785-789, 1965.

Laffan, R.J., High, J.P., and Burke, J.C.: The prolonged action of fluphenazine enanthate after depot injection. *Int. J. Neuropsychiatry* 1: 300-306, 1965.

Lambert, P.A., and Marcou, G.: Fluphenazine enanthate given to inpatients and outpatients. *Dis. Nerv. Syst.* (Suppl.) 31: 63-65, 1970.

de Lamerens, S., Tuttle, A.H., and Aballi, A.J.: Neonatal bilirubin levels after use of phenothiazine derivatives for obstetric analgesia. *J. Pediatrics* 65: 925-928, 1964.

Laska, E., Varga, E., Wanderling, J., Simpson, G., Logemann, G.W., and Shaw, B.K.: Patterns of psychotropic use for schizophrenia. *Dis. Nerv. Syst.* 34: 294-305, 1973.

Learoyd, B.M.: Psychotropic drugs and the elderly patient. *Med. J. Australia* 1: 1131-1133, 1972.

Leestma, J.E., and Koenig, K.L.: Sudden death and phenothiazines; a current controversy. *Arch. Gen. Psychiatry* 18: 137-148, 1968.

Leff, J.P., and Wing, J.K.: Trial of maintenance therapy in schizophrenia. *Br. Med. J.* 3: 559-664, 1971.

Lehmann, H.E.: Psychopharmacological treatment of schizophrenia. *Schizophrenia Bulletin,* Issue No. 13, 1975.

Letemendia, F.J., Harris, A.D., and Willems, J.A.: Effects on chronic patients of administrative changes. *Br. J. Psychiatry*, 1967.

Levenson, A.J., Burnett, G.B., Nottingham, J.D., Sermas, C.E., and Thornby, J.I.: Speed and rate of remission of acute schizophrenia: a comparison of intramuscularly administered fluphenazine HCl with thiothixene and haloperidol. *Curr. Ther. Res.* 20: 695-700, 1976.

Levenson, A.J., and Dunbar, P.W.: The L-D trend oriented psychiatric record. *Dis. Nerv. Syst.* 38: 465-467, 1977.

Lindstedt, G., Nilsson, L., Walinder, J., Skott, A., and Ohman, R.: On the prevalence, diagnosis and management of lithium-induced hypothyroidism in psychiatric patients. *Brit. J. Psychiatry* 130: 452-458, 1977.

Linnoila, M., Saario, I., and Maki, M.: Effect of treatment with diazepam or lithium and alcohol on psychomotor skills related to driving. *Eur. J. Clin. Pharmacol.* 7: 337-342, 1974.

Litkey, L.J., and Feniczy, P.: An approach to the control of homosexual practices. *Int. J. Neuropsychiatry* 3: 20-29, 1967.

Litvak, R., and Kaebling, R.: Agranulocytosis, leukopenia and psychotropic drugs. *Arch. Gen. Psychiatry* 24: 265-267, 1971.

London, P.: *Behavior Control* New York: Harper & Row, 1969, pp. 11-17 and 204-209.

Ludwig, A.: Beyond psychotropic drugs. *Highlights of 18th Annual Conference, Veterans Administration Studies in Mental Health and Behavioral Sciences*, New Orleans, La., March 28-30, 1973.

MacKay, A.V.P., Loose, R., and Glen, A.I.M.: Labor on lithium. *Brit. Med. J.* 1: 878, 1976.

MacNeil, S., and Jenner, F.A.: Lithium and polyuria. In: Johnson, F.N. (Ed.) *Lithium Research and Therapy.* New York: Academic Press, pp. 473-484, 1975.

Maltbie, A.A., and Cavenar, J.O.: Akathisia diagnosis: an objective test. *Psychosomatics.* 18: 36-39, 1977.

Man, P.L., and Chen, C.H.: Rapid tranquilization of acutely psychotic patients with intramuscular haloperidol and chlorpromazine. *Psychosomatics.* 14: 59-63, 1973.

Mandel, A., and Gross, M.: Agranulocytosis and phenothiazines. *Dis. Nerv. Syst.* 29: 32-36, 1968.

Marder, J., Soylu, D., DiMascio, A., and Stuecks, R.N.: Nursing costs in administering drugs: multiple vs. b.i.d. dosage schedules. *Hosp. Formulary Management* 6: 21, 1971.

Marder, J.E., and DiMascio, A.: Improving scheduling and reducing costs of psychotropic drugs for outpatients. *Hosp. and Community Psychiat.* 24: 556-557, 1973.

Marshall, E.J.: Why patients do not take their medication. *Amer. J. Psychiatry* 138: 148, 1971.

Marsden, C.D., Tarsy, D., and Baldessarini, R.J.: Spontaneous and drug-induced movement disorders in psychotic patients. In: Benson, D.F., and Blumer, D., (Eds.) *Psychiatric Aspects of Neurologic Disease*. New York: Grune & Stratton, pp. 219-266, 1975.

Mason, A.S., Forrest, I.S., and Butler, H.: Adherence to maintenance therapy and rehospitalization. *Dis. Nerv. Syst.* 24: 103-104, 1963.

Mason, A.S.: Basic principles in the use of antipsychotic agents. *Hosp. and Community Psychiatry* 24: 825-829, 1973.

Mason, A.S., and DeWolfe, A.S.: Usage of psychotropic drugs in a mental hospital: 1. As needed (PRN) Antipsychotic medications. *Curr. Ther. Res.* 16: 853-860, 1974.

Mason, A.S.: The psychotropic drug summary, *Dis. Nerv. Syst.* 36: 44-45, 1975.

Mason, A.S.: Toward rational antipsychotic drug therapy: avoidance of multiple dose schedules. *J. Kentucky Med. Assoc.* 74: 453-455, 1976.

Mason, A.S., and Granacher, R.P.: Basic principles of rapid neuroleptization. *Dis. Nerv. Syst.* 37: 547-551, 1976.

Mason, A.S., Nerviano, V., DeBurger, R.A.: Patterns of antipsychotic drug use in four southeastern state hospitals. *Dis. Nerv. Syst.* 38: 541-545, 1977a.

Mason, A.S., Nerviano, V., DeBurger, R.A.: Patients of antipsychotic drug usage: results of a one-year educational campaign. *Hosp. and Community Psychiatry* 29: 100-101, 1977b.

Matuk, F., and Kalyanaraman, K.: Syndrome of inappropriate secretion of antidiuretic hormone in patients treated with psychotherapeutic drugs. *Arch. Neurol.* 34: 374-375, 1977.

May, P.R.A.: Rational treatment for an irrational disorder: what does the schizophrenic patient need? *Am. J. Psychiatry* 133: 1008-1012, 1976.

McClellan, T.A. and Cowan, G.: Use of antipsychotic and antidepressant drugs by chronically ill patients. *Am. J. Psychiatry* 126: 1171-1173, 1970.

McClelland, H.A., Farguharson, R.G., Leyburn, P., Furness, J.A., Schiff, A.A.: Very high dose fluphenazine decanoate. A controlled trial in chronic schizophrenia. *Arch. Gen. Psychiatry* 33: 1435-1439, 1976.

McDowell, F.H., and Lee, J.E.: Extrapyramidal diseases. In: Baker, A.B. and Baker, L.H. (Eds.) *Clinical Neurology*. New York: Harper & Row, Chapter 26, 1976.

McGeer, P.L., McGeer, E.G., and Suzuk, J.S.: Aging and extrapyramidal function. *Arch. Neurol.* 34: 33-35, 1977.

Mellin, G.: Drugs in the first trimester of pregnancy and the fetal life of homo sapiens. *Am. J. Obst. Gynec.* 90: 1169-1180, 1964.

Meltzer, H.Y., and Fang, V.S.: The effect of neuroleptics on serum prolactin in schizophrenic patients. *Arch. Gen. Psychiatry* 33: 279-286, 1976.

Mendels, J.: Lithium in the acute treatment of depressive states. In: Johnson, F.N. (Ed.) *Lithium Research and Therapy*. New York: Academic Press, pp. 43-62, 1975.

Mendlewicz, J., Fieve, R.R., Stallone, F., and Fleiss, J.L.: Genetic history as a predictor of lithium response in manic depressive illness. *Lancet* 1: 599-600, 1972.

Merlis, S., Sheppard, C., Collins, L., et al.: Polypharmacy in psychiatry: patterns of differential treatment. *Am. J. Psychiatry* 126: 1647-1651, 1970.

Merlis, S., Beyel, V., Fiorentino, D., et al.: Polypharmacy in psychiatry: empiricism, efficacy and rationale. In: Masserman, J.H. (Ed.), *Current Psychiatric Therapies*. New York: Grune & Stratton, 1972.

Mesard, L., Wrigley, A., and Gee, S.: The ordering of antipsychotic drugs for the treatment of psychotic patients in VA hospitals. Report and Statistics Services, Office of the Comptroller, Veterans Administration Central Office, Washington, D.C. 1976.

Morgan, R., and Cheadle, J.: Maintenance treatment of chronic schizophrenia with neuroleptic drugs. *Acta. Psychiat. Scand.* 50: 78-85, 1974.

Mountain, H.E.: Crash tranquilization in a millieu therapy setting. *J. of Fort Logan Mental Health Center.* 11: 42-44, 1963.

National Institute of Mental Health—Pharmacology Service Center, Collaborative Study Group: Phenothiazine treatment in acute schizophrenia. *Arch. Gen. Psychiatry* 10: 246-261, 1964.

Neff, K.E., Denney, D., and Blachely, P.H.: Control of severe agitation with droperidol. *Dis.*

Nerv. Syst. 33: 594-597, 1972.

Neil, J.F., Himmelhoch, J.M., and Licata, S.M.: Emergence of myasthenia gravis during treatment with lithium carbonate. *Arch. Gen. Psychiatry* 33: 1090-1092, 1976.

Nelson, M.M., and Forfar, J.O.: Association between drugs administered during pregnancy and congenital abnormalities of the fetus. *Br. Med. J.*, 1: 523-527, 1971.

Netter, K.H., and Bergheim, P.: Some characteristics of human placental cytochrome P-450. In: Morselli, P.L., Garattini, S., and Sereni, F. (Eds.) *Basic and Therapeutic Aspects of Perinatal Pharmacology.* New York: Raven Press, pp. 39-52, 1975.

Neve, H.K.: Demonstration of Largactil (Chlorpromazine) urine. *J. Ment. Sci.* 104: 488-490, 1958.

Nilson, J.A.: Immediate treatment expedites hospital release. *Hosp. and Community Psychiatry* 20: 36-38, 1969.

Noonan, J.P.A., and Burnstein, M.H., Ananth, J., and Clark, R.: Sex and neuroleptic medication. *Psychiatric Journal of the University of Ottawa,* 1: 86-87, 1977.

Nursing Home Care in the United States: Supporting paper No. 2, drugs in nursing homes, misuse, high costs and kickbacks. Washington, D.C.: U.S. Government Printing Office, 1974.

O'Connell, R.A.: Leukocytosis during lithium carbonate treatment. *Int. J. Pharmacopsychiatry* 4: 30-34, 1970.

O'Donoghue, S.E.F.: Distribution of pethidine and chlorpromazine in maternal, fetal, and neonatal biological fluids. *Nature* (London) 229: 124-125, 1971.

Office of the Secretary for H.E.W.: Interim report on nursing home survey, Washington, D.C.: U.S. Government Printing Office, 1975.

Oldham, A.J., and Bott, M.: Management of excitement in a general hospital psychiatric ward by high dose haloperidol. *Acta. Psychiat. Scand.* 47: 369-376, 1971.

Ordy, J.M., Samorajski, R.L., Collins, R.L., and Rolsten, C.: Prenatal chlorpromazine effects on liver, survival, and behavior of mice offspring. *J. Pharm. Exp. Ther.* 151: 110-125, 1966.

Orlov, P., Kasparian, G., DiMascio, A., and Cole, J.O.: Withdrawal of antiparkinson drugs. *Arch. Gen. Psychiatry* 25: 410-412, 1971.

Ota, K.Y., Kurland, A.A., Rocha, J., and Block, B.A.: A comparison of the relative clinical efficacy of two chlorpromazine preparations. *Curr. Ther. Res.* 16: 1014-1021, 1974.

Overall, J.E., Hollister, L.E., Meyer, F., Kimbell, I., and Shelton, J.: Imipramine and thioridazine in depressed and schizophrenic patients. *J.A.M.A.* 189: 93-96, 1964.

Owens, D.: The use of fluphenazines in a continuing-care program. *Hosp. and Community Psychiatry* 29: 115-118, 1978.

Ozarin, L.D.: *Address at Sixth World Congress of Psychiatry,* Honolulu, Hawaii, Nov. 1977.

Palestine, M.L., and Alatorre, E.: Control of acute alcohol withdrawal. *Curr. Ther. Res.* 20: 289-299, 1976.

Palmer, E.D.: Dysphagia in parkinsonism, *J.A.M.A.* 229: 1349, 1974.

Pandey, G.N., Goel, I. and Davis, J.M.: Effect of neuroleptic drugs on lithium uptake by the human erythrocyte. *Clin. Pharm. Ther.* 26: 96-101, 1979.

Park, L.C., and Lipman, R.S.: A comparison of patient dosage deviation reports with pill counts. *Psychopharmacologia.* 6: 299-302, 1964.

Parkes, C.M., Brown, C.W., and Monch, E.M.: The general practitioner and the schizophrenic patient. *Br. Med. J.* 1: 972-976, 1962.

Paulson, G.W., Rizvi, C.A., and Crane, G.E.: Tardive dyskinesia as a possible sequel of long term therapy with phenothiazines. *Clin. Ped.* 14: 953, 1975.

Pecknold, J.C., Ananth, J.V., Ban, T.A., and Lehmann, H.E.: Lack of indication for use of antiparkinson medication. *Dis. Nerv. Syst.* 32: 538-541, 1971.

Peele, R., and Van Loetzen, I.S.: Phenothiazine deaths: a critical review. *Am. J. Psychiatry* 130: 306-309, 1973.

Peet, M.: Lithium in the acute treatment of mania. In: Johnson, F.N. (Ed.) *Lithium Research and Therapy,* New York: Academic Press, pp. 25-41, 1975.

Pelkonen, O., Korhonen, P., Jouppila, P., and Karki, N.T.: Placental transfer and fetal metabolism of drugs. In: Morselli, P.L., Garattini, S., and Sereni, F. (Eds.) *Basic and*

Therapeutic Aspects of Perinatal Pharmacology, New York: Raven Press, pp. 65-74, 1975.

Penna-Ramos, A.: Thioridazine HCl vs. Chlordiazepoxide HCl in controlling symptoms attributable to alcohol withdrawal. *Dis. Nerv. Syst.* 38: 144-147, 1977.

Peroutka, S.J., U'Prichard, D.C., Greenberg, P.A., and Snyder, S.H.: Neuroleptic drug interaction with norepinephrine alpha-receptor binding sites in rat brain. *Neuropharmacology* 16: 549-556, 1977.

Physicians' Desk Reference, Oradell, N.J.: Medical Economics Company, 1977.

Physicians' Desk Reference, Oradell, N.J.: Medical Economics Company, 1979.

Polak, P., and Laycob, L.: Rapid Tranquilization. *Amer. J. Psychiatry* 118: 300-307, 1971.

Polizos, P., Engelhardt, D.M., and Hoffman, S.P.: CNS consequences of psychotropic drug withdrawal in schizophrenic children. *Psychopharmacol. Bull.* 9: 34-35, 1973.

Pollack, B.: The validity of the Forrest Reagent Test for the detection of chlorpromazine or other phenothiazines in the urine. *Am. J. Psychiatry* 115: 77-78, 1958.

Polvan, N., Yagcioglu, V., Itil, M.: High and very high dose fluphenazine in the treatment of chronic psychosis. In: Cerletti, A., and Bare, F.J. (Eds.) *The Present Status of Psychotropic Drugs, Pharmacological and Clinical Aspects: Proceedings of the Sixth International Congress of the Collegium Internationale Neuropsycho-Pharmacologicum*, Tarragona, Spain, April, 1968. Amsterdam: Excerpta Medica, International Congress Series, No. 180, 1969.

Prien, R.F.: The clinical effectiveness of lithium: comparison with other drugs. In: Johnson, F.N. (Ed.) *Lithium Research and Therapy*, New York: Academic Press, 1975.

Prien, R.F., and Cole, J.O.: High dose chlorpromazine therapy in chronic schizophrenia. *Arch. Gen. Psychiatry* 18: 482-495, 1968.

Prien, R.F., Levine, J., and Cole, J.O.: High dose trifluoperazine therapy in chronic schizophrenia. *Am. J. Psychiatry* 126: 53-61, 1969.

Prien, R.F., Levine, J., and Cole, J.O.: Indications for high dose chlorpromazine therapy in chronic schizophrenia. *Dis. Nerv. Syst.* 31: 739-745, 1970.

Prien, R.F., and Klett, C.J.: An appraisal of long-term use of tranquilizing medication with hospitalized chronic schizophrenics. *Schizophrenia Bull.* 5: 64-73, 1972.

Prien, R.F., Gillis, R., and Caffey, E.M.: Intermittent drug therapy in hospitalized chronic schizophrenics. *Hosp. and Community Psychiatry* 24: 317-322, 1973a.

Prien, R.F., Klett, C.L.J., and Caffey, E.M.: Lithium carbonate and imipramine in prevention of affective episodes. *Arch. Gen. Psychiatry* 29: 420-425, 1973b.

Prien, R.F., Klett, C.J., and Caffey, E.M.: Lithium prophylaxis in recurrent affective illness. *Am. J. Psychiatry* 131: 198-203, 1974.

Prien, R. and Caffey, E.: Guidelines for antipsychotic drug use. *Resident and Staff Physician* 9: 165-172, 1975.

Prockop, L.D., and Marcus, D.J.: Cerebrospinal fluid lithium: passive transfer kinetics. *Life Sci.* 11: 859-868, 1972.

Quitkin, F., Rifkin, A., and Klein, D.F.: Very high dosage vs. standard dosage fluphenazine in schizophrenia—a double-blind study of nonchronic treatment—refractory patients. *Arch. Gen. Psychiatry* 32: 1276-1281, 1975.

Quitkin, F., Rifkin, A., and Klein, D.F.: Prophylaxis of affective disorders. *Arch. Gen. Psychiatry* 33: 337-341, 1976.

Quitkin, F., Rifkin, A., Gochfield, L., and Klein, D.F.: Tardive dyskinesia—are first signs reversible? *Am. J. Psychiatry* 134: 84-87, 1977.

Ramsey, T.A., Mendels, J., Stokes, J.W., and Fitzgerald, R.G.: Lithium carbonate and kidney function. *J.A.M.A.* 219: 1446-1449, 1972.

Raskind, M.A., Alvarez, C., Pietrzyk, M., Westerlund, K., and Herlin, S.: Helping the elderly psychiatric patient in crisis. *Geriatrics*, 31: 41-56, 1976.

Redlich, F.C., and Freedman, D.X.: *The Theory and Practice of Psychiatry*. New York, Basic Books, 1966.

Richardson, H.L., Gaupner, K.I., and Richardson, M.E.: Intramyocardial lesions in patients dying suddenly and unexpectedly. *J.A.M.A.* 195: 114-120, 1966.

Rickels, K.: Use of antianxiety agents in anxious outpatients. *Psychopharmacology*, 58: 1-17,

1978.

Rifkin, A., Quitkin, F., Carillo, C., Klein, D.F., and Oaks, G.: Very high dose fluphenazine for nonchronic treatment-refractory patients. *Arch. Gen. Psychiatry* 25: 398-403, 1971.

Rifkin, A., Quitkin, F., and Klein, D.F.: Akinesia. *Arch. Gen. Psychiatry* 32: 672-674, 1975.

Rifkin, A., Quitkin, F., Kane, J., et al.: Long-term use of antipsychotic drugs. In: Klein, D., and Gittelman-Klein, R. (Eds.) *Progress in Psychiatric Drug Treatment.* New York: Brunner/Mazel, 1976.

Rifkin, A., Quitkin, F., Kane, J., Struve, F., and Klein, D.F.: Are prophylactic antiparkinson drugs necessary? A controlled study of procyclidine withdrawal. *Arch. Gen. Psychiatry* 35: 483-489, 1978.

Rivera-Calimlim, L.: Chlorpromazine-trihexiphendyl interaction. *Drug Therapy,* pp. 196-197, Nov. 1976.

Rivera-Calimlim, L., Griesbach, P.H., and Perlmutter, R.: Plasma chlorpromazine concentrations in children with behavioral disorders and mental illness. *Clin. Pharm. Ther.* 26: 114-121, 1979.

Roisin, L., True, C., and Knight, M.: Structural effects of tranquilizers. *Res. Publ. Assoc. Nerv. Ment. Dis.* 37: 285, 1959.

Ropert, R., Levy, L., and Ropert, M.: Problems posses par les essais d'employ des neuroleptiquies a action prolonge's (NAP) dans les syndrome psychiatrique argus. *Ann. Psychol.* (Paris) 1: 259-267, 1973.

Rosati, D.: Hypotensive side effects of phenothiazines and their management. *Dis. Nerv. Syst.* 25: 366-369, 1964.

Rosenberger, P.B., Wheelden, J.A., and Kaltokin, M.: Effect of haloperidol on stuttering. *Am. J. Psychiatry* 133: 331-334, 1976.

Rubinstein, A., Eidelman, A.I., Melamed, J., Gartner, L.M., and Kandall, S.: Possible effect of maternal promethazine therapy on neonatal immunologic functions. *J. Pediatrics* 89: 136-138, 1976.

Rumeau-Rouquette, C., Goujard, J., and Hel, G.: Possible teratogenic effect of phenothiazines in human beings. *Teratology* 15: 57-64, 1977.

Samet, J.M., and Surawicz, B.: Cardiac function in patients treated with phenothiazines. Comparison with quinidine. *J. Clin. Pharmacol.* 14: 588-596, 1974.

Sangiovanni, F., Taylor, M.A., Abrams, R., Gaztanaga, P.: Rapid control of psychotic excitement states with intramuscular haloperidol. *Am. J. Psychiatry* 130: 1155-1156, 1973.

Sanseigne, A.: Chemistry and pharmacology of fluphenazine decanoate. *Dis. Nerv. Syst.* (Suppl.) 31. 10-11, 1070.

Schou, M.. Lithium in psychiatric therapy and prophylaxis. *J. Psychiatr. Res.* 6: 67-95, 1968.

Schou, M., Amidsen, A., and Thomsen, K.: The effect of lithium on the normal mind. In: Baudis, P., Petrova, E., and Sedivec, V. (Eds.) *Psychiatric Progrediens.* Pizen. 1968a.

Schou, M., Amidsen, A., and Trap-Jensen, J.: Lithium poisoning. *Am. J. Psychiatry* 125: 520-527, 1968b.

Schou, M.: Lithium: elimination rate, dosage, control, poisoning, goiter, mode of action. *Acta. Psychiatr. Scand.* 207 (Suppl.) 49: 54, 1969.

Schou, M., Baastrup, P.C., Groff, P., Weis, P., and Angst, J.: Pharmacological and clinical problems of lithium prophylaxis. *Brit. J. Psychiatry* 116: 615-619, 1970.

Schou, M., personal communication, Louisville, KY, Feb., 1976.

Schroeder, N.H., Caffey, E.M., and Loeri, T.W.: Antipsychotic drug use: Physician prescribing practices in relation to current recommendations. *Dis. Nerv. Syst.* 38: 114-116, 1977.

Schukit, M.A.: Drugs in combination with other therapies for alcoholics. In: Greenblatt, M. (Ed.) *Drugs in Combination With Other Therapies.* New York: Grune & Stratton, 1975.

Scokel, P.W., and Jones, W.N.: Infant jaundice after phenothiazine drugs for labor: an enigma. *Obst. Gynec.* 20: 124, 1962.

Shader, R.I., and DiMascio, A.: *Psychotropic Drug Side Effects.* Baltimore: Williams & Wilkins, 1970.

Shader, R.I., and Greenblatt, D.J.: The pharmacologic treatment of anxiety states. In: Shader, R.I., (Ed.) *Manual of Psychiatric Therapeutics.* Boston: Little, Brown & Co., 1975.

Shader, R.I., and Jackson, A.H.: Approaches to schizophrenia. In: Shader, R.I. (Ed.) *Manual of Psychiatric Therapeutics.* Boston: Little, Brown & Co., 1975.

Shader, R.I., Elkins, R., and Ciraulo, D.: On guidelines for maximum dosages. *Am. J. Psychiatry* 135: 499-500, 1977.

Shapiro, A.K., Shapiro, E., Wayne, H., and Clarkin, J.: The psychopathology of Gilles de la Tourette's Syndrome. *Am. J. Psychiatry* 129: 427-434, 1972.

Shapiro, A.K., Shapiro, E., Wayne, H.: Treatment of Tourette's Syndrome with haloperidol, a review of 34 cases. *Arch. Gen. Psychiatry* 28: 92-97, 1973.

Shapiro, A.K., and Shapiro, E.: Treatment of Gilles de la Tourette syndrome. *J.A.M.A.* 283: 29, 1977.

Shapiro, A., Shapiro, E., Brunn, R., and Sweet, R.: *Gilles de la Tourette syndrome.* New York: Raven Press, 1978.

Shaw, E.B., Dermott, R.V., Lee, R., and Burbridge, T.N.: Phenothiazines as a cause of severe seizures. *Pediatrics* 23: 485-492, 1959.

Sheppard, C., Collins, L., Fiorentio, D., Fracchia, J., and Merlis, S.: Polypharmacy in psychiatric treatment: 1. Incidence at a state hospital. *Curr. Ther. Res.* 11: 765-774, 1969.

Sheppard, C., Beyel, V., Fracchia, J., et al.: Polypharmacy in psychiatry: a multi-state comparison of psychotropic drug combinations. *Dis. Nerv. Syst.* 35: 183-189, 1974.

Shields, K.G., Ballinger, C.M., and Hathaway, B.N.: Antiemetic effectiveness of haloperidol in human volunteers challenged with apomorphine. *Anesth. Analg. Curr. Res.* 50: 1017-1024, 1971.

Shopsin, B., Johnson, G., and Gershon, S.: Neurotoxicity with lithium. *Int. Pharmacopsychiatry* 170-182, 1970.

Shopsin, B., and Gershon, S.: Cogwheel rigidity related to lithium maintenance. *Am. J. Psychiatry* 132: 536-537, 1975.

Shuttleworth, E., Wise, G., and Paulson, G.W.: Choreoathetosis and diphenylhydantoin intoxication. *J.A.M.A.* 230: 1170-1171, 1974.

Sider, R.C., Rubin, R.R., and Fligsten, K.E.: Psychiatrists and psychotropic drug costs. *Comprehensive Psychiat.* 17: 723-733, 1976.

Silverman, J.A., Winters, R.N., and Strande, C.: Lithium carbonate therapy during pregnancy: apparent lack of effect upon the fetus. *Am. J. Obst. Gyn.* 109: 934-936, 1971.

Simpson, G.M., Amin, M., Angus, J.W.S., Edwards, J.G., Go, S.H., and Lee, J.H.: Role of antidepressants and neuroleptics in the treatment of depression. *Arch. Gen. Psychiatry* 27: 337-345, 1972.

Simpson, G.M., Varga, E., Reiss, M., Cooper, T.B., Bergner, P.E., and Lee, J.H.: Bioequivalency of generic and brand-named chlorpromazine. *Clin. Pharm. Ther.* 15: 631-641, 1974.

Simpson, G.M., Branchey, M.H., Lee, J.H., Viotashevsky, A., and Zoubok: Lithium in tardive dyskinesia. *Pharmakopsychiatr. Neuropsychopharmakol.* 9: 76-80, 1976.

Simpson, G.M., Viotashevsky, A., Young, M.A., and Lee, J.H.: Deanol in the treatment of tardive dyskinesia. *Psychopharmacology* 52: 257-261, 1977.

Singer, I., and Rotenberg, D.: Mechanisms of lithium action. *New Eng. J. Med.* 289: 254-260, 1973.

Singh, M.M., and Smith, J.M.: Reversal of some therapeutic effects of an antipsychotic agent by an antiparkinson drug. *J. Nerv. Ment. Dis.* 157: 50-58, 1973.

Singh, M.M., and Kay, S.R.: A comparative study of haloperidol and chlorpromazine in terms of clinical effects and therapeutic reversal with benztropine in schizophrenia. Theoretical implications for potency differences among neuroleptics. *Psychopharmacologia* 43: 103-113, 1975.

Sletten, K.W., Lang, W.J., Brown, M.L., Ballou, S.R., and Gershon, S.: Chronic chlorpromazine administration. *Clin. Pharm. Ther.* 6:575-586, 1965.

Slotnick, V.B.: Management of the acutely agitated psychotic patient with parenteral neuroleptics; a comparative symptom effectiveness profile of haloperidol and chlorpromazine. Paper presented at the Fifth World Congress of Psychiatry, Mexico City, Nov. 1971.

Smith, J.W., Seidl, L.G., and Cluff, L.E.: Studies on the epidemiology of adverse drug reactions V. Clinical factors influencing susceptibility. *Ann. Intern. Med.* 65: 629-640, 1966.

Snyder, S., Greenberg, D., and Yamamura, H.T.: Antischizophrenic drugs and the brain cholinergic receptors. *Arch. Gen. Psychiatry* 31: 58-61, 1974.

Solomon, K.: Maintenance antipsychotic dosage and tardive dyskinesia. *Am. J. Psychiatry* 134: 1314-1315, 1977a.

Solomon, K.: Phenothiazine-induced bulbar palsy-like syndrome and sudden death. *Am. J. Psychiatry* 134: 308-311, 1977b.

Sovner, R., DiMascio, A., Berkowitz, D., and Randolph, P.: Tardive dyskinesia and informed consent. *Psychosomatics* 19: 172-177, 1978.

Spalding, J.M.K., and Nelson, E.: The autonomic nervous system. In: Baker, A.B., and Baker, L.H. (Eds.) *Clinical Neurology*, New York: Harper & Row, 1976.

Spiegel, J., and Bell, N.: The family of the psychiatric patient. In: Arieti, S. (Ed.) *American Handbook of Psychiatry*, New York: Basic Books, Vol. I, pp. 114-149, 1959.

Sprague, R.L.: Research findings and their impact upon FDA Pediatric Advisory Panel. Paper presented at the 99th Annual Meeting of the American Association on Mental Deficiency, Portland, Oregon, May, 1975.

Stein, L.I., and Test, M.A.: Training in community living: one-year evaluation. *Am. J. Psychiatry* 133: 917-918, 1976.

Stein, R.S., Beamen, C., Ali, M.Y., Hansen, R., et al.: Lithium carbonate attenuation of chemotherapy-induced neutropenia. *New Eng. J. Med.* 297: 430-431, 1977.

Stevens, J.R.: An anatomy of schizophrenia. *Arch. Gen. Psychiatry* 29: 177-189, 1973.

Stewart, T.S.: Spinal cord injury: a role for the psychiatrist. *Am. J. Psychiatry* 134: 538-541, 1977.

Stokes, H.B.: Trifluoperazine for the symptomatic treatment of chorea, *Dis. Nerv. Syst.* 36: 102-105, 1975.

Stotsky, B.A.: Relative efficacy of parenteral haloperidol and thiothixene for emergency treatment of acutely excited and agitated patients. *Dis. Nerv. Syst.* 38: 967-973, 1977.

Strothers, J.K., Wilson, D.W., and Royston, J.: Lithium toxicity in the newborn. *Brit. Med. J.* 3: 233-234, 1973.

Swedburg, K., and Winblad, B.: Heart failure as a complication of lithium treatment: Preliminary report of a fatal case. *Acta. Med. Scand.* 196: 279-280, 1974.

Swett, C.: Outpatient phenothiazine use and bone marrow suppression. *Arch. Gen. Psychiatry* 32: 1416-1418, 1975.

Swett, C., Cole, J.O., Shapiro, S., and Slone, D.: Extrapyramidal side effects in chlorpromazine recipients: Emergence according to benztropine prophylaxis. *Arch. Gen. Psychiatry* 34: 661-663, 1977.

Swett, C.O., and Shader, R.I.: Cardiac side effects and sudden death in hospitalized psychiatric patients. *Dis. Nerv. Syst.* 38: 69-72, 1977.

Talso, P.J., and Clarke, R.W.: Excretion and distribution of lithium in the dog. *Am. J. Physiol.* 166: 202-208, 1951.

Tamer, A., McKey, R., Arias, D., et al.: Phenothiazine-induced extrapyramidal dysfunction in the neonate. *J. Pediatr.* 75: 479-480, 1969.

Tangedahl, T.N., and Gau, G.T.: Myocardial irritability associated with lithium carbonate therapy. *New Eng. J. Med.* 287: 867-869, 1972.

Tarsy, D., and Baldessarini, R.J.: The tardive dyskinesia syndrome. In: Klawans, H., (Ed.) *Clinical Neuropharmacology*, Vol. I, New York: Raven Press, pp. 21-61, 1976.

Tarsy, D., Granacher, R., and Bralower, M.: Tardive dyskinesia in young adults. *Am. J. Psychiatry* 134: 1032-1034, 1977.

Taylor, M.A., and Abrams, R.: Acute mania. Clinical and genetic study of responders and non-responders to treatments. *Arch. Gen. Psychiatry* 32: 863-865, 1975.

Thomsen, K. and Schou, M.: Renal lithium excretion in man. *Amer. J. Physiol.* 215: 823-827, 1968.

Thomsen, K., and Schou, M.: The treatment of lithium poisoning. In: Johnson, F.N. (Ed.) *Lithium Research and Therapy*. New York: Academic Press, 1975.

Thornburg, J.E., and Moore, K.E.: Pharmacologically induced modifications of behavioral and neurochemical development. In: Mirkin, B.L. (Ed.) *Perinatal Pharmacology and Therapeutics*. New York: Academic Press, pp. 270-354, 1976.

Thornton, W.E., and Thornton, B.P.: Crisis psychopharmacology techniques. *Dis. Nerv. Syst.*

34: 32-34, 1974.

Thornton, W.E.: Combining antipsychotic agents. *Am. J. Psychiatry* 132: 302, 1975.

Tibbets, J.C.N.: Single daily doses of chlorpromazine. *Lancet* 1: 689, 1958.

Treffert, D.A.: Psychiatry's image. *Psychiatric News*, 11: 16-18, 1978.

Trent, C.L., and Muhl, W.P.: Professional liability insurance and the American psychiatrist. *Am. J. Psychiatry* 132: 1312-1314, 1976.

Tseng, H.L.: Interstitial myocarditis probably related to lithium carbonate intoxication. *Arch. Path.* 92: 444-448, 1971.

Turek, I.S.: Drug-induced dyskinesia: reality or myth? *Dis. Nerv. Syst.* 36: 397-399, 1975.

Vacaflor, L., Lehmann, H.E., and Ban, T.A.: Side effects and teratogenicity of lithium carbonate treatment. *J. Clin. Pharm.* 10: 387-389, 1970.

Vacaflor, L.: Lithium side effects and toxicity: The clinical picture. In: Johnson, F.N. (Ed.) *Lithium Research and Therapy*, New York: Academic Press, pp. 211-225, 1975.

Van der Velde, C.D.: Toxicity of lithium carbonate in elderly patients. *Am. J. Psychiatry* 127: 1075-1977, 1971.

Van Leeuwen, A.M.H., Molders, J., Sterkmans, P., Mielants, P., Martens, C.P., Toussaintic, Hovent, A.M., Desseilles, M.F., Koch, H., Devroye, A., and Parrent, M.: Droperidol in acutely agitated patients. *J. Nerv. Ment. Dis.* 164: 280-283, 1977.

van Praag, H.M., and Dols, L.C.W.: Fluphenazine enanthate and fluphenazine decanoate: A comparison of their duration of action and motor side effects. *Am. J. Psychiatry* 130: 801-804, 1973.

van Praag, H.M.: *Psychotropic Drugs*, New York: Brunner/Mazel, 1978.

Van Putten, T.: Milieu therapy: Contra-indications. *Arch. Gen. Psychiatry* 29: 640-642, 1973.

Van Putten, T.: Why do schizophrenic patients refuse to take their drugs? *Arch. Gen. Psychiatry* 31: 67-73, 1974.

Van Putten, T.: The many faces of akathisia. *Comp. Psychiatry* 16: 43-47, 1975.

Van Putten, T., Crumpton, E., and Yale, C.: Drug refusal in schizophrenia and the wish to be crazy. *Arch. Gen. Psychiatry* 33: 1443-1446, 1976.

Van Putten, T., and May, P.R.A.: "Akinetic depression" in schizophrenia. *Arch. Gen. Psychiatry* 35: 1101-1107, 1978.

Van Thiel, D.: Esophageal disease and bowel dysfunction. Presented at Practical Medicine for the General Psychiatrist, Pittsburgh, Pa., Nov. 7, 1977.

Vendsborg, P.B., Bech, P., and Rafaelsen, O.J.: Lithium treatment and weight gain. *Acta. Psychiat. Scand.* 53: 139-147, 1976.

Vendsborg, P.B., and Rafaelsen, O.J.: Lithium in man: effect on glucose tolerance and serum electrolytes. *Acta. Psychiat. Scand.* 49: 601-610, 1973.

Vendsborg, P.B., and Prytz, S.: Glucose tolerance and serum lipids in man after long-term lithium administration. *Acta. Psychiat. Scand.* 53: 64-69, 1976.

Viol, G.W., Grof, P., and Daigle, L.: Renal tubular function in patients on long-term lithium therapy. *Am. J. Psychiatry* 132: 68-70, 1976.

Wallerstein, R.O.: Blood. In: Drupp, M.A., and Chatton, M.J. (Eds.) *Current Medical Diagnosis and Treatment*, Los Altos, Ca.: Lange, 1975.

Warnes, H., Lehman, H.E., and Ban, T.A.: A dynamic ileus during psychoactive medication: A report of three fatal and five severe cases. *Canadian Med. Assoc. J.* 96: 1112-1113, 1967.

Weiner, W.J., Goetz, C.G., Nausieda, P.A., and Klawans, H.L.: Respiratory dyskinesias: extrapyramidal dysfunction and dyspnea. *Ann. Int. Med.* 88: 327-331, 1978.

Weinstein, M.R., and Goldfield, M.D.: Administration of lithium during pregnancy. In: Johnson, F.N. (Ed.) *Lithium Research and Therapy*, New York: Academic Press, pp. 237-264, 1975.

Wells, C.E.: Chronic brain disease: An overview. *Am. J. Psychiatry* 135: 1-12, 1978.

Wellens, H.J., Cats, V.K., and Duren, D.R.: Symptomatic sinus node abnormalities following lithium carbonate therapy. *Am. J. Med.* 59: 285-287, 1975.

Werry, J., and Aman, M.: Methylphenidate and haloperidol in children. Effects on attention, memory and activity. *Arch. Gen. Psychiatry* 32: 790-795, 1975.

White, J.H.: *Pediatric Psychopharmacology*, Baltimore: Williams & Wilkins, 1977.

Whittier, J.R., and Korenyi, C.: Effect of oral fluphenazine on Huntington's Chorea. *Int. J. Neoropsychiat.* 4: 1-3, 1968.

Wilbanks, G.D., Bressler, B., Petter, C.H., Cherny, W.B., and London, W.L.: Toxic effects of lithium carbonate in a mother and newborn infant. *J.A.M.A.* 213: 865-867, 1970.

Wilcox, D.R.C., Gillan, R.W., and Hare, E.H.: Do psychotic patients take their drugs? *Brit. Med. J.* 2: 790-795, 1965.

Wilson, J.H.P., Donker, A.J.M., Hem, G.K., Van der and Wientjes, J.: Peritoneal dialysis for lithium poisoning. *Brit. Med. J.* 2: 749-750, 1976a.

Wilson, J.R., Kraus, E.S., Bailas, M.M., and Rakita, L.: Reversible sinus node abnormalities due to lithium carbonate therapy. *New Eng. J. Med.* 294: 1223-1224, 1976b.

Winkleman, N.W.: An appraisal of chlorpromazine. *Am. J. Psychiatry* 113: 961-971, 1957.

Winsberg, B.G., and Yepes, L.E.: Antipsychotics. In: Werry, J.S. (Ed.) *Pediatric Psychopharmacology.* New York: Brunner/Mazel, 1978, pp. 234-272.

Woodrow, K.M., Gilles de la Tourette's Disease—A review. *Am. J. Psychiatry* 131: 1000-1003, 1974.

Wysenbeek, H., Steiner, K., and Goldberg, S.C.: Trifluoperazine: Comparison between regular and high doses. *Psychopharmacologia.* 36: 147-150, 1974.

Yaffe, S.J. and Stern, L.: Clinical implications of perinatal pharmacology. In: Mirkin, B.L. (Ed.) New York: Academic Press, 355-428, 1976.

Yepes, L.E., and Winsberg, B.G.: Vomiting during neuroleptic withdrawal in children. *Am. J. Psychiatry* 134: 574, 1977.

Yesavage, J.A., and Freeman, A.M.: Acute phencyclidine (PCP) intoxication. Psychopathology and prognosis. *J. Clin. Psychiatry* 43: 664-666, 1978.

Zavodnick, S.: Suggestions for a rational approach to the chemotherapy of schizophrenia. *Dis. Nerv. Syst.* 37: 671-675, 1977.

Zimmerman, H.J.: The differential diagnosis of jaundice. *M. Clin. N. Amer.* 52, 1968.

Zucker, G., Eisinger, R.P., Floch, M.H., and Singer, M.M.: Treatment of shock and prevention of ischemic necrosis with levarteranol-phentolamine mixtures. *Circulation* 22: 935-937, 1960.

Subject Index

Name Index

324